MAN ⦀⦀⦀⦀⦀⦀⦀⦀⦀⦀⦀ HORITY
D1347753

clinical evidence

Cardiovascular Disorders

The international source of the best available evidence for cardiovascular health care

Manchester NHS Informatics Library

T02130

BMJ
Publishing
Group

Reprinted from *Clinical Evidence*, Issue 6, 2001, published by the BMJ Publishing Group.

Editorial Office
BMJ Publishing Group, BMA House, Tavistock Square, London, WC1H 9JR, UK.
Tel: +44 (0)20 7387 4499; Fax: +44 (0)20 7383 6242 www.bmjpg.com

Clinical Evidence Cardiovascular Disorders
Please email us at CEfeedback@bmjgroup.com to register interest in future updates of *Clinical Evidence Cardiovascular Disorders* or complete the feedback card provided in this book.

Subscription prices for Clinical Evidence
The full edition of *Clinical Evidence* is published six monthly (June/December) by BMJ Publishing Group in print, online, and CD-ROM formats. The annual subscription rates for Issues 6 and 7 (December 2001 and June 2002) are:

Individual: £75 • US$110 • Can$160
Institutional: £160 • US$240 • Can$345
Student/Nurse: £35 • US$50 • Can$75

For further subscription information please visit the subscription page of our website www.clinicalevidence.com or email us at cesubscriptions@bmjgroup.com (UK and ROW) or clinevid@pmds.com (Americas). You may also telephone us or fax us on the following numbers:

UK and ROW Tel: +44 (0)20 7383 6270 • Fax: +44 (0)20 7383 6402
Americas Tel: +1 800 373 2897/240 646 7000 • Fax: +1 240 646 7005

Bulk subscriptions for societies and organisations
The Publishers offer discounts for any society or organisation buying bulk quantities for their members/customers. Please contact Miranda Lonsdale, Sales Manager, at mlonsdale@bmjgroup.com

Contributors
If you are interested in becoming a contributor to *Clinical Evidence* please contact us at clinicalevidence@bmjgroup.com

Rights
For information on translation rights, please contact Daniel Raymond-Barker at draymond-barker@bmjgroup.com

Copyright
© 2002 BMJ Publishing Group
All rights reserved. No part of this publication may be reproduced, stored in a retrieval system, or transmitted, in any form or by any means, electronic, mechanical, photocopying, recording and/or otherwise, without the permission of the publishers.

British Library Cataloguing in Publication Data
A CIP catalogue record for this book can be obtained from the British Library:
ISBN 0 7279 1720 X

Permission to reproduce
Please contact Josephine Woodcock at jwoodcock@bmjgroup.com when requesting permission to reprint all or part of any contribution in *Clinical Evidence*.

Legal Disclaimer
Care has been taken to confirm the accuracy of the information presented and to describe generally accepted practices. However, the authors, editors, and publishers are not responsible for errors or omissions or for any consequences from application of the information in this book and make no warranty, expressed or implied, with respect to the contents of the publication.

Categories presented in *Clinical Evidence* indicate a judgement about the strength of the evidence available and the relative importance of benefits and harms. The categories do not indicate whether a particular treatment is generally appropriate or whether it is suitable for individuals.

Printed and bound in Great Britain by Thanet Press Ltd, Margate, Kent.

Team and Advisors

Editor Stuart Barton **Section Advisor for Cardiovascular Disorders** Cindy Mulrow **Deputy Editor** Giselle Jones **Clinical Editors** Luis Gabriel Cuervo Amore, Anjana Patel, Charles Young **Quality Assurance Editor** James Woodcock **North American Editor** David Goldmann **Editorial Manager** Josephine Woodcock **Publishing Assistant** Polly Brown **Freelance Editors** Anna Donald, Martin Duerden, David Lewis, Vivek Muthu, Steve Reid **Information Specialists** Olwen Beaven, Sarah Greenley, Karen Pettersen, Sam Vincent **Production Editor** Samantha Bedser **Production Assistant** Claire Folkes **Digital Production** Karen Caillé, Kourosh Mojar, Palm Springs **Print Production** Charlotte Pestridge **Business Manager** Lisette Cleyndert **New Product Development Manager** Maysoon Nasser **Knowledge Systems Manager** Jonathan Fistein **Marketing and Sales (UK)** Diane Harris, Miranda Lonsdale, Daniel Raymond-Barker **Marketing and Sales (USA)** Diane McCabe **Department Administrator** Hannah Lawrence

EDITORIAL BOARD

Janet Allan, USA • Anarfi Asmoa-Baah, Switzerland • Don Berwick, USA • Warren Browner, USA • Iain Chalmers, UK • Nicky Cullum, UK •Tony Dixon, Hong Kong • David Eddy, USA • Paul Glasziou, Australia• Peter Gøtzsche, Denmark • Trisha Greenhalgh, UK • Andy Haines, UK • Brian Haynes, Canada • Alex Jadad, Canada • Ryuki Kassai, Japan • Duncan Keeley, UK • Marcia Kelsen, UK • Ilkka Kunnamo, Finland • Joseph Lau, USA • Rosanne Leipzig, USA • Alessandro Liberati, Italy • John Martin, UK • David Matchar, USA • Donna Mead, Wales • Ruairidh Milne, UK • Cindy Mulrow, USA • Andy Oxman, Norway • Miroslav Palat, Czech Republic • Neil Powe, USA • Drummond Rennie, USA • Susan Ross, USA • HPS Sachdev, India • Deborah Saltman, Australia • Martin Shipley, UK • Eleanor Wallace, USA • David Wilkinson, Australia • Steve Woolf, USA •Jeremy Wyatt, UK

Contents

Clinical Evidence Cardiovascular Disorders

Welcome to this collection of cardiovascular reprints from *Clinical Evidence,* a compendium of the best available evidence to guide clinical practice in specific cardiovascular disorders. This book is aimed primarily at cardiologists, clinical pharmacologists, generalist physicians, nurses, and physicians' assistants who care for people with cardiovascular disorders or who promote the prevention of cardiovascular disease. In addition, we believe that this book will be useful for adults with cardiovascular conditions, as well as for healthcare managers involved in organising cardiovascular services.

We decided to publish a *Clinical Evidence* version devoted solely to cardiovascular disorders for several reasons. Despite multiple advances in prevention and treatment, cardiovascular disorders remain the leading cause of morbidity, disability, and mortality in most western countries. Cardiovascular experts have long been stalwart standard bearers for rigorous evaluations of treatments. Literally, thousands of randomised controlled trials have evaluated hundreds of different prevention and treatment options for various cardiovascular disorders. New treatments are constantly being developed and tested, and some old treatments are discarded if better alternatives are found. Practitioners need quick, reliable knowledge about the optimum treatments for cardiovascular disorders, but they are overwhelmed by the variety of available options and the rapid accumulation of research evidence. We hope to help practicing clinicians who care for people with cardiovascular conditions by finding, sorting, critiquing, and summarising the best available research evidence.

About Clinical Evidence

Clinical Evidence is a continuously updated international source of evidence on the effects of clinical interventions. It summarises the current state of knowledge, ignorance, and uncertainty about the prevention and treatment of clinical conditions, based on thorough searches and appraisal of the literature. It purposely emphasises rigorous evidence about treatment and prevention that has been derived from randomised controlled trials and systematic reviews of the trials. It is neither a textbook of medicine nor a book of guidelines. It describes the best available evidence, and where there is no good evidence it says so. *Clinical Evidence* is regularly expanded to include new summaries of evidence on additional diseases, syndromes, and clinical questions.

A UNIQUE RESOURCE
Clinical Evidence has several unique features:
- Its contents are driven by questions rather than by the availability of research evidence. Rather than start with the evidence and summarise what is there, important clinical questions are identified and the literature searched for the best available evidence to answer them.
- It identifies but does not try to fill important gaps in the evidence. We believe that it is helpful for clinicians to know when uncertainty stems from gaps in the evidence rather than gaps in their own knowledge.
- It is updated every 6 months in print and on CD-ROM, and monthly online. This means that you can rely on it to keep you up-to-date in the areas that are covered.
- It specially aims not to make recommendations because differences in individual patients' baseline risks and preferences, and in the local availability of interventions, will always mean that the evidence must be individually interpreted rather than applied across the board. *Clinical Evidence* provides the raw material for developing locally applicable clinical practice guidelines, and for clinicians and patients to make up their own minds on the best course of action. We identify and summarise the evidence, you apply it and make the decisions.

A WORK IN PROGRESS

Clinical Evidence is an evolving project. We knew before we started that we were undertaking an enormous task, and the more we worked the more we realised its enormity. We recognise that there is some mismatch between what we aim to eventually achieve and what we have achieved so far. Although we make conscientious efforts to ensure that our literature searches are comprehensive and current and that appraisals of studies are systematic and objective, we inevitably miss some important studies. In order not to make unjustified claims about the accuracy of the information, we use phrases such as "we found no systematic review" rather than "there is no systematic review". In order to be as explicit as possible about the methods used for each contribution, we have asked each set of contributors to provide a brief methods section, describing the searches that were performed and how individual studies were selected.

For more information about our methods and processes, visit our website at www.clinicalevidence.com.

Cindy Mulrow
Section Advisor for Cardiovascular Disorders
Professor of Medicine

A guide to this book

The book is arranged by common cardiovascular topics. We include evidence relevant to both prevention and treatment of cardiovascular disease, and address a variety of associated risk factors such as dyslipidaemia, sedentary lifestyle, tobacco use, hypertension, unhealthy diets, and obesity.

SUMMARY PAGE
The summary page for each topic presents questions addressed, a list of the interventions covered (categorised according to whether they have been found to be effective or not), and some key messages. We have developed the categories of effectiveness from one of the Cochrane Collaboration's first and most popular products, *A guide to effective care in pregnancy and childbirth*.[1] The categories we now use are explained in the table below:

TABLE	Categorisation of treatment effects in *Clinical Evidence*.
Beneficial	Interventions whose effectiveness has been demonstrated by clear evidence from randomised controlled trials, and expectation of harms that is small compared with the benefits.
Likely to be beneficial	Interventions for which effectiveness is less well established than for those listed under "beneficial".
Trade off between benefits and harms	Interventions for which clinicians and patients should weigh up the beneficial and harmful effects according to individual circumstances and priorities.
Unknown effectiveness	Interventions for which there are currently insufficient data or data of inadequate quality.
Unlikely to be beneficial	Interventions for which lack of effectiveness is less well established than for those listed under "likely to be ineffective or harmful".
Likely to be ineffective or harmful	Interventions whose ineffectiveness or harmfulness has been demonstrated by clear evidence.

CATEGORISING THE EVIDENCE
Categorising the effectiveness of interventions is not straightforward. First, evidence is often limited. Interventions may have been tested only in narrow groups of people, such as those who are at particularly high risk for an outcome. Interventions may have been tested in tightly controlled circumstances that are not easily replicable in general practice, and direct comparisons of important alternative treatments may not be available. Second, finding no good evidence that a treatment works is not the same as saying that the treatment doesn't work. Statements of effectiveness necessarily are a reflection of currently available evidence and ideally distinguish between lack of benefit and lack of evidence of benefit. Third, several dimensions must be considered simultaneously when making decisions about effectiveness. These include the following: types, magnitudes, and frequency of expected benefits; types, magnitudes, and frequency of expected harms; level or rigor of evidence relevant to expected benefits and harms; and degree of certainty around expected benefits and harms.

INFORMATION ABOUT THE CONDITION

After each summary page, we present up-to-date, quantified, and referenced information about the condition. We define the clinical problem or condition of interest; describe its incidence, aetiology, risk factors, and prognosis; state the primary aims of treatment and/or prevention; and delineate the major outcomes of interest. Clinical outcomes, such as survival, heart attacks and strokes, symptoms, disability, and quality of life are emphasised. We then note the methods of our summaries, including the dates of the most recent searches and appraisal of evidence for each topic.

THE FILTERED EVIDENCE

The meat of *Clinical Evidence* follows. We present pertinent clinical questions and list multiple different therapeutic and/or preventive options. High quality evidence regarding the potential benefits and harms associated with the different options is summarised. Comments are supplied on the quality of the evidence, applicability of the results for different subgroups of people, and on any trials that are known to be in progress. Finally, we define important terms in glossaries and list the selected references.

Decisions about treatment and prevention require judgements about the trade offs between benefits and harms, and between alternative priorities. The best people to make these decisions are individuals and their personal healthcare providers; therefore, we talk about the effects of interventions, both positive and negative, rather than the effectiveness. For each question or intervention option we present evidence on benefits and harms under separate headings. We make no systematic attempt to provide information on drug dosages, formulations, indications, and contraindications. For this information, we refer readers to their national drug formularies. We also do not include information on cost or cost effectiveness of interventions as costs can vary greatly both within and between countries.

FEEDBACK

We hope that clinicians find *Clinical Evidence Cardiovascular Disorders* useful. We value your feedback on *Clinical Evidence Cardiovascular Disorders,* and in particular whether you would like to receive regular updates in print. Please email us at CEfeedback@bmjgroup.com or complete and return the feedback card provided in this book.

REFERENCES

1. Enkin M, Keirse M, Renfrew M, et al. *A guide to effective care in pregnancy and childbirth*. Oxford: Oxford University Press, 1998.

Glossary

Absolute risk (AR) This is the probability that an individual will experience the specified outcome during a specified period. It lies in the range 0 to 1, or is expressed as a percentage. In contrast to common usage, the word "risk" may refer to adverse events (such as myocardial infarction) or desirable events (such as cure).

Absolute risk increase (ARI) The absolute difference in risk between the experimental and control groups in a trial. It is used when the risk in the experimental group exceeds the risk in the control group, and is calculated by subtracting the AR in the control group from the AR in the experimental group. This figure does not give any idea of the proportional increase between the two groups; for this, relative risk increase (RRI) is needed (see below).

Absolute risk reduction (ARR) The absolute difference in risk between the experimental and control groups in a trial. It is used when the risk in the control group exceeds the risk in the experimental group, and is calculated by subtracting the AR in the experimental group from the AR in the control group. This figure does not give any idea of the proportional reduction between the two groups; for this, relative risk reduction (RRR) is needed (see below).

Baseline risk The risk of the event occurring without the active treatment. Estimated by the baseline risk in the control group.

Bias Systematic deviation of study results from the true results, because of the way(s) in which the study is conducted.

Blinding/ blinded A trial is blinded if all the people involved are unaware of the treatment group to which trial participants are allocated until after the interpretation of results. This includes trial participants and everyone involved in administering treatment or recording trial results.

Case control study A study design that examines a group of people who have experienced an event (usually an adverse event) and a group of people who have not experienced the same event, and looks at how exposure to suspect (usually noxious) agents differed between the two groups. This type of study design is most useful for trying to ascertain the cause of rare events, such as rare cancers.

Clinically significant A finding that is clinically important. Here, "significant" takes its everyday meaning of "important" (compared with statistically significant; see below). Where the word "significant" or "significance" is used without qualification in the text, it is being used in its statistical sense.

Cluster randomisation A cluster randomised study is one in which a group of participants are randomised to the same intervention together. Examples of cluster randomisation include allocating together people in the same village, hospital, or school. If the results are then analysed by individuals rather than the group as a whole bias can occur.

Cohort study A non-experimental study design that follows a group of people (a cohort), and then looks at how events differ among people within the group. A study that examines a cohort, which differs in respect to exposure to some suspected risk factor (e.g. smoking), is useful for trying to ascertain whether exposure is likely to cause specified events (e.g. lung cancer). Prospective cohort studies (which track participants forward in time) are more reliable than retrospective cohort studies.

Completer analysis Analysis of data from only those participants who remained at the end of the study. Compare with intention to treat analysis, which uses data from all participants who enrolled (see below).

Confidence interval (CI) The 95% confidence interval (or 95% confidence limits) would include 95% of results from studies of the same size and design in the same population. This is close but not identical to saying that the true size of the effect (never exactly known) has a 95% chance of falling within the confidence interval. If the 95%

confidence interval for a relative risk (RR) or an odds ratio (OR) crosses 1, then this is taken as no evidence of an effect. The practical advantages of a confidence interval (rather than a P value) is that they present the range of likely effects.

Controls in a randomised controlled trial (RCT) refer to the participants in its comparison group. They are allocated either to placebo, no treatment, or a standard treatment.

Crossover randomised trial A trial in which participants receive one treatment and have outcomes measured, and then receive an alternative treatment and have outcomes measured again. The order of treatments is randomly assigned. Sometimes a period of no treatment is used before the trial starts and in between the treatments (washout periods) to minimise interference between the treatments (carry over effects). Interpretation of the results from crossover randomised controlled trials (RCTs) can be complex.

Cross sectional study A study design that involves surveying a population about an exposure, or condition, or both, at one point in time. It can be used for assessing prevalence of a condition in the population.

Effect size (standardised mean differences) In the literature, effect size is used to refer to a variety of measures of treatment effect. In *Clinical Evidence* it refers to a standardised mean difference, a statistic for combining continuous variables (such as pain scores or height), from different scales.

Event The occurrence of a dichotomous outcome that is being sought in the study (such as myocardial infarction, death, or a four-point improvement in pain score).

Experimental study A study in which the investigator studies the effect of intentionally altering one or more factors under controlled conditions.

Factorial design A factorial design attempts to evaluate more than one intervention compared with control in a single experiment.

False negative A person with the target condition (defined by the gold standard) who has a negative test result.

False positive A person without the target condition (defined by the gold standard) who has a positive test result.

Fixed effects The "fixed effects" model of meta-analysis considers, often unreasonably, that the variability between the studies is exclusively because of a random sampling variation around a fixed effect (see random effects below).

Hazard ratio (HR) This is broadly equivalent to relative risk (RR), but is useful when the risk is not constant with respect to time. It uses information collected at different times. The term is typically used in the context of survival over time. If the HR is 0.5 then the relative risk of dying in one group is half the risk of dying in the other group.

Heterogeneity In the context of meta-analysis, heterogeneity means dissimilarity between studies. It can be because of the use of different statistical methods (statistical heterogeneity), or evaluation of people with different characteristics, treatments, or outcomes (clinical heterogeneity). Heterogeneity may render pooling of data in meta-analysis unreliable or inappropriate.

Homogeneity Similarity (see heterogeneity above).

Incidence The number of new cases of a condition occurring in a population over a specified period of time.

Intention to treat analysis Analysis of data for all participants based on the group to which they were randomised and not based on the actual treatment they received.

Likelihood ratio The ratio of the probability that an individual with the target condition has a specified test result to the probability that an individual without the target condition has the same specified test result.

Meta-analysis A statistical technique that summarises the results of several studies in a single weighted estimate, in which more weight is given to results of studies with more events and sometimes to studies of higher quality.

Morbidity Rate of illness but not death.

Mortality Rate of death.

Negative likelihood ratio (NLR) The ratio of the probability that an individual with the target condition has a negative test result to the probability that an individual without the target condition has a negative test result. This is the same as the ratio (1-sensitivity/specificity).

Negative predictive value (NPV) The chance of not having a disease given a negative test result (not to be confused with specificity, which is the other way round; see below).

Not significant/non-significant (NS) In *Clinical Evidence*, not significant means that the observed difference, or a larger difference, could have arisen by chance with a probability of more than one in 20 (i.e. 5%), assuming that there is no underlying difference. This is not the same as saying there is no effect, just that this experiment does not provide convincing evidence of an effect. This could be because the trial was not powered to detect an effect that does exist, because there was no effect, or because of the play of chance.

Number needed to harm (NNH) One measure of treatment harm. It is the average number of people from a defined population you would need to treat with a specific intervention for a given period of time to cause one additional adverse outcome. NNH can be calculated as 1/ARI. In *Clinical Evidence*, these are usually rounded downwards.

Number needed to treat (NNT) One measure of treatment effectiveness. It is the number of people you would on average need to treat with a specific intervention for a given period of time to prevent one additional adverse outcome or achieve one additional beneficial outcome. NNT can be calculated as 1/ARR (see appendix 2). In *Clinical Evidence*, NNTs are usually rounded upwards.

NNT for a meta-analysis Absolute measures are useful at describing the effort required to obtain a benefit, but are limited because they are influenced by both the treatment and also by the baseline risk of the individual. If a meta-analysis includes individuals with a range of baseline risks, then no single NNT will be applicable to the people in that meta-analysis, but a single relative measure (odds ratio or relative risk) may be applicable if there is no heterogeneity. In *Clinical Evidence* an NNT is provided for meta-analysis, based on a combination of the summary odds ratio (OR) and the mean baseline risk observed in the control group.

Odds The odds of an event happening is defined as the probability that an event will occur, expressed as a proportion of the probability that the event will not occur.

Odds ratio (OR) One measure of treatment effectiveness. It is the odds of an event happening in the experimental group expressed as a proportion of the odds of an event happening in the control group. The closer the OR is to one, the smaller the difference in effect between the experimental intervention and the control intervention. If the OR is greater (or less) than one, then the effects of the treatment are more (or less) than those of the control treatment. Note that the effects being measured may be adverse (e.g. death or disability) or desirable (e.g. survival). When events are rare the OR is analagous to the relative risk (RR), but as event rates increase the OR and RR diverge.

Odds reduction The complement of odds ratio (1-OR), similar to the relative risk reduction (RRR) when events are rare.

P value The probability that an observed difference occurred by chance, if it is assumed that there is in fact no real difference between the effects of the interventions. If this probability is less than one in 20 (which is when the P value is less than 0.05), then the result is conventionally regarded as being "statistically significant".

Placebo A substance given in the control group of a clinical trial, which is ideally identical in appearance and taste or feel to the experimental treatment and believed to lack any disease specific effects. In the context of non-pharmacological interventions, placebo is usually referred to as sham treatments (see sham treatment below).

Positive likelihood ratio (LR+) The ratio of the probability that an individual with the target condition has a positive test result to the probability that an individual without the target condition has a positive test result. This is the same as the ratio (sensitivity/1-specificity).

Positive predictive value (PPV) The chance of having a disease given a positive test result (not to be confused with sensitivity, which is the other way round; see below).

Power A study has adequate power if it can reliably detect a clinically important difference (i.e. between two treatments) if one actually exists. The power of a study is increased when it includes more events or when its measurement of outcomes is more precise.

Pragmatic study An RCT designed to provide results that are directly applicable to normal practice (compared with explanatory trials that are intended to clarify efficacy under ideal conditions). Pragmatic RCTs recruit a population that is representative of those who are normally treated, allow normal compliance with instructions (by avoiding incentives and by using oral instructions with advice to follow manufacturers instructions), and analyse results by "intention to treat" rather than by "on treatment" methods.

Prevalence The proportion of people with a finding or disease in a given population at a given time.

Publication bias Occurs when the likelihood of a study being published varies with the results it finds. Usually, this occurs when studies that find a significant effect are more likely to be published than studies that do not find a significant effect, so making it appear from surveys of the published literature that treatments are more effective than is truly the case.

Randomised controlled trial (RCT) Typically a trial in which participants are randomly assigned to two groups: one (the experimental group) receiving the intervention that is being tested and the other (the comparison or control group) receiving an alternative treatment or placebo. This design allows assessment of the relative effects of interventions. Sometimes, RCTs have more than one experimental group.

Random effects The "random effects" model assumes a different underlying effect for each study and takes this into consideration as an additional source of variation, which leads to somewhat wider confidence intervals than the fixed effects model. Effects are assumed to be randomly distributed, and the central point of this distribution is the focus of the combined effect estimate (see fixed effects above).

Regression analysis Given data on a dependent variable and one or more independent variables, regression analysis involves finding the "best" mathematical model to describe or predict the dependent variable as a function of the independent variable(s). There are several regression models that suit different needs. Common forms are linear, logistic, and proportional hazards.

Relative risk (RR) The number of times more likely (RR greater than 1) or less likely (RR less than 1) an event is to happen in one group compared with another. It is the ratio of the absolute risk (AR) for each group. It is analogous to the odds ratio (OR) when events are rare.

Relative risk increase (RRI) The proportional increase in risk between experimental and control participants in a trial.

Relative risk reduction (RRR) The proportional reduction in risk between experimental and control participants in a trial. It is the complement of the relative risk (1-RR).

Sensitivity The chance of having a positive test result given that you have a disease (not to be confused with positive predictive value [PPV], which is the other way around; see above).

Sensitivity analysis Analysis to test if results from meta-analysis are sensitive to restrictions on the data included. Common examples are large trials only, higher quality trials only, and more recent trials only. If results are consistent this provides stronger evidence of an effect and of generalisability.

Sham treatment An intervention given in the control group of a clinical trial, which is ideally identical in appearance and feel to the experimental treatment and believed to lack any disease specific effects (e.g. detuned ultrasound or random biofeedback).

Significant By convention, taken to mean statistically significant at the 5% level (see statistically significant below). This is the same as a 95% confidence interval not including the value corresponding to no effect.

Specificity The chance of having a negative test result given that you do not have a disease (not to be confused with negative predictive value [NPV], which is the other way around; see above).

Standardised mean difference (SMD) A measure of effect size used when outcomes are continuous (such as height, weight, or symptom scores) rather than dichotomous (such as death or myocardial infarction). The mean differences in outcome between the groups being studied are standardised to account for differences in scoring methods (such as pain scores). The measure is a ratio; therefore, it has no units.

Statistically significant Means that the findings of a study are unlikely to be because of chance. Significance at the commonly cited 5% level ($P < 0.05$) means that the observed difference or greater difference would occur by chance in only one in 20 similar cases. Where the word "significant" or "significance" is used without qualification in the text, it is being used in this statistical sense.

Subgroup analysis Analysis of a part of the trial/meta-analysis population in which it is thought the effect may differ from the mean effect.

Systematic review A review in which specified and appropriate methods have been used to identify, appraise, and summarise studies addressing a defined question. It can, but need not, involve meta-analysis. In *Clinical Evidence*, the term systematic review refers to a systematic review of RCTs unless specified otherwise.

True negative A person without the target condition (defined by the gold standard) who has a negative test result.

True positive A person with the target condition (defined by the gold standard) who also has a positive test result.

Validity The soundness or rigour of a study. A study is internally valid if the way it is designed and carried out means that the results are unbiased and it gives you an accurate estimate of the effect that is being measured. A study is externally valid if its results are applicable to people encountered in regular clinical practice.

Weighted mean difference (WMD) A measure of effect size used when outcomes are continuous (such as symptom scores or height) rather than dichotomous (such as death or myocardial infarction). The mean differences in outcome between the groups being studied are weighted to account for different sample sizes and differing precision between studies. The WMD is an absolute figure and so takes the units of the original outcome measure.

Search date January 2001

Gregory YH Lip and Sridhar Kamath

INTERVENTIONS

Key Messages

- We found little direct evidence from RCTs that included people solely with acute atrial fibrillation. Most of the available evidence is extrapolated from RCTs that include people with other types of atrial fibrillation.

- We found limited evidence from two small RCTs that β blockers increase the chance of returning to sinus rhythm compared with verapamil.

- We found three small RCTs of rate limiting calcium antagonists versus placebo. One RCT found that verapamil was much less effective than amiodarone at restoring sinus rhythm.

- Three RCTs have found good evidence that digoxin is no better than placebo at restoring sinus rhythm in people with acute atrial fibrillation, but digoxin lowered the ventricular rate in the short term more than placebo.

DEFINITION   Acute atrial fibrillation refers to the sudden onset of rapid, irregular and chaotic atrial activity, and the 48 hours after that onset. It includes both the first symptomatic onset of persistent atrial fibrillation and episodes of paroxysmal atrial fibrillation. It is sometimes difficult to distinguish episodes of new onset atrial fibrillation from newly diagnosed atrial fibrillation. Atrial fibrillation within 72 hours of onset is sometimes called recent onset atrial fibrillation. In this review, we have excluded episodes of atrial fibrillation that arise during or soon after cardiac surgery.

INCIDENCE/   We found limited evidence of the incidence or prevalence of acute
PREVALENCE   atrial fibrillation. Extrapolation from the Framingham study[1] suggests an incidence in men of 3 per 1000 person years at age 55 years, rising to 38 per 1000 person years at 94 years. In women, the incidence was 2 per 1000 person years at age 55 years, and 32.5 per 1000 person years at 94 years. The prevalence of atrial fibrillation ranged from 0.5% for people aged 50–59 years to 8.8% in people aged 80–89 years. Among acute emergency medical admissions in the UK, 3–6% have atrial fibrillation, and about 40% were newly diagnosed.[2,3] Among acute hospital admissions in New Zealand, 10.4% (95% CI 8.6% to 11.5%) had documented atrial fibrillation.[4]

AETIOLOGY/   Paroxysms of atrial fibrillation are more common in athletes.[5] Age
RISK FACTORS   increases the risk of developing acute atrial fibrillation. Men are more likely to develop atrial fibrillation than women (38 year follow up from the Framingham Study, RR after adjustment for age and known predisposing conditions 1.5).[6] Atrial fibrillation can occur in association with underlying disease (both cardiac and non-cardiac) or can arise in the absence of any other condition. Epidemiological surveys have found that risk factors for the development of acute atrial fibrillation include ischaemic heart disease, hypertension, heart failure, valve disease, diabetes, alcohol abuse, thyroid disorders, and disorders of the lung and pleura.[1] In a UK survey of acute hospital admissions with atrial fibrillation, a history of ischaemic heart disease was present in 33%, heart failure in 24%, hypertension in 26%, and rheumatic heart disease in 7%.[3] In some populations, the acute effects of alcohol explain a large proportion of the incidence of acute atrial fibrillation.

PROGNOSIS   We found no evidence about the proportion of people with acute atrial fibrillation who develop more chronic forms of atrial fibrillation (e.g. paroxysmal, persistent, or permanent atrial fibrillation). Observational studies and placebo arms of RCTs have found that over 50% of people with acute atrial fibrillation revert spontaneously within 24–48 hours, especially atrial fibrillation associated with an identifiable precipitant such as alcohol or myocardial infarction. We found little evidence about the effects on mortality and morbidity of acute atrial fibrillation where no underlying cause is found. Acute atrial fibrillation during myocardial infarction is an independent predictor of both short term and long term mortality.[7] Onset of atrial fibrillation reduces cardiac output by 10–20% irrespective of the underlying ventricular rate[8,9] and can contribute to heart failure. People with acute atrial fibrillation who present with heart failure have worse prognosis. Acute atrial fibrillation is associated with a risk of imminent stroke.[10-13] One case series used transoesophageal echocardiography in people who had developed acute atrial fibrillation within the preceding 48 hours; it found that 15% had atrial thrombi.[14] An ischaemic stroke associated with atrial fibrillation is more likely to be fatal, have a recurrence, and leave a serious functional deficit among survivors, than a stroke not associated with atrial fibrillation.[15]

AIMS
To reduce symptoms, morbidity and mortality, with minimum adverse effects.

OUTCOMES
Major outcomes include measures of symptoms, recurrent stroke or transient ischaemic attack, thromboembolism, death, and major bleeding. Proxy measures include heart rhythm, ventricular rate, timing to restoration of sinus rhythm. Frequent spontaneous reversion to sinus rhythm makes it difficult to interpret short term studies of rhythm; treatments may accelerate restoration of sinus rhythm without increasing the proportion of people who eventually convert. The clinical importance of changes in mean heart rate is also unclear.

METHODS
Clinical Evidence search and appraisal January 2001. Current Contents, textbooks, review articles and recent abstracts were reviewed. Many studies were not solely in people with acute atrial fibrillation. The text indicates where results have been extrapolated from studies of paroxysmal, persistent, or permanent atrial fibrillation. Atrial fibrillation that follows coronary surgery has been excluded.

QUESTION **What are the effects of treatments for acute atrial fibrillation?**

OPTION **β BLOCKERS**

One small RCT found that timolol versus placebo reduced ventricular rate. A small comparative RCT found that esmolol versus verapamil increased the chance of returning to sinus rhythm.

Benefits:
We found no systematic review. **Versus placebo:** We found one RCT (61 people with atrial fibrillation of unspecified duration, ventricular rate > 120/minute), which compared intravenous timolol (1 mg) versus intravenous placebo given immediately and repeated twice at 20 minute intervals if sinus rhythm was not achieved.[16] It found that 20 minutes after the last injection, intravenous timolol versus placebo significantly increased the proportion of people who had a ventricular rate below 100 a minute (41% with timolol v 3% with placebo; P < 0.01), and increased the proportion of people who converted to sinus rhythm, although the increase was not significant (5/29 [17%] v 2/32 [6%], P = 0.18). **Versus verapamil:** We found one RCT (31 people with onset of atrial fibrillation or atrial flutter [see glossary, p 6] within the previous 48 hours), which found that esmolol versus verapamil increased the proportion of people who returned to sinus rhythm (50% v 12%; P < 0.03) but had no significant effect on the final ventricular rate (100/minute with esmolol v 98/minute with verapamil).[17]

Harms: β Blockers may exacerbate heart failure and hypotension in acute atrial fibrillation. β Blockers plus rate limiting calcium channel blockers (diltiazem, verapamil) may increase the risk of asystole and sinus arrest.[18-20] β Blockers can precipitate bronchospasm.[21] In the RCT, both esmolol and verapamil were associated with mild hypotension.

Comment: Esmolol is a rapidly acting intravenous β blocker. In addition to the evidence from people with acute atrial fibrillation, we found one systematic review of β blockers versus placebo in people with either acute or chronic atrial fibrillation.[22] It found that in seven of 12 comparisons at rest and in all during exercise, β blockers reduced ventricular rate compared with placebo. We found no RCTs that reported quality of life, functional capacity, or mortality.

OPTION	RATE LIMITING CALCIUM CHANNEL ANTAGONISTS (VERAPAMIL AND DILTIAZEM)

We found three small RCTs of rate limiting calcium antagonists versus placebo. One RCT found that verapamil was much less effective than amiodarone at restoring sinus rhythm.

Benefits: We found no systematic review in people with acute atrial fibrillation. **Versus placebo:** We found three RCTs.[23-25] The first RCT (21 men with atrial fibrillation and a rapid ventricular rate, age 37–70 years) was a crossover comparison of intravenous verapamil versus saline.[23] It found that intravenous verapamil versus saline reduced ventricular rate within 10 minutes (reduction > 15% of the initial rate: 17/20 [85%] with verapamil v 2/14 [14%] with saline). It also found that three people converted to sinus rhythm, but it is not clear from the results whether these effects can be attributed to verapamil or saline. The second RCT (double blind crossover study of 20 people with atrial fibrillation or atrial flutter [see glossary, p 6] for 2 hours to 2 years) compared intravenous low dose verapamil versus placebo.[24] A positive response was defined as conversion to sinus rhythm or a decrease of the ventricular response to less than 100 a minute, or by more than 20% of the initial rate. If a positive response did not occur within 10 minutes, then a second bolus injection was given (placebo for people who initially received verapamil, verapamil for people who initially received placebo). The response rate was not significantly different between low dose verapamil and placebo arms. With the first bolus injection, verapamil versus placebo significantly reduced ventricular rate (mean heart rate 118/minute with verapamil arm v 138/minute with placebo), and more people converted to sinus rhythm within 30 minutes but the difference was not significant (3/20 with verapamil v 0/15 with placebo, P = 0.12). The third RCT (113 people with either acute or chronic atrial fibrillation or flutter, mean age 64, 83% male, ventricular rate > 120/minute) found that intravenous diltiazem versus placebo significantly improved the proportion of people who achieved the combined outcome of conversion to sinus rhythm or ventricular rate less than 100 a minute or ventricular rate reduced by more than 20% of the initial rate (93% v 12%, P < 0.001).[25] **Versus amiodarone:** We found one RCT (24 consecutive people with acute paroxysms of atrial fibrillation lasting

20 minutes to 48 hours, 15 male, mean age 71 years, mean ventricular rate 125/minute) of intravenous verapamil versus intravenous amiodarone.[26] It found that amiodarone converted more people to sinus rhythm than verapamil in the 3 hours after the injection (77% with amiodarone v 0% with verapamil; P < 0.001). **Versus digoxin:** We found one RCT (30 consecutive people, 10 male, mean age 72 years, 26 with acute atrial fibrillation, 4 with atrial flutter, unspecified duration) comparing intravenous diltiazem versus intravenous digoxin versus both.[27] It found significant reductions of ventricular rate by diltiazem within 5 minutes, and by digoxin only after 3 hours. No additional benefit was found with the combination of digoxin and diltiazem. **Versus other calcium channel blockers:** We found no systematic reviews or large RCTs. We found one double blind crossover RCT (7 people with acute atrial fibrillation and 2 with atrial flutter),[28] which compared intravenous diltiazem versus verapamil, and found no significant differences in rate control or measures of systolic function.

Harms: Rate limiting calcium antagonists may exacerbate heart failure and hypotension. In people with Wolff Parkinson White syndrome (see glossary, p 6), verapamil may increase the ventricular rate and can cause ventricular arrhythmias.[29]

Comment: The evidence suggests that rate limiting calcium channel blockers such as verapamil and diltiazem reduce ventricular rate in acute or recent onset atrial fibrillation, but they are probably no better than placebo in restoring sinus rhythm. We found no studies of the effect of rate limiting calcium channel blockers on exercise tolerance in people with acute or recent onset atrial fibrillation, but studies in people with chronic atrial fibrillation have found improved exercise tolerance.

OPTION   DIGOXIN

Three RCTs have found that digoxin is no better than placebo at restoring sinus rhythm in people with acute atrial fibrillation, but digoxin lowered the ventricular rate in the short term more than placebo.

Benefits: **Versus placebo:** We found no systematic review of digoxin for acute atrial fibrillation but found three RCTs.[30-32] The first RCT (239 people with atrial fibrillation within 7 days of onset, mean age 66 years, mean ventricular rate 122/minute)[30] found that intravenous digoxin (mean 0.88 mg) versus placebo did not increase the restoration of sinus rhythm by 16 hours (51% with digoxin v 46% with placebo). It found a rapid and clinically important reduction in ventricular rate at 2 hours (to 105/minute with digoxin v 117/minute with placebo; P = 0.0001). Similar findings were reported in two smaller RCTs.[31,32] One RCT (40 people within 7 days of the onset of atrial fibrillation, mean age 64 years, 23 male) compared high dose intravenous digoxin (1.25 mg) versus placebo. Restoration to sinus rhythm was not significantly different (9/19 [47%] with digoxin v 8/20 [40%] with placebo, P = 0.6). The ventricular rate after 30 minutes was significantly lower compared with placebo (P < 0.02).[31] The second RCT (36 people within 7 days of the onset of atrial fibrillation) compared oral digoxin versus placebo.

Conversion to sinus rhythm by 18 hours was not significantly different (50% with digoxin v 44% with placebo; ARR +6%, 95% CI −11% to +22%).[32]

Harms: Digoxin at toxic doses may result in visual, gastrointestinal and neurological symptoms, heart block, and arrhythmias.

Comment: The peak action of digoxin is delayed, taking 6–12 hours to reduce mean ventricular rate below 100 a minute. We found one systematic review and RCTs of digoxin versus placebo in people with chronic atrial fibrillation, which found that control of the ventricular rate control during exercise was poor unless a β blocker or rate limiting calcium antagonist (verapamil or diltiazem) was used in combination.[22,33,34] The evidence suggests that digoxin is no better than placebo at restoring sinus rhythm in people with recent onset atrial fibrillation.

GLOSSARY

Atrial flutter A similar arrhythmia to atrial fibrillation but the atrial electrical activity is less chaotic and has a characteristic saw tooth appearance on an electrocardiogram.

Wolff Parkinson White syndrome Occurs when an additional electrical pathway exists between the atria and the ventricles as a result of anomalous embryonic development. The extra pathway may cause rapid arrhythmias. Worldwide it affects about 0.2% of the general population. In people with Wolff Parkinson White syndrome, β blockers, calcium channel blockers, and digoxin can increase the ventricular rate and cause ventricular arrhthmias.

REFERENCES

1. Benjamin EJ, Wolf PA, Kannel WA. The epidemiology of atrial fibrillation. In: Falk RH, Podrid P, eds. *Atrial fibrillation: mechanisms and management*. 2nd ed. Philadelphia; Lippincott-Raven Publishers, 1997:1–22.

2. Lip GYH, Tean KN, Dunn FG. Treatment of atrial fibrillation in a district general hospital. *Br Heart J* 1994;71:92–95.

3. Zarifis J, Beevers DG, Lip GYH. Acute admissions with atrial fibrillation in a British multiracial hospital population. *Br J Clin Pract* 1997;51:91–96.

4. Stewart FM, Singh Y, Persson S, Gamble GD, Braatvedt GD. Atrial fibrillation: prevalence and management in an acute general medical unit. *Aust N Z J Med* 1999;29:51–58.

5. Furlanello F, Bertoldi A, Dallago M, et al. Atrial fibrillation in elite athletes. *J Cardiovasc Electrophysiol* 1998;9(8 suppl):63–68.

6. Kannel WB, Wolf PA, Benjamin EJ, Levy D. Prevalence, incidence, prognosis, and predisposing conditions for atrial fibrillation: population-based estimates. *Am J Cardiol* 1998;82:2N–9N.

7. Pedersen OD, Bagger H, Kober L, Torp-Pedersen C. The occurrence and prognostic significance of atrial fibrillation/flutter following acute myocardial infarction. TRACE Study group. TRAndolapril Cardiac Evalution. *Eur Heart J* 1999;20:748–754.

8. Clark DM, Plumb VJ, Epstein AE, Kay GN. Hemodynamic effects of an irregular sequence of ventricular cycle lengths during atrial fibrillation. *J Am Coll Cardiol* 1997;30:1039–1045.

9. Schumacher B, Luderitz B. Rate issues in atrial fibrillation: consequences of tachycardia and therapy for rate control. *Am J Cardiol* 1998;82:29N–36N.

10. Peterson P, Godfredson J. Embolic complications in paroxysmal atrial fibrillation. *Stroke* 1986;17:622–626.

11. Sherman DG, Goldman L, Whiting RB, Jurgensen K, Kaste M, Easton JD. Thromboembolism in patients with atrial fibrillation. *Arch Neurol* 1984;41:708–710.

12. Wolf PA, Kannel WB, McGee DL, Meeks SL, Bharucha NE, McNamara PM. Duration of atrial fibrillation and imminence of stroke: the Framingham study. *Stroke* 1983;14:664–667.

13. Corbalan R, Arriagada D, Braun S, et al. Risk factors for systemic embolism in patients with paroxysmal atrial fibrillation. *Am Heart J* 1992;124:149–153.

14. Stoddard ME, Dawkins PR, Prince CR, Ammash NM. Left atrial appendage thrombus is not uncommon in patients with acute atrial fibrillation and a recent embolic event: a transesophageal echocardiographic study. *J Am Coll Cardiol* 1995;25:452–459.

15. Lin HJ, Wolf PA, Kelly-Hayes M, et al. Stroke severity in atrial fibrillation. The Framingham Study. *Stroke* 1996;27:1760–1764.

16. Sweany AE, Moncloa F, Vickers FF, Zupkis RV, Rahway NJ. Antiarrhythmic effects of intravenous timolol in supraventricular arrhythmias. *Clin Pharmacol Ther* 1985;37:124–127.

17. Platia EV, Michelson EL, Porterfield JK, Das G. Esmolol versus verapamil in the acute treatment of atrial fibrillation or atrial flutter. *Am J Cardiol* 1989;63:925–929.

18. Lee TH, Salomon DR, Rayment CM, Antman EM. Hypotension and sinus arrest with exercise-induced hyperkalemia and combined verapamil/propranolol therapy. *Am J Med* 1986;80:1203–1204.

19. Misra M, Thakur R, Bhandari K. Sinus arrest caused by atenolol-verapamil combination. *Clin Cardiol* 1987;10:365–367.

20. Yeh SJ, Yamamoto T, Lin FC, Wang CC, Wu D. Repetitive sinoatrial exit block as the major mechanism of drug-provoked long sinus or atrial pause. *J Am Coll Cardiol* 1991;18:587–595.

21. Doshan HD, Rosenthal RR, Brown R, Slutsky A, Applin WJ, Caruso FS. Celiprolol, atenolol and propranolol: a comparison of pulmonary effects in asthmatic patients. *J Cardiovasc Pharmacol* 1986; 8(suppl 4):105–108.

22. Segal JB, McNamara RL, Miller MR, et al. The evidence regarding the drugs used for ventricular rate control. *J Fam Pract* 2000;49:47–59.

23. Aronow WS, Ferlinz J. Verapamil versus placebo in atrial fibrillation and atrial flutter. *Clin Invest Med* 1980;3:35–39.

24. Waxman HL, Myerburg RJ, Appel R, Sung RJ. Verapamil for control of ventricular rate in paroxysmal supraventricular tachycardia and atrial fibrillation or flutter: a double-blind randomized cross-over study. *Ann Intern Med* 1981;94:1–6

25. Salerno DM, Dias VC, Kleiger RE, et al. Efficacy and safety of intravenous diltiazem for treatment of atrial fibrillation and atrial flutter: the Diltiazem-Atrial Fibrillation/Flutter Study Group. *Am J Cardiol* 1989;63:1046–1051.

26. Noc M, Stajer D, Horvat M. Intravenous amiodarone versus verapamil for acute conversion of paroxysmal atrial fibrillation to sinus rhythm. *Am J Cardiol* 1990;65:679–680.

27. Schreck DM, Rivera AR, Tricarico VJ. Emergency management of atrial fibrillation and flutter: intravenous diltiazem versus intravenous digoxin *Ann Emerg Med* 1997;29:135–140.

28. Phillips BG, Gandhi AJ, Sanoski CA, Just VL, Bauman JL. Comparison of intravenous diltiazem and verapamil for the acute treatment of atrial fibrillation and atrial flutter. *Pharmacotherapy* 1997;17:1238–1245.

29. Strasberg B, Sagie A, Rechavia E, et al. Deleterious effects of intravenous verapamil in Wolff-Parkinson-White patients and atrial fibrillation. *Cardiovasc Drugs Ther* 1989;2: 801–806.

30. DAAF trial group. Intravenous digoxin in acute atrial fibrillation. Results of a randomized, placebo-controlled multicentre trial in 239 patients. The Digitalis in Acute AF (DAAF) Trial Group. *Eur Heart J* 1997;18:649–654.

31. Jordaens L, Trouerbach J, Calle P, et al. Conversion of atrial fibrillation to sinus rhythm and rate control by digoxin in comparison to placebo. *Eur Heart J* 1997;18:643–648.

32. Falk RH, Knowlton AA, Bernard SA, Gotlieb NE, Battinelli NJ. Digoxin for converting recent-onset atrial fibrillation to sinus rhythm. *Ann Intern Med* 1987;106:503–506.

33. Farshi R, Kistner D, Sarma JS, Longmate JA, Singh BN. Ventricular rate control in chronic atrial fibrillation during daily activity and programmed exercise: a crossover open-label study of five drug regimens. *J Am Coll Cardiol* 1999;33:304–310.

34. Klein HO, Pauzner H, Di Segni E, David D, Kaplinsky E. The beneficial effects of verapamil in chronic atrial fibrillation. *Arch Intern Med* 1979; 139:747–749.

Gregory YH Lip

Professor of Cardiovascular Medicine

Sridhar Kamath

Haemostasis Thrombosis and Vascular Biology Unit
University Department of Medicine
City Hospital
Birmingham
UK

Competing interests: GL is UK principal investigator for the ERAFT Trial (Knoll) and has been reimbursed by various pharmaceutical companies for attending several conferences, and running educational programmes and research projects. SK, none declared.

Cardiorespiratory arrest in children

Search date June 2001

David Creery and Kate Ackerman

QUESTIONS

INTERVENTIONS

*Although we found no direct evidence to support their use, widespread consensus holds that (on the basis of indirect evidence and extrapolation from adult data) these interventions should be universally applied to children who have arrested. Placebo controlled trials would be considered unethical.

See glossary, p 14

Key Messages

- Outcome following out-of-hospital cardiorespiratory arrest in children is poor, and it is unclear at what stage intervention becomes futile.

- Prospective and retrospective observational studies have consistently found that out-of-hospital cardiorespiratory arrest in children, where the cause is uncertain (such as in fatal and near miss sudden infant death syndrome), has a far worse prognosis than arrest from any other cause.

- It is widely accepted that cardiopulmonary resuscitation and ventilation should be undertaken in children who have arrested. Placebo controlled trials would be considered unethical. We found no prospective evidence on the effects of training parents to perform cardiopulmonary resuscitation.

- One RCT found no evidence that endotracheal intubation improved survival or neurological outcome compared with bag-mask ventilation in children who have arrested in the community.

- We found no prospective evidence on the effects of bicarbonate, calcium, different doses of adrenaline (epinephrine), or direct current cardiac shock to improve the outcome of non-submersion out-of-hospital cardiorespiratory arrest in children.

DEFINITION   Non-submersion out-of-hospital cardiorespiratory arrest in children is a state of pulselessness and apnoea occurring outside of a medical facility and not caused by submersion in water.[1]

INCIDENCE/ We found 12 studies (3 prospective, 9 retrospective) reporting the
PREVALENCE incidence of non-submersion out-of-hospital cardiorespiratory arrest in children (see table 1, p 15).[2-13] Eleven studies reported the incidence in both adults and children, and eight reported the incidence in children.[2-9,11-13] Incidence of arrests in the general population ranged from 2.2–5.7/100 000 people a year (mean 3.1, 95% CI 2.1 to 4.1). Incidence of arrests in children ranged from 6.9–18.0/100 000 children a year (mean 10.6, 95% CI 7.1 to 14.1).[8] One prospective study (300 children) found that about 50% of out-of-hospital cardiorespiratory arrests occurred in children under 12 months, and about two thirds occurred in children under 18 months.[11]

AETIOLOGY/ We found 26 studies reporting the causes of non-submersion
RISK FACTORS pulseless arrests (see glossary, p 14) in a total of 1574 children. commonest causes of arrest were undetermined causes as in sudden infant death syndrome (see glossary, p 14) (39%), trauma (18%), chronic disease (7%), and pneumonia (4%) (see table 2, p 16).[1,3-12,14-28]

PROGNOSIS   We found no systematic review that investigated non-submersion arrests alone. We found 27 studies (5 prospective, 22 retrospective; total of 1754 children) that reported only on out-of-hospital arrest.[1-12,14-28] The overall survival rate following out-of-hospital arrest was 5% (87 children). Nineteen of these studies (1140 children) found that of the 48 surviving children, 12 (25%) had no or mild neurological disability and 36 (75%) had moderate or severe neurological disability. We found one systematic review (search date 1997), which reported outcomes after cardiopulmonary resuscitation for both in-hospital and out-of-hospital arrests of any cause, including submersion in children.[29] Studies were excluded if they did not report survival. The review found evidence from prospective and retrospective observational studies that out-of-hospital arrest of any cause in children carries a poorer prognosis than arrest within hospital (132/1568 children [8%] survived to hospital discharge after out-of-hospital arrest *v* 129/544 children [24%] after in-hospital arrests). About half of the survivors were involved in studies that reported neurological outcome. Of these, survival with "good neurological outcome" (i.e. normal or mild neurological deficit) was higher in children who arrested in hospital compared with those who arrested elsewhere (60/77 surviving children [78%] in hospital *v* 28/68 [41%] elsewhere).[29]

AIMS   To improve survival and minimise neurological sequelae in children suffering non-submersion out-of-hospital cardiorespiratory arrest.

OUTCOMES   Out-of-hospital death rate; rate of death in hospital without return of spontaneous circulation; return of spontaneous circulation with subsequent death in hospital; and return of spontaneous circulation with successful hospital discharge with mild, moderate, severe, or no neurological sequelae; adverse effects of treatment.

METHODS   *Clinical Evidence* search and appraisal June 2001. In addition, we searched citation lists of retrieved articles and relevant review articles. Studies reporting out-of-hospital arrest in adults that listed "adolescent" as a MeSH heading were also reviewed. Both authors reviewed the retrieved studies independently and differences were resolved by discussion. We selected studies reporting out-of-hospital cardiorespiratory arrests in children. Studies were excluded if data relating to submersion could not be differentiated from non-submersion data (except where we found no data relating exclusively to non-submersion arrest; in such cases we have included studies that did not differentiate these types of arrest, and have made it clear that such evidence is limited by this fact). Some features of cardiorespiratory arrest in adults appear to be different from arrest in children, so studies were excluded if data for adults could not be differentiated from data for children.

QUESTION **What are the effects of treatments for non-submersion out-of-hospital cardiorespiratory arrest?**

OPTION **AIRWAY MANAGEMENT AND VENTILATION**

It is widely accepted that good airway management and rapid ventilation should be undertaken in a child who has arrested, and it would be considered unethical to test its role in a placebo controlled trial.

Benefits: We found no studies comparing airway management and ventilation versus no intervention.

Harms: We found insufficient information.

Comment: It would be considered unethical to test the role of airway management and ventilation in a placebo controlled trial.

OPTION **INTUBATION VERSUS BAG-MASK VENTILATION**

One controlled trial found no evidence of a difference in survival or neurological outcome between bag-mask ventilation and endotracheal intubation in children requiring airway management in the community.

Benefits: We found no systematic review. We found one high quality controlled trial (830 children requiring airway management in the community, including 98 children who had arrested after submersion) comparing (using alternate day allocation) bag-mask ventilation versus endotracheal intubation (given by paramedic staff trained in these techniques).[30] Treatments were not randomised; each was allocated on alternate days. Analysis was by intention to treat (see comment below). The trial found no significant difference in rates of survival or good neurological outcome (normal, mild deficit, or no change from baseline function) between the two treatment groups (105/349 [30%] survived after bag-mask ventilation v 90/373 [24%] after intubation; OR 1.36, 95% CI 0.97 to 1.89; good neurological outcome achieved in 80/349 [23%] of children after bag-mask ventilation v 70/373 [19%] after intubation; OR 1.27, 95% CI 0.89 to 1.83; OR for non-submersion cardiorespiratory arrest calculated by author).

Harms: The trial found that time spent at the scene of the arrest was longer when intubation was intended, and this was the only significant determinant of a longer total time from dispatch of paramedic team to arrival at hospital (mean time at scene 9 min with bag-mask v 11 min with intubation, P < 0.001; mean total time 20 min with bag-mask v 23 min with intubation, P < 0.001).[30] However, the trial found no significant difference between bag-mask ventilation and intubation for complications common to both treatments (complications in 727 children for whom data were available, bag-mask v intubation: gastric distension 31% v 7%, P = 0.20; vomiting 14% v 14%, P = 0.82; aspiration 14% v 15%, P = 0.84; oral or airway trauma 1% v 2%, P = 0.24). A total of 186 children across both treatment groups were thought by paramedical staff to be successfully intubated. Of these, oesophageal intubation occurred in three children (2%); the tube became dislodged in 27 children (14%; unrecognised in 12 children, recognised in 15); right main bronchus intubation occurred in 33 children (18%); and an incorrect size of tube was used in 44 children (24%). Death occurred in all but one of the children with oesophageal intubation or unrecognised dislodging of the tube.[30]

Comment: **Population characteristics:** The baseline characteristics of children did not differ significantly between groups in age, sex, ethnicity, or cause of arrest. The trial did not report the frequency of pulseless arrest (see glossary, p 14) versus respiratory arrest (see glossary, p 14). **Intention to treat:** Intubation and bag-mask ventilation are not mutually exclusive. The study protocol allowed bag-mask ventilation before intubation and after unsuccessful intubation. Of 420 children allocated to intubation, 115 received bag-mask ventilation before intubation, 128 received bag-mask ventilation after attempted intubation, four were lost to follow up, and the remainder received intubation that was believed to be successful. Of 410 children allocated to bag-mask ventilation, 10 children were intubated successfully (although in violation of study protocol), nine received bag-mask ventilation after attempted intubation, six were lost to follow up, and the remainder received bag-mask ventilation in accordance with study protocol.[30]

OPTION   **INTRAVENOUS ADRENALINE (EPINEPHRINE)**

Intravenous adrenaline (epinephrine) at "standard dose" (0.01 mg/kg) is a widely accepted treatment for establishing return of spontaneous circulation. We found no prospective evidence comparing adrenaline (epinephrine) versus placebo, or comparing standard or single doses versus high or multiple doses of adrenaline (epinephrine), in children who have arrested in the community.

Benefits: We found no systematic review, no RCTs, and no prospective observational studies.

Harms: We found no prospective data in this context.

Comment: **Versus placebo:** Standard dose adrenaline (epinephrine) is a widely accepted treatment for arrests in children. Placebo controlled trials would be considered unethical. **High versus low dose:** Two small retrospective studies (128 people) found no evidence of

Cardiorespiratory arrest in children

a difference in survival to hospital discharge between low or single dose and high or multiple dose adrenaline (epinephrine), although the studies were too small to rule out an effect.[8,12]

OPTION   INTRAVENOUS BICARBONATE

We found no RCTs on the effects of intravenous bicarbonate in out-of-hospital cardiorespiratory arrest in children.

Benefits: We found no RCTs.

Harms: We found insufficient evidence.

Comment: Bicarbonate is widely believed to be effective in arrest associated with hyperkalaemic ventricular tachycardia or fibrillation, but we found no prospective evidence supporting this.

OPTION   INTRAVENOUS CALCIUM

We found no RCTs on the effects of intravenous calcium in out-of-hospital cardiorespiratory arrest in children.

Benefits: We found no RCTs.

Harms: We found insufficient evidence.

Comment: Calcium is widely believed to be effective in arrest associated with hyperkalaemic ventricular tachycardia or fibrillation, but we found no prospective evidence supporting this.

OPTION   BYSTANDER CARDIOPULMONARY RESUSCITATION

It is widely accepted that cardiopulmonary resuscitation and ventilation should be undertaken in children who have arrested. Placebo controlled trials would be considered unethical. We found no RCTs on the effects of training parents to perform cardiopulmonary resuscitation. One systematic review of observational studies has found that children who were witnessed having an arrest and who received bystander cardiopulmonary resuscitation were more likely to survive to hospital discharge.

Benefits: We found no RCTs. We found one systematic review (search date 1997) of prospective and retrospective studies. This concluded that survival was improved in children who were witnessed to arrest and received cardiopulmonary resuscitation from a bystander. Of 150 witnessed arrests outside hospital, 28 of 150 (19%) survived to hospital discharge. Of those children who received bystander cardio-pulmonary resuscitation, 20 of 76 (26%) survived to discharge.[29] The review did not report survival rates in children whose arrests were not witnessed, but the overall survival rate for out-of-hospital cardiac arrest was 8%. **Training parents to perform cardiopulmonary resuscitation:** We found no systematic review and no RCTs examining the effects of training parents to perform cardiopulmonary resuscitation in children who have arrested out-side hospital.

Harms: Potential harms include those resulting from unnecessary chest compression after respiratory arrest with intact circulation.

Comment: The review of observational studies found that children who received bystander cardiopulmonary resuscitation had a hospital discharge rate of 26% (20/76) versus 11% (8/74) for children who also had their arrests witnessed but had not received cardiopulmonary resuscitation. Cardiopulmonary resuscitation was not randomly allocated and children resuscitated may be systematically different from those who did not receive resuscitation. The apparent survival rates for witnessed arrests and arrests with bystander initiated cardiopulmonary resuscitation may be artificially high because of inappropriate evaluation of true arrest. However, assuming confounding variables were evenly distributed between groups, then the best estimate of the benefit of cardiopulmonary resuscitation is a 15% absolute increase in the probability that children will be discharged alive from hospital.

OPTION	DIRECT CURRENT CARDIAC SHOCK

It is widely accepted that children who arrest outside hospital and are found to have ventricular fibrillation or pulseless ventricular tachycardia should receive direct current cardiac shock treatment. Placebo controlled trials would be considered unethical. We found no RCTs on the effects of direct current cardiac shock in children who have arrested in the community, regardless of the heart rhythm.

Benefits: We found no systematic review and no RCTs.

Harms: We found insufficient evidence.

Comment: **In children with ventricular fibrillation:** One retrospective study (29 children with ventricular fibrillation who had arrested out-of-hospital from a variety of causes, including submersion) found that of 27 children who were defibrillated, 11 survived (5 with no sequelae, 6 with severe disability). The five children with good outcome all received defibrillation within 10 minutes of arrest (time to defibrillation not given for those who died). Data on the two children who were not defibrillated were not presented.[31] **In children with asystole:** One retrospective study in 90 children with asystole (see glossary, p 14) (including those who had arrested after submersion) found that 49 (54%) had received direct current cardiac shock treatment. None of the children survived to hospital discharge, regardless of whether or not direct current cardiac shock was given.[32] We found one systematic review (search date 1997) of observational studies (1420 children who had arrested outside hospital) that recorded electrocardiogram rhythm. Bradyasystole (see glossary, p 14) or pulseless electrical activity (see glossary, p 14) were found in 73%, whereas ventricular fibrillation pulseless ventricular tachycardia (see glossary, p 14) were found 10%.[29] The review found that survival after ventricular fibrillation or ventricular tachycardia arrest was higher than after asystolic arrest in children. Survival to discharge reported in the systematic review was 5% (39/802) for children with initial rhythm asystole (see glossary, p 14) and 30% (29/97) with initial rhythm ventricular fibrillation (see glossary, p 14) or ventricular tachycardia.[29]

Cardiovascular disorders

GLOSSARY

Asystole The absence of cardiac electrical activity

Bradyasystole Bradycardia clinically indistinguishable from asystole

Initial rhythm asystole The absence of cardiac electrical activity at initial determination

Initial rhythm ventricular fibrillation Electrical rhythm is ventricular fibrillation at initial determination

Pulseless arrest Absence of palpable pulse

Pulseless electrical activity The presence of cardiac electrical activity in absence of a palpable pulse

Pulseless ventricular tachycardia Electrical rhythm of ventricular tachycardia in absence of a palpable pulse

Respiratory arrest Absence of respiratory activity

Sudden infant death syndrome The sudden unexpected death of a child, usually between the ages of 1 month and 1 year, for which a thorough postmortem examination does not define an adequate cause of death. Near miss sudden infant death syndrome refers to survival of a child after an unexpected arrest of unknown cause

REFERENCES

1. Schindler MB, Bohn D, Cox PN, et al. Outcome of out-of-hospital cardiac or respiratory arrest in children. *N Engl J Med* 1996;335:1473–1479.

2. Broides A, Sofer S, Press J. Outcome of out of hospital cardiopulmonary arrest in children admitted to the emergency room. *Isr Med Assoc J* 2000;2:672–674.

3. Eisenberg M, Bergner L, Hallstrom A. Epidemiology of cardiac arrest and resuscitation in children. *Ann Emerg Med* 1983;12:672–674.

4. Applebaum D, Slater PE. Should the Mobile Intensive Care Unit respond to pediatric emergencies? *Clin Pediatr (Phila)* 1986;25: 620–623.

5. Tsai A, Kallsen G. Epidemiology of pediatric prehospital care. *Ann Emerg Med* 1987;16: 284–292.

6. Thompson JE, Bonner B, Lower GM. Pediatric cardiopulmonary arrests in rural populations. *Pediatrics* 1990;86:302–306.

7. Safranek DJ, Eisenberg MS, Larsen MP. The epidemiology of cardiac arrest in young adults. *Ann Emerg Med* 1992;21:1102–1106.

8. Dieckmann RA, Vardis R. High-dose epinephrine in pediatric out-of-hospital cardiopulmonary arrest. *Pediatrics* 1995;95:901–913.

9. Kuisma M, Suominen P, Korpela R. Paediatric out-of-hospital cardiac arrests — epidemiology and outcome. *Resuscitation* 1995;30:141–150.

10. Ronco R, King W, Donley DK, Tilden SJ. Outcome and cost at a children's hospital following resuscitation for out-of-hospital cardiopulmonary arrest. *Arch Pediatr Adolesc Med* 1995;149: 210–214.

11. Sirbaugh PE, Pepe PE, Shook JE, et al. A prospective, population-based study of the demographics, epidemiology, management, and outcome of out-of-hospital pediatric cardiopulmonary arrest. *Ann Emerg Med* 1999; 33:174–184.

12. Friesen RM, Duncan P, Tweed WA, Bristow G. Appraisal of pediatric cardiopulmonary resuscitation. *Can Med Assoc J* 1982;126: 1055–1058.

13. Hu SC. Out-of-hospital cardiac arrest in an Oriental metropolitan city. *Am J Emerg Med* 1994; 12:491–494.

14. Barzilay Z, Somekh E, Sagy M, Boichis H. Pediatric cardiopulmonary resuscitation outcome. *J Med* 1988;19:229–241.

15. Bhende MS, Thompson AE. Evaluation of an end-tidal CO_2 detector during pediatric cardiopulmonary resuscitation. *Pediatrics* 1995; 95:395–399.

16. Brunette DD, Fischer R. Intravascular access in pediatric cardiac arrest. *Am J Emerg Med* 1988;6: 577–579.

17. Clinton JE, McGill J, Irwin G, Peterson G, Lilja GP, Ruiz E. Cardiac arrest under age 40: etiology and prognosis. *Ann Emerg Med* 1984;13:1011–1015.

18. Hazinski MF, Chahine AA, Holcomb GW, Morris JA. Outcome of cardiovascular collapse in pediatric blunt trauma. *Ann Emerg Med* 1994;23: 1229–1235.

19. Losek JD, Hennes H, Glaeser P, Hendley G, Nelson DB. Prehospital care of the pulseless, nonbreathing pediatric patient. *Am J Emerg Med* 1987;5:370–374.

20. Ludwig S, Kettrick RG, Parker M. Pediatric cardiopulmonary resuscitation. A review of 130 cases. *Clin Pediatr (Phila)* 1984;23:71–75.

21. Nichols DG, Kettrick RG, Swedlow DB, Lee S, Passman R, Ludwig S. Factors influencing outcome of cardiopulmonary resuscitation in children. *Pediatr Emerg Care* 1986;2:1–5.

22. O'Rourke PP. Outcome of children who are apneic and pulseless in the emergency room. *Crit Care Med* 1986;14:466–468.

23. Rosenberg NM. Pediatric cardiopulmonary arrest in the emergency department. *Am J Emerg Med* 1984;2:497–499.

24. Sheikh A, Brogan T. Outcome and cost of open- and closed-chest cardiopulmonary resuscitation in pediatric cardiac arrests. *Pediatrics* 1994;93: 392–398.

25. Suominen P, Rasanen J, Kivioja A. Efficacy of cardiopulmonary resuscitation in pulseless paediatric trauma patients. *Resuscitation* 1998; 36:9–13.

26. Suominen P, Korpela R, Kuisma M, Silfvast T, Olkkola KT. Paediatric cardiac arrest and resuscitation provided by physician-staffed emergency care units. *Acta Anaesthesiol Scand* 1997;41:260–265.

27. Torphy DE, Minter MG, Thompson BM. Cardiorespiratory arrest and resuscitation of children. *Am J Dis Child* 1984;138: 1099–1102.

28. Walsh R. Outcome of pre-hospital CPR in the pediatric trauma patient [abstract]. *Crit Care Med* 1994;22:A162.

29. Young KD, Seidel JS. Pediatric cardiopulmonary resuscitation: a collective review. *Ann Emerg Med* 1999;33:195–205. Search date 1997; primary sources Medline and bibliographic search.

30. Gausche M, Lewis RJ, Stratton SJ, et al. Effect of out-of-hospital pediatric endotracheal intubation on survival and neurological outcome. *JAMA* 2000;283:783–790.

31. Mogayzel C, Quan L, Graves JR, Tiedeman D, Fahrenbruch C, Herndon P. Out-of-hospital ventricular fibrillation in children and adolescents: causes and outcomes. *Ann Emerg Med* 1995;25:484–491.

32. Losek JD, Hennes H, Glaeser PW, Smith DS, Hendley G. Prehospital countershock treatment of pediatric asystole. *Am J Emerg Med* 1989;7:571–575.

David Creery
Children's Hospital of Eastern Ontario
Ottawa
Canada

Kate Ackerman
The Children's Hospital
Boston
USA

Competing interests: None declared.

| TABLE 1 | Incidence of non-submersion out-of-hospital cardiorespiratory arrest in children* (see text, p 9). |

Reference	Location	Year	Incidence per 100 000 people in total population	Incidence per 100 000 children
12	Manitoba, Canada	1982	2.9	ND
3	King County, USA	1983	2.4	9.9
4	Jerusalem, Israel	1986	2.5	6.9
5	Fresno, USA	1987	5.7	ND
6	Midwestern USA	1990	4.7	ND
7	King County, USA	1992	2.4	10.1
13	Taipei, Taiwan	1994	1.3	ND
8	San Francisco, USA	1995	2.2	16.1
9	Helsinki, Finland	1995	1.4	9.1
10	Birmingham, USA	1995	ND	6.9
11	Houston, USA	1999	4.9	18.0
2	Southern Israel	2000	3.5	7.8

* Incidence represents arrests per 100 000 population per year. ND, no data.

TABLE 2 Causes of non-submersion out-of-hospital cardiorespiratory arrest in children* (see text, p 9).

Cause	Number of arrests (%)	Number of survivors (%)
Undetermined	691 (43.9)	1 (0.1)
Trauma	311 (19.8)	10 (3.2)
Chronic disease	126 (8.0)	9 (7.1)
Pneumonia	75 (4.8)	6 (8.0)
Non-accidental injury	23 (1.5)	2 (8.7)
Aspiration	20 (1.3)	0 (0)
Overdose	19 (1.2)	3 (15.8)
Other	309 (19.6)	28 (9.1)
Total	**1574 (100)**	**59 (3.7)**

*Figures represent the numbers of arrests/survivors in children with each diagnosis.

QUESTIONS

INTERVENTIONS

Key Messages

- Diabetes mellitus increases the risk of cardiovascular disease. Cardiovascular risk factors in people with diabetes include conventional risk factors (age, prior cardiovascular disease, cigarette smoking, hypertension, dyslipidaemia, sedentary lifestyle, family history of premature cardiovascular disease), and more diabetes specific risk factors (elevated urinary protein excretion, poor glycaemic control).

- We found no good evidence on the effects of screening people with diabetes for high cardiovascular risk.

- We found no direct evidence on the effects of promoting smoking cessation in people with diabetes. Observational evidence and extrapolation from people without diabetes suggest that promotion of smoking cessation is likely to reduce cardiovascular events.

RCTs have found:

- Antihypertensive treatment in people with diabetes reduces cardiovascular events.
- Aggressive blood pressure control with target diastolic blood pressures of ≤ 80 mmHg compared with less tight control reduces cardiovascular morbidity and mortality.
- Weak and conflicting evidence comparing the effects of angiotensin enzyme (ACE) inhibitors with other antihypertensive treatments.
- Statins and fibrates are effective in primary and secondary prevention of cardiovascular disease in people with diabetes and dyslipidaemia.
- Aspirin is effective in primary and secondary prevention of cardiovascular disease in people with diabetes.
- Aggressive control of blood glucose with insulin and oral agents, or both, does not increase the risk of cardiovascular disease, and may decrease this risk.
- Coronary artery bypass grafting (CABG) reduces the death rate more than percutaneous transluminal coronary angioplasty (PTCA) in people with diabetes and multivessel coronary artery disease.
- In people with diabetes and acute myocardial infarction (AMI), one RCT found that PTCA significantly reduced the risk of death or cardiovascular events within 30 days of treatment.
- The combination of stent and glycoprotein IIb/IIIa inhibition in people with diabetes undergoing percutaneous coronary revascularisation reduces restenosis rates and serious morbidity.

DEFINITION   **Diabetes mellitus:** See definition under glycaemic control in diabetes, p 58. **Cardiovascular disease:** Atherosclerotic disease of the heart and/or the coronary, cerebral, or peripheral vessels leading to clinical events such as AMI, congestive heart failure, sudden cardiac death, stroke, gangrene, and/or need for revascularisation procedures.

INCIDENCE/   Diabetes mellitus is a major risk factor for cardiovascular disease. In
PREVALENCE the USA, 60–75% of people with diabetes die from cardiovascular causes.[1] The annual incidence of cardiovascular disease is increased in diabetic men (RR 2–3) and in diabetic women (RR 3–4) after adjusting for age and other cardiac risk factors.[2] About 45% of middle aged and older white people with diabetes have evidence of coronary artery disease, compared with about 25% of people without diabetes in the same populations.[2] In a population based cohort study of 1059 diabetic and 1373 non-diabetic Finnish adults aged 45–64 years, the 7 year risk of AMI was as high in adults with diabetes without previous cardiac disease as it was in people without diabetes with previous cardiac disease.[3]

AETIOLOGY/   Conventional risk factors for cardiovascular disease contribute to
RISK FACTORS increasing its relative risk in people with diabetes to about the same extent as in those without diabetes (see aetiology under primary prevention, p 130). The absolute risk of cardiovascular disease is

almost the same in diabetic women as in diabetic men. Cardiovascular risk factors relatively specific to people with diabetes include longer duration of diabetes during adulthood (the years of exposure to diabetes before age 20 add little to risk of cardiovascular disease);[4] raised blood glucose concentrations (reflected in fasting blood glucose or HbA1c); and microalbuminuria (albuminuria 30–299 mg/24 hours). People with diabetes and microalbuminuria have a higher risk of coronary morbidity and mortality than people with normal levels of urinary albumin and a similar duration of diabetes (RR 2–3).[5,6] Clinical proteinuria increases the risk of major cardiac events in type 2 diabetes (RR 3)[7] and in type 1 diabetes (RR 9),[4,8,9] compared with individuals with the same type of diabetes having normal albumin excretion. Physical inactivity is a significant risk factor for cardiovascular events in both men and women. A cohort study of diabetic women found that participation in little or no physical activity (< 1 hour per week) compared with participation in physical activity for at least 7 hours a week was associated with doubling of the risk of a cardiovascular event.[10] A cohort study of 1263 diabetic men (mean follow up 12 years) found that low baseline cardiorespiratory fitness compared with moderate or high fitness increased overall mortality (RR 2.9); and overall mortality was higher in those reporting no recreational exercise in the previous 3 months compared with those reporting any recreational physical activity in the same period (RR 1.7).[11]

PROGNOSIS Diabetes mellitus increases the risk of mortality or serious morbidity after a coronary event (RR 1.5–3).[2,3,12,13] This excess risk is partly accounted for by increased prevalence of other cardiac risk factors in people with diabetes. A systematic review found that "stress hyperglycaemia" in diabetic people on admission to hospital for AMI compared with diabetic people with lower glucose levels was associated with increased mortality in hospital (RR 1.7, 95% CI 1.2 to 2.4).[14]

AIMS To reduce mortality and morbidity from cardiovascular disease, with minimum adverse effects.

OUTCOMES Incidence of fatal or non-fatal AMI; congestive heart failure; sudden cardiac death; coronary revascularisation; stroke; gangrene; angiographic evidence of coronary, cerebral vascular, or peripheral arterial stenosis.

METHODS *Clinical Evidence* search and appraisal December 2000. We searched for systematic reviews and RCTs with at least 10 confirmed clinical cardiovascular events among people with diabetes. Studies reporting only intermediate end points (e.g. regression of plaque on angiography, lipid changes) were not considered.

QUESTION **What are the effects of screening for high cardiovascular risk in people with diabetes?**

We found no good evidence about screening people with diabetes for cardiovascular risk.

Benefits: We found no systematic review and no large RCTs.

Harms: We found inadequate evidence.

Comment: Screening for conventional risk factors as well as regular determination of HbA1c (see glossary, p 30), lipid profile, and urinary albumin excretion will identify people at high risk.[15,16] Consensus opinion in the USA recommends screening for cardiovascular disease with exercise stress testing in previously sedentary adults with diabetes who are planning to undertake vigorous exercise programmes.[15,17] We found no evidence that such testing prevents cardiac events.

QUESTION   **What are the effects of promoting smoking cessation in people with diabetes?**

Observational studies have found that cigarette smoking is associated with increased cardiovascular death in people with diabetes. In non-diabetic people, smoking cessation has been found to be associated with reduced risk.

Benefits: We found no systematic review or RCTs of the promotion of smoking cessation specifically in people with diabetes.

Harms: We found no evidence of harms.

Comment: People with diabetes are likely to benefit from smoking cessation at least as much as people who do not have diabetes but have other risk factors for cardiovascular events (see smoking cessation under secondary prevention of ischaemic cardiac events, p 179).

QUESTION   **What are the effects of antihypertensive drugs in people with diabetes?**

OPTION   **ANTIHYPERTENSIVE TREATMENT VERSUS NO ANTIHYPERTENSIVE TREATMENT**

Systematic reviews of RCTs have found that diuretics, ACE inhibitors, and β blockers reduce cardiovascular events in people with diabetes and no previous cardiovascular events. One large RCT found that an ACE inhibitor reduced subsequent cardiovascular events and overall mortality in people with diabetes aged over 55 with additional cardiac risk factors, previously diagnosed coronary vascular disease (CVD), or both. No class of medication had significant adverse effects on metabolism or quality of life at the doses used in the trials reviewed.

Benefits: **Primary prevention:** See table 1, p 33. We found one systematic review (published 1997, 2 RCTs included a subgroup of 1355 people with diabetes who had no previous cardiovascular events)[18] and one subsequent RCT.[19] The systematic review found that active treatment (stepped care beginning with a diuretic) versus less active treatment (either placebo[20] or referral to usual care in the community[21]) significantly reduced cardiovascular morbidity and mortality (OR for morbidity and mortality 0.64, 95% CI 0.50 to 0.82; for overall mortality 0.85, 95% CI 0.62 to 1.17) and major cardiovascular events (AR 27% with control v 19% with active treatment over 5 years; NNT 13 middle aged and older adults with diabetes for 5 years). The subsequent RCT (4695 people, 495 with diabetes, aged ≥ 60 years with blood pressure 165–220/ < 95 mmHg) found that active treatment (beginning with nitrendipine) versus placebo reduced all cardiovascular events over a median of 2 years (AR 13/252 [5.2%] for active treatment v 31/240 [12.9%] for controls; ARR 8%, 95% CI 3% to 10%; RR 0.4, 95% CI 0.21 to 0.75; NNT 13, 95% CI 10 to 31) but had no significant effect on overall mortality (AR 16/252 for active treatment v 26/240 for controls; ARR +4.5%, 95% CI –0.7% to +7.4%; RR 0.96, 95% CI 0.32 to 1.06).[19] **Primary and secondary prevention:** See table 3, p 37. We found one systematic review (search date not stated, 4 RCTs, 1100 people with diabetes out of 15 843 people aged > 55 years)[22] and one subsequent RCT.[23] The systematic review found that diuretics (1008 people) versus placebo reduced the risk of major CVD events (fatal or non-fatal coronary events or stroke, sudden death, or death from embolism; RR 0.8). No conclusion was reached regarding initial treatment with β blockers because so few people with diabetes (92 people) received them.[22] The subsequent RCT (3577 diabetic people out of 9541 people aged ≥ 55 years with at least 1 of the following risk factors: diagnosed CVD, current smoker, hypercholesterolaemia, hypertension, or microalbuminuria) compared ramipril (10 mg) versus placebo and vitamin E versus placebo over 4.5 years in a 2 x 2 factorial design (see table 3, p 37).[23] Compared with placebo, ramipril reduced major cardiovascular events (CVD death, AMI, or stroke 277/1808 with ramipril v 351/1769 with placebo; RR 0.75, 95% CI 0.64 to 0.88; ARR 4.5%; NNT 22 older people with diabetes and additional risk factors treated for 4.5 years to prevent 1 major cardiovascular event, 95% CI 14 to 43), and death from any cause (196/1808 v 248/1769; RR 0.76, 95% CI 0.67 to 0.92; ARR 3.2%; NNT 32, 95% CI 19 to 98). The relative effect of ramipril was present in all subgroups regardless of hypertensive status, microalbuminuria, type of diabetes, and nature of diabetes treatment (diet, oral agents, or insulin). Vitamin E treatment had no effect on morbidity or mortality.[23] **Secondary prevention:** See table 2, p 35. We found one systematic review (7 RCTs with follow up ≥ 1 year; 2564 people with diabetes and previous cardiovascular events).[18] It found that both ACE inhibitors and β blockers reduced the risk of subsequent cardiac events in people with diabetes and previous myocardial infarction, with or without hypertension. Active treatment versus placebo significantly reduced overall mortality (6 RCTs, 2402 people; OR 0.82, 95% CI 0.69 to 0.99). Cardiovascular morbidity plus mortality was reduced by a similar amount, but was reported by only two RCTs in the systematic review and the reduction was not significant (2 RCTs, 654 people; OR 0.82, 95% CI 0.60 to 1.13).

Harms: No class of medication had significant adverse effects on metabolism or quality of life at the doses used in the trials reviewed. More people allocated to ramipril than to placebo withdrew because of cough (7% v 2%). This was the only adverse effect occurring more frequently in the ACE inhibitor recipients than in controls.[22]

Comment: None.

OPTION   **DIFFERENT ANTIHYPERTENSIVE DRUGS**

One systematic review of large RCTs has found that ACE inhibitors versus calcium channel blockers as initial therapy for hypertension significantly reduce cardiovascular events in people with type 2 diabetes aged 50–65 years. We found no clear evidence directly comparing ACE inhibitors and diuretics. One large RCT found that an ACE inhibitor versus a β blocker had similar effect on cardiovascular events. One large RCT has found that doxazosin (an α blocker) versus chlortalidone (chlorthalidone) (a diuretic) increases the risk of congestive heart failure.

Benefits: We found one systematic review (search date 2000, 4 RCTs, 2180 people with diabetes)[24] and two subsequent RCTs.[25,26] The systematic review compared ACE inhibitors (1133 people) versus other antihypertensive drugs (diuretics, β blockers, or calcium channel blockers; 1047 people).[24] **ACE inhibitors versus calcium channel blockers:** We found one systematic review,[24] which found two RCTs[27,28] comparing ACE inhibitors versus calcium channel blockers in people with diabetes, and one subsequent RCT[25] comparing ACE inhibitors versus calcium channel antagonists versus conventional treatment (β blockers or hydrochlorothiazide plus amiloride). The two RCTs in the systematic review found that ACE inhibitors versus calcium channel blockers significantly reduced cardiovascular events (34/424 [8%] with ACE inhibitor v 151/526 [16%] with calcium channel blocker; ARR 8%, 95% CI 4% to 13%; RR 0.49, 95% CI 0.33 to 0.72; NNT 13, 95% CI 7 to 25). ACE inhibitors versus calcium channel blockers also reduced the three outcomes of death, AMI, and stroke, but the reductions were not significant. The subsequent RCT (6614 people, 719 with diabetes, mean age 76 years, mean blood pressure 190/99 mmHg) found (among the subgroup of people with diabetes) no significant difference in the incidence of major cardiovascular events over 4 years (64.2 events/1000 person years with ACE inhibitors v 67.7 with calcium antagonists v 75.0 with conventional agents).[25] **ACE inhibitors versus diuretics:** We found one systematic review,[24] which found no RCTs specifically comparing ACE inhibitors versus diuretics in people with diabetes, but found one RCT (572 people, 6.1 years) comparing ACE inhibitors versus alternative treatment that included β blockers, combination β blockers and diuretics, and diuretics in people with and without diabetes. Fewer people allocated to captopril experieinced AMI, stroke or death compared to diuretics or β blockers (43/263 [18%] with diuretics/β blockers v 30/309 [10%] with captopril; ARR 6.6%, 95 CI 1.1% to 12.2%; NNT 15).[24] **ACE inhibitors versus β blockers:** We found one systematic review, which included one RCT (758 people, 456 cardiovascular events) comparing an ACE inhibitor (captopril) versus a β blocker (atenolol) over 8.4 years.[29] The RCT found that captopril versus atenolol did not significantly reduce the number of cardiovascular events (102/400 [25.5%] with captopril v 75/358 [20.9%] with atenolol; ARI +5%, 95% CI −1% to +11%; RR 1.22, 95% CI 0.94 to 1.58). **Other comparisons:** We found no systematic review but found one RCT[26] (age ≥ 55 years, with hypertension and either previous CVD or at least 1 additional CVD risk factor) comparing chlortalidone, doxazosin, amlodipine, and lisinopril. After 3.3 years of follow up there was no difference between doxazosin

(3183 people with diabetes) and chlortalidone (5481 people) in the primary outcome (fatal coronary heart disease [CHD] or non-fatal AMI), but the doxazosin arm was terminated because of an excess risk of combined CVD events (coronary heart disease death, non-fatal AMI, stroke, revascularisation procedures, angina, congestive heart failure, and peripheral vascular disease) compared with chlortalidone (OR 1.24, 95% CI 1.12 to 1.38). The RCT is still in progress.[26]

Harms: In one RCT, people taking atenolol gained more weight than those taking captopril (3.4 kg with atenolol v 1.6 kg with captopril, P = 0.02).[29] Over the first 4 years of the trial, people allocated to atenolol had higher mean HbA1c (7.5% v 7.0%, P = 0.004), but there was no difference between groups over the subsequent 4 years. There was no difference between atenolol and captopril in rates of hypoglycaemia, lipid concentrations, tolerability, blood pressure lowering, or prevention of disease events.

Comment: We found evidence that ACE inhibitors are superior to calcium channel blockers as initial therapy. We found no clear evidence directly comparing ACE inhibitors and diuretics. It is unclear whether ACE inhibitors or β-blockers are superior to each other. In most trials, combination therapy with more than one agent was required to achieve target blood pressures.

OPTION	DIFFERENT TARGET BLOOD PRESSURE

RCTs have found that setting lower target blood pressures reduces cardiovascular events.

Benefits: We found several recent trials with large numbers of participants with diabetes (see table 1, p 33, and table 3, p 37). In two large RCTs, tighter control of blood pressure reduced the risk of major cardiovascular events.[29-31] In one, people with diabetes who were randomised to target diastolic blood pressure ≤ 80 mmHg had half the risk of major cardiovascular events compared with their counterparts randomised to target blood pressure ≤ 90 mmHg.[31] In the other large RCT, people with hypertension and type 2 diabetes randomised to tight blood pressure control (< 150/< 85 mmHg) with atenolol (358 people) or captopril (400 people) had reduced incidence of "any diabetes related end point" deaths (primarily cardiovascular deaths), stroke, and microvascular disease.[29,30]

Harms: We found no good evidence of a threshold below which it is harmful to lower blood pressure.

Comment: Aggressive lowering of blood pressure in people with diabetes and hypertension reduces cardiovascular morbidity and mortality. In most trials, combination therapy with more than one agent was required to achieve target blood pressures.

QUESTION	What are the effects of lipid lowering agents in people with diabetes?

Subgroup analyses of results for people with diabetes enrolled into large RCTs of statins or fibrates versus placebo have found benefit in primary and secondary prevention of AMI.

Cardiovascular disease in diabetes

Benefits: **Primary prevention:** We found no systematic review. Three large RCTs with significant numbers of diabetic participants have compared lipid lowering agents with placebo, and found reductions in the risk of cardiovascular events (see table 1, p 33). In the first, men aged 45–73 years and women aged 55–73 years were randomised to diet plus lovastatin 20–40 mg/day or diet plus placebo, and followed for a mean of 5.2 years.[32] Only people with total cholesterol 4.65–6.82 mmol/l, low density lipoprotein cholesterol (LDL-C) 3.36–4.91 mmol/l, high density lipoprotein cholesterol (HDL-C) ≤ 1.16 mmol/l (men) or ≤ 1.22 mmol/l (women), and triglycerides ≤ 4.52 mmol/l were included in the trial. The second RCT (4081 Finnish men aged 40–55 years) compared gemfibrozil 600 mg twice daily versus placebo over 5 years. Required baseline lipid concentrations were (total minus HDL-C) ≥ 5.2 mmol/l; participants were not excluded on the basis of triglyceride level.[33] The third RCT (164 men and women with type 2 diabetes aged 35–65 years) compared bezafibrate versus placebo for 3 years.[34] Required baseline lipids included one or more of the following: total cholesterol 5.2 to 8.0 mmol/l, serum triglyceride 1.8–8.0 mmol/l, HDL-C ≤ 1.1 mmol/l, or total to HDL-C ratio ≥ 4.7. **Secondary prevention:** We found no systematic review but found four RCTs involving people with diabetes (see table 2, p 35). One RCT (4444 men and women aged 35–70 years with previous AMI or angina pectoris, total cholesterol concentrations of 5.5–8.0 mmol/l, and triglycerides ≤ 2.5 mmol/l) compared simvastatin versus placebo over a median of 5.4 years.[35] Simvastatin dosage was initially 20 mg daily, with blinded dosage titration up to 40 mg daily, according to cholesterol response during the first 6–18 weeks. The relative risk of main end points in people with diabetes treated with simvastatin were as follows: total mortality 0.57 (95% CI 0.30 to 1.08), major cardiovascular events 0.45 (95% CI 0.27 to 0.74), and any atherosclerotic event 0.63 (95% CI 0.43 to 0.92).[23] The second RCT (4159 men and women aged 21–75 years, 3–20 months after MI and with total cholesterol < 6.2 mmol/l, triglycerides < 3.92 mmol/l, and LDL-C 3.0–4.5 mmol/l) compared pravastatin 40 mg/day versus placebo over a median of 5 years.[36] Among the people with diabetes, the relative risk of major coronary events (death from coronary disease, non-fatal AMI, CABG, or PTCA) was 0.75 (95% CI 0.57 to 1.0). The third RCT (9014 men and women aged 31–75 with AMI or unstable angina, plasma total cholesterol 4.0–7.0 mmol/l, and plasma triglycerides < 5.0 mmol/l) compared pravastatin 40 mg daily versus placebo for a mean of 6.1 years.[37] Among the 782 participants with diabetes, the relative risk of CHD death or non-fatal AMI was 0.84 (95% CI 0.59 to 1.10). The fourth RCT (2531 men aged < 74 with previous CVD, AMI, angina, revascularisation, or angiographically documented coronary stenosis), (HDL-C ≤ 1.0 mmol/l, LDL-C ≤ 3.6 mmol/l and triglycerides ≤ 3.4 mmol/l) compared gemfibrozil 1200 mg daily with placebo for a median of 5.1 years (treatment was intended to raise HDL-C levels rather than reduce LDL-C).[38] Among the 627 participants with diabetes, the relative risk of CHD death or non-fatal MI was 0.76 (95% CI 0.57 to 1.0).

Harms: None reported.

Comment: Most published clinical trials with sufficient statistical power to detect effects on cardiovascular events have enrolled comparatively small numbers of diabetic people or excluded them altogether. The available evidence is therefore based almost entirely on subgroup analyses of larger trials. Several large ongoing trials are evaluating the effects of fibrates in people with diabetes.

QUESTION | **What are the effects of blood glucose control on cardiovascular disease in people with diabetes?**

In most cohort studies, higher average concentrations of blood glucose in people with diabetes were associated with a higher incidence of cardiovascular disease. RCTs provide modest support for glucose lowering with insulin, sulphonylureas, or metformin in primary prevention of cardiovascular disease, and strong support for intensive insulin treatment after AMI.

Benefits: **Primary prevention:** See table 1, p 33. We found no systematic review. In people with diabetes, higher average levels of blood glucose are associated with a higher incidence of cardiovascular disease. We found two RCTs.[39-42] Both found that intensive hypoglycaemic treatment reduced the risks of microvascular diabetic complications in both type 1 and type 2 diabetes, although neither trial found that intensive glycaemic control significantly reduced cardiovascular risk. In the first trial, 1441 people with type 1 diabetes aged 13–39 years and free of cardiovascular disease, hypertension, hypercholesterolaemia, and obesity at baseline, were randomly assigned to conventional or intensive diabetes treatment and followed for a mean of 6.5 years.[41,42] Major macrovascular events were almost twice as frequent in the conventionally treated group (40 events) as in the intensive treatment group (23 events), although the differences were not significant (ARR 2.2%; RR 0.59, 95% CI 0.32 to 1.1). In the second trial, 3867 people aged 25–65 years (median 54 years) with type 2 diabetes that was inadequately controlled on diet alone, were randomised to conventional treatment (diet only, 1138 people, drugs added only if needed to keep fasting glucose < 15.0 mmol/l), intensive treatment with a sulphonylurea (1573 people), or insulin (1156 people).[39] People who were $\geq$ 120% of ideal body weight were randomised to conventional treatment (411 people), metformin (342 people), sulphonylureas (542 people), or insulin (409 people).[40] Intensive treatment beginning with a sulphonylurea or insulin improved glycaemic control (HbA1c 7.9% with conventional treatment compared with 7% with intensive treatment). Compared with conventional treatment, intensive treatment reduced diabetes related end points (RR 0.88, 95% CI 0.80 to 0.99; NNT 39 for 5 years to prevent 1 additional diabetes related end point) and the risk of AMI (ARs 14.7/1000 person years for intensive v 17.4/1000 person years for conventional; RR 0.84, 95% CI 0.71 to 1.0). Risks of stroke and amputation did not differ significantly among groups.[39] **Secondary prevention:** See table 3, p 37. We found no systematic review but found two RCTs. One small RCT (153 men with type 2 diabetes, mean age 60 years, many of whom had previous cardiovascular events) compared standard insulin (once daily) with intensive treatment with a stepped plan designed to achieve near normal blood

Cardiovascular disorders

sugar levels.[43] After 27 months, the rate of new cardiovascular events was not significantly different between the groups (24/75 [32%] with intensive therapy v 16/80 [20%] with standard insulin; RR 1.6, 95% CI 0.92 to 2.5). In the second trial, 620 people (mean age 68 years, 63% men, 84% with type 2 diabetes) with random blood glucose ≥ 11 mmol/l were randomised within 24 hours of an AMI to either standard treatment or intensive insulin treatment.[44,45] The intensive insulin group received an insulin glucose infusion for 24 hours followed by subcutaneous insulin four times daily for at least 3 months. The standard treatment group received insulin only when it was clinically indicated. HbA1c fell significantly with intensive insulin treatment (absolute fall of 1.1% with intensive treatment v 0.4% with standard treatment at 3 months and 0.9% v 0.4% at 12 months). Intensive treatment lowered mortality (ARs 19% v 26% at 1 year and 33% v 44% at a mean of 3.4 years; RR 0.72, 95% CI 0.55 to 0.92; NNT 9 treated for 3.4 years to prevent 1 additional premature death). The absolute reduction in the risk of mortality was particularly striking in people who were not previously taking insulin and had no more than one of the following risk factors before the AMI that preceded randomisation: age ≥ 70 years, history of previous AMI, history of congestive heart failure, current treatment with digitalis. In this low risk subgroup, the ARR was 15% (NNT 7 for 3.4 years).

Harms: Sulphonylureas and insulin, but not metformin, increased the risks of weight gain and hypoglycaemia. On an intention to treat basis, the proportions of people per year with severe hypoglycaemic episodes were 0.7%, 1.2%, 1%, 2%, and 0.6% for conventional, chlorpropamide, glibenclamide, insulin, and metformin groups. These frequencies of hypoglycaemia were much lower than those observed with intensive treatment in people with type 1 diabetes in the first primary prevention RCT.[41,42] One RCT found no evidence that any specific treatment (insulin, sulphonylurea, or metformin) increased overall risk of cardiovascular disease.[39,40]

Comment: The role of intensive glucose lowering in primary prevention of cardiovascular events remains unclear. However, such treatment clearly reduces the risk of microvascular disease and does not increase the risk of cardiovascular disease. The potential of the second and larger primary prevention RCT to demonstrate an effect of tighter glycaemic control was limited by the small difference achieved in median HbA1c between intensive and conventional treatment. In contrast, in the first primary prevention trial, a larger 1.9% difference in median HbA1c was achieved between groups, but the young age of the participants and consequent low incidence of cardiovascular events limited the power of the study to detect an effect of treatment on incidence of cardiovascular disease.[41,42] The study of insulin in type 2 diabetes[43] included men with a high baseline risk of cardiovascular events and achieved a 2.1% absolute difference in HbA1c. The RCT was small and the observed difference between groups could have arisen by chance. The design of the trial of intensive versus standard glycaemic control following AMI does not distinguish whether the early insulin infusion or the later intensive subcutaneous insulin treatment was the more important determinant of improved survival in the intensively treated group. The larger primary prevention trial found no evidence that oral hypoglycaemics increase cardiovascular mortality,[39,40] but the possibility that oral hypoglycaemics may be harmful after AMI cannot be ruled out.

QUESTION **What is the effect of aspirin in people with diabetes?**

Very large RCTs of primary and mixed primary and secondary prevention, and a systematic review of secondary prevention, support a cardioprotective role for aspirin.

Benefits:
Primary prevention: We found no systematic review but found two RCTs. In the only large primary prevention RCT comparing aspirin versus placebo and reporting results for people with diabetes, 22 701 US male physicians aged 40–85 years were assigned to aspirin 325 mg every other day or to placebo, and followed for an average of 5 years.[46] The trial found that, after 5 years, among the 533 physicians with diabetes, aspirin versus placebo reduced the risk of AMI (11/275 [4%] with aspirin v 26/258 [10.1%] with placebo; RR 0.39, 95% CI 0.20 to 0.79; NNT 16, 95% CI 12 to 47). A second RCT comparing aspirin with placebo did not specify the number of people with diabetes, but it did report that aspirin reduced AMI to a similar degree in the subgroup of people with diabetes and in the overall trial population (RR 0.85).[31] **Primary and early secondary prevention:** We found one RCT. The largest RCT of aspirin prophylaxis in people with diabetes involved 3711 diabetic men and women (30% with type 1 diabetes, 48% with prior cardiovascular disease).[47] It compared aspirin (650 mg/day) with placebo and followed the participants for a mean of 5 years. It found a non-significant reduction in overall mortality in those treated with aspirin (RR 0.91, 95% CI 0.75 to 1.11). AMI occurred in 289 people (16%) in the aspirin group and 336 (18%) in the placebo group (ARR 2%, 95% CI 0.1% to 4.9%). Fifty people would need to be treated for 5 years with aspirin 650 mg/day to prevent one additional AMI. **Secondary prevention:** We found one systematic review (search date 1990, 145 RCTs of antiplatelet treatment, primarily aspirin).[48] Results for people with diabetes are tabulated (see table 3, p 37).

Harms:
In the large trial comparing aspirin versus placebo for primary and secondary prevention, fatal or non-fatal stroke occurred in 5% on aspirin and 4.2% on placebo (P = NS).[47] There was no significant increase with aspirin in the risks of vitreous, retinal, gastrointestinal, or cerebral haemorrhage. In the systematic review, doses of aspirin ranged from 75–1500 mg/day. Most trials used 75–325 mg/day of aspirin. Doses higher than 325 mg/day increased the risk of haemorrhagic adverse effects without improving preventive efficacy. No difference in efficacy or adverse effects was found in the dose range 75–325 mg.[48]

Comment:
We found insufficient evidence to define precisely which people with diabetes should be treated with aspirin. The risk of cardiovascular disease is very low before age 30; most white diabetic adults aged over 30 are at increased risk of cardiovascular disease. Widely accepted contraindications to aspirin treatment include aspirin allergy, bleeding tendency, anticoagulant treatment, recent gastrointestinal bleeding, and clinically active liver disease.[15,49]

Cardiovascular disease in diabetes

QUESTION **What are the effects of treating proteinuria in people with diabetes?**

Elevated urinary protein excretion is a risk factor for cardiovascular disease. One large RCT has found that an ACE inhibitor reduces cardiovascular risk compared with placebo in people with or without microalbuminuria.

Benefits: We found no good evidence.

Harms: We found no good evidence.

Comment: One large RCT found that the ACE inhibitor ramipril, which reduces urinary protein excretion, also reduced cardiovascular morbidity and mortality in older diabetic people with other cardiac risk factors.[23] However, the relative cardioprotective effect was present to the same extent in people with or without microalbuminuria.

QUESTION **Coronary artery bypass graft versus percutaneous transluminal coronary angioplasty in people with diabetes**

One RCT has found that coronary artery bypass graft (CABG) reduces the death rate more than percutaneous transluminal coronary angioplasty (PTCA) in people with diabetes and multivessel coronary artery disease.

Benefits: We found no systematic review but found one RCT (1829 people with two or three vessel coronary disease, 353 with diabetes; mean age 62 years) comparing CABG with PTCA, without stenting or glycoprotein IIb/IIIa blockade (see table 3, p 37).[50] After a mean 7.7 years, fewer diabetic people assigned to CABG than PTCA died or suffered Q-wave myocardial infarction (85/170 [50%] with PTCA v 60/173 [34.7%] with CABG; ARR 15%, 95% CI 5% to 26%; RR 0.69, 95% CI 0.54 to 0.89; NNT 7, 95% CI 4 to 20). This survival benefit was confined to those receiving at least one internal mammary graft.

Harms: In the RCT, in-hospital mortality among people with diabetes was 1.2% after CABG versus 0.6% after PTCA. Myocardial infarction during the initial hospitalisation was three times more common after CABG than after PTCA (5.8% v 1.8%). None of these differences was significant.

Comment: Adjunctive therapies (heparin or abciximab) were not used in the RCT.

QUESTION **What are the effects of primary coronary angioplasty versus thrombolysis for acute myocardial infarction in people with diabetes?**

One RCT has found that treatment of AMI in diabetic people with primary coronary angioplasty rather than thrombolytic therapy results in a non-significant reduction of death and cardiovascular events at 30 days.

Benefits: We found no systematic review. One RCT (1138 people with AMI presenting within 12 hours of chest pain onset, 177 with diabetes, mean age of diabetic people 65 years) compared primary angio-plasty with thrombolysis (alteplase) (see table 3, p 37).[51] At 30 days, fewer diabetic people assigned to primary angioplasty experienced the composite end point of death, reinfarction or disabling stroke, but the difference was not significant (11/99 [11%] with primary angioplasty v 13/78 [17%] with alteplase; ARR +5.6%, 95% CI −4.8 to +15.9%). In the RCT, 30 day mortality among people with diabetes was eight of 99 people (81%) after angioplasty versus five of 78 people (6.4%) after alteplase. This difference was not significant.

Harms: See harms of CABG versus PTCA, p 28.

Comment: None.

QUESTION **Glycoprotein IIb/IIIa inhibitors and intracoronary stenting (as adjunct to percutaneous coronary revascularisation) in people with diabetes**

Two RCTs have that the combination of stent and glycoprotein IIb/IIIa inhibition (abciximab) reduces restenosis rates and serious morbidity in people with diabetes undergoing percutaneous coronary angioplasty.

Benefits: We found no systematic review but found two RCTs (see table 3, p 37).[52-55] The first RCT (2792 people, 638 with diabetes, mean age 61 years, 38% female, all undergoing PTCA or directional atherectomy without stenting) compared placebo plus standard dose heparin versus abciximab plus standard dose heparin versus abciximab plus low dose heparin. Abciximab was given as a bolus plus 12 hour infusion. The primary indications for intervention were unstable angina (51%), stable ischaemia (33%), and recent AMI (16%). A total of 44% had a prior coronary intervention, 56% had multivessel disease, and 74% a history of hypertension. Compared with placebo, abciximab reduced the combined end point of death or AMI in both standard dose and low dose heparin arms (at 30 days by over 60% and at 6 months by over 50%). Abciximab reduced the rate of restenosis in people without diabetes (hazard ratio 0.78) but not in people with diabetes. The second RCT (2401 people, 491 with diabetes, mean age 60 years, 29% female, 69% hypertensive, 30% recent smokers, 48% prior AMI, 10% prior CABG) compared stent plus placebo (173 people) versus stent plus abciximab (162 people) versus balloon angioplasty plus abciximab (156 people). At 12 months, death or large AMI occurred in 13.9% of those receiving stent and placebo, 8.3% with PTCA and abciximab, and 4.9% with stent and abciximab. Subsequent revascularisation rates following stent and abciximab (13.7%) were much lower than those following stent and placebo (22.4%) or PTCA and abciximab (25.3%).[53-55] For both outcomes, the difference between the stent plus abciximab group and the other two groups was significant. We found an analysis of individual person results of these two trials and a third, earlier trial.[56] In the 1462 diabetic people, abciximab reduced overall mortality (26/540 [4.8%] v 21/844 [2.5%]; ARR 2.3%; NNT 43, 95% CI 23 to 421).

Harms: There was slightly more bleeding in people given abciximab than in those given placebo (4.3% v 3.0% for major bleeding; 6.9% v 6.3% for minor bleeding; 0% v 0.17% for intracranial haemorrhage). None of these differences were significant.[57]

Comment: For people with diabetes undergoing percutaneous procedures, the combination of stent and glycoprotein IIb/IIIa inhibition reduces restenosis rates and serious morbidity. It is unclear whether these adjunctive therapies would reduce morbidity, mortality, and restenosis associated with percutaneous revascularisation procedures to the levels seen with CABG. There was imbalance of the baseline characteristics among the study groups of the second RCT.[53] However, in a multivariate analysis, the treatment effects remained after adjusting for baseline differences.

GLOSSARY

HbA1c The haemoglobin A1c test is the commonest laboratory test of glycated haemoglobin (haemoglobin that has glucose irreversibly bound to it). HbA1c provides an indication of the "average" blood glucose over the last 3 months. The HbA1c is a weighted average over time of the blood glucose level; many different glucose profiles can produce the same level of HbA1c.

REFERENCES

1. Geiss LS, Herman WH, Smith PJ. Mortality in non-insulin-dependent diabetes. In: Harris MI, ed. *Diabetes in America.* 2nd ed. Bethesda, MD: National Institutes of Health, 1995:233–255.
2. Wingard DL, Barrett-Connor E. Heart disease and diabetes. In: Harris MI, ed. *Diabetes in America.* 2nd ed. Bethesda, MD: National Institutes of Health, 1995:429–448.
3. Haffner SM, Lehto S, Ronnemaa T, et al. Mortality from coronary heart disease in subjects with type 2 diabetes and in nondiabetic subjects with and without prior myocardial infarction. *N Engl J Med* 1998;339:229–234.
4. Krolewski AS, Warram JH, Freire MB. Epidemiology of late diabetic complications. A basis for the development and evaluation of preventive programs. *Endocrinol Metab Clin North Am* 1996; 25:217–242.
5. Messent JW, Elliott TG, Hill RD, et al. Prognostic significance of microalbuminuria in insulin-dependent diabetes mellitus: a twenty-three year follow-up study. *Kidney Int* 1992;41:836–839.
6. Dinneen SF, Gerstein HC. The association of microalbuminuria and mortality in non-insulin-dependent diabetes mellitus: a systematic overview of the literature. *Arch Intern Med* 1997; 157:1413–1418. Search date 1995; primary sources Medline 1966 to 1994, Scisearch, hand-searching of bibliographies.
7. Valmadrid CT, Klein R, Moss S E, Klein BE. The risk of cardiovascular disease mortality associated with microalbuminuria and gross proteinuria in persons with older-onset diabetes mellitus. *Arch Intern Med* 2000;160:1093–1100.
8. Borch Johnsen K, Andersen PK, Deckert T. The effect of proteinuria on relative mortality in type 1 (insulin-dependent) diabetes mellitus. *Diabetologia* 1985;28:590–596.
9. Warram JH, Laffel LM, Ganda OP, et al. Coronary artery disease is the major determinant of excess mortality in patients with insulin-dependent diabetes mellitus and persistent proteinuria. *J Am Soc Nephrol* 1992;3(suppl 4):104–110.
10. Hu FB, Stampfer MJ, Solomon C, et al. Physical activity and risk for cardiovascular events in diabetic women. *Ann Intern Med* 2001;134: 96–105.
11. Wei M, Gibbons LW, Kampert JB, Nichaman MZ, Blair SN. Low cardiorespiratory fitness and physical inactivity as predictors of mortality in men with type 2 diabetes. *Ann Intern Med* 2000;132: 605–611.
12. Behar S, Boyko V, Reicher-Reiss H, et al. Ten-year survival after acute myocardial infarction: comparison of patients with and without diabetes. SPRINT Study Group. Secondary Prevention Reinfarction Israeli Nifedipine Trial. *Am Heart J* 1997;133:290–296.
13. Mak KH, Moliterno DJ, Granger CB, et al. Influence of diabetes mellitus on clinical outcome in the thrombolytic era of acute myocardial infarction: GUSTO-I Investigators: global utilization of streptokinase and tissue plasminogen activator for occluded coronary arteries. *J Am Coll Cardiol* 1997;30:171–179.
14. Capes SE, Hunt D, Malmberg K, Gerstein HC. Stress hyperglycaemia and increased risk of death after myocardial infarction in patients with and without diabetes: a systematic overview. *Lancet* 2000;355:773–778. Search date 1998; primary sources Medline, Science Citation Index, hand searches of bibliographies of relevant articles, and contact with experts in the field.
15. Meltzer S, Leiter L, Daneman D, et al. Clinical practice guidelines for the management of diabetes in Canada. *Can Med Assoc J* 1998; 159(suppl 8):1–29.
16. American Diabetes Association. Clinical practice recommendations 2000. *Diabetes Care* 2000; 23(suppl 1):1–116.
17. American Diabetes Association. Diabetes mellitus and exercise. *Diabetes Care* 2000;23(suppl 1):50–54.
18. Fuller J, Stevens LK, Chaturvedi N, et al. Antihypertensive therapy in preventing cardiovascular complications in people with diabetes mellitus. In: The Cochrane Library, Issue 4, 2000. Oxford, Update Software. Search date not given; primary sources Medline; Embase; and hand searches of speciality journals in cardiovascular disease, stroke, renal disease, and hypertension.
19. Tuomilehto J, Rastenyte D, Birkenhäger WH, et al. Effects of calcium-channel blockade in older patients with diabetes and systolic hypertension. *N Engl J Med* 1999;340:677–684.
20. Curb JD, Pressel SL, Cutler JA, et al. Effect of diuretic-based antihypertensive treatment on cardiovascular disease risk in older diabetic patients with isolated systolic hypertension. Systolic Hypertension in the Elderly Program Cooperative Research Group. *JAMA* 1996;276: 1886–1892.

21. Davis BR, Langford HG, Blaufox MD, et al. The association of postural changes in systolic blood pressure and mortality in persons with hypertension: the Hypertension Detection and Follow-up Program experience. *Circulation* 1987; 75:340–346.

22. Lievre M, Guyffier F, Ekomb T, et al. Efficacy of diuretics and β blockers in diabetic hypertensive patients. *Diabetes Care* 2000;23:B65–B71. Search date not stated; primary source Individual Data Analysis of Antihypertensive Drug Interventions (INDANA) project database.

23. Heart Outcomes Prevention Evaluation (HOPE) Study Investigators. Effects of ramipril on cardiovascular and microvascular outcomes in people with diabetes mellitus: results of the HOPE study and the MICRO-HOPE substudy. *Lancet* 2000;355:253–259.

24. Pahor M, Psaty BM, Alderman MH, Applegate WB, Williamson JD, Furberg CD. Therapeutic benefits of ACE inhibitors and other antihypertensive drugs in patients with type 2 diabetes. *Diabetes Care* 2000;23:888–892. Search date January 2000; primary source Medline.

25. Lindholm LH, Hansson L, Ekbom T, et al. Comparison of antihypertensive treatment in preventing cardiovascular events in elderly diabetic patients: results from the Swedish trial in old patients with hypertension–2. *J Hypertens* 2000; 18:1671–1675.

26. ALLHAT Collaborative Research Group. Major cardiovascular events in hypertensive patients randomised to doxazosin vs chlorthalidone: the antihypertensive and lipid-lowering treatment to prevent heart attack trial (ALLHAT). *JAMA* 2000; 283:1967–1975.

27. Estacio RO, Jeffers BW, Hiatt WR, et al. The effect of nisoldipine as compared with enalapril on cardiovascular events in patients with non-insulin-dependent diabetes and hypertension. *N Engl J Med* 1998;338:645–652.

28. Tatti P, Pahor M, Byington RP, et al. Outcome results of the Fosinopril versus Amlodipine Cardiovascular Events randomised Trial (FACET) in patients with hypertension and NIDDM. *Diabetes Care* 1998;21:597–603.

29. UK Prospective Diabetes Study Group. Efficacy of atenolol and captopril in reducing risk of macrovascular and microvascular complications in type 2 diabetes: UKPDS 39. *BMJ* 1998;317: 713–720.

30. UK Prospective Diabetes Study Group. Tight blood pressure control and risk of macrovascular and microvascular complications in type 2 diabetes: UKPDS 38. *BMJ* 1998;317:703–713.

31. Hansson L, Zanchetti A, Carruthers SG, et al. Effects of intensive blood-pressure lowering and low-dose aspirin in patients with hypertension: principal results of the Hypertension Optimal Treatment (HOT) randomised trial. *Lancet* 1998; 351:1755–1762.

32. Downs JR, Clearfield M, Weis S, et al. Primary prevention of acute coronary events with lovastatin in men and women with average cholesterol levels: results of AFCAPS/TexCAPS. Air Force/Texas Coronary Atherosclerosis Prevention Study. *JAMA* 1998;279:1615–1622.

33. Koskinen P, Manttari M, Manninen V, et al. Coronary heart disease incidence in NIDDM patients in the Helsinki Heart Study. *Diabetes Care* 1992;15:820–825.

34. Elkeles RS, Diamond JR, Poulter C, et al. Cardiovascular outcomes in type 2 diabetes. A double-blind placebo-controlled study of bezafibrate: the St Mary's, Ealing, Northwick Park

35. Pyorala K, Pedersen TR, Kjekshus J, et al. Cholesterol lowering with simvastatin improves prognosis of diabetic patients with coronary heart disease. A subgroup analysis of the Scandinavian Simvastatin Survival Study (4S). *Diabetes Care* 1997;20:614–620.

36. Sacks FM, Pfeffer MA, Moye LA, et al. The effect of pravastatin on coronary events after myocardial infarction in patients with average cholesterol levels. Cholesterol and Recurrent Events Trial investigators. *N Engl J Med* 1996;335: 1001–1009.

37. The Long-term Intervention with Pravastatin in Ischemic Disease (LIPID) Study Program. Prevention of cardiovascular events and death with pravastatin in patients with coronary heart disease and a broad range of initial cholesterol levels. *N Engl J Med* 1998;339:1349–1357.

38. Rubins HB, Robins SJ, Collins D, et al. Gemfibrozil for the secondary prevention of coronary heart disease in men with low levels of high-density lipoprotein cholesterol. Veterans Affairs High-Density Lipoprotein Cholesterol Intervention Trial Study Group. *N Engl J Med* 1999;341:410–418.

39. UK Prospective Diabetes Study Group. Intensive blood-glucose control with sulphonylureas or insulin compared with conventional treatment and risk of complications in patients with type 2 diabetes (UKPDS 33). *Lancet* 1998;352: 837–853.

40. UK Prospective Diabetes Study Group. Effect of intensive blood-glucose control with metformin on complications in overweight patients with type 2 diabetes (UKPDS 34). *Lancet* 1998;352: 854–865.

41. DCCT Research Group. The effect of intensive treatment of diabetes on the development and progression of long-term complications in insulin-dependent diabetes mellitus. *N Engl J Med* 1993; 329:977–986.

42. DCCT Research Group. Effect of intensive diabetes management on macrovascular events and risk factors in the Diabetes Control and Complications Trial. *Am J Cardiol* 1995;75:894–903.

43. Abraira C, Colwell J, Nuttall F, et al. Cardiovascular events and correlates in the Veterans Affairs Diabetes Feasibility Trial: Veterans Affairs Cooperative Study on glycemic control and complications in type II diabetes. *Arch Intern Med* 1997;157:181–188.

44. Malmberg K, Ryden L, Efendic S, et al. Randomised trial of insulin-glucose infusion followed by subcutaneous insulin treatment in diabetic patients with acute myocardial infarction (DIGAMI study): effects on mortality at 1 year. *J Am Coll Cardiol* 1995;26:57–65.

45. Malmberg K. Prospective randomised study of intensive insulin treatment on long term survival after acute myocardial infarction in patients with diabetes mellitus. DIGAMI (Diabetes Mellitus, Insulin Glucose Infusion in Acute Myocardial Infarction) Study Group. *BMJ* 1997;314: 1512–1515.

46. Steering Committee of the Physicians' Health Study Research Group. Final report on the aspirin component of the ongoing Physicians' Health Study. *N Engl J Med* 1989;321:129–135.

47. ETDRS Investigators. Aspirin effects on mortality and morbidity in patients with diabetes mellitus. *JAMA* 1992;268:1292–1300.

48. Collaborative overview of randomised trials of antiplatelet therapy–I: Prevention of death, myocardial infarction, and stroke by prolonged antiplatelet therapy in various categories of

patients. Antiplatelet Trialists' Collaboration. *BMJ* 1994;308:81–106. Search date March 1990; primary sources Medline; Current Contents; manual searches of journals; reference lists from clinical trial and review articles; inquiry among colleagues, and manufacturers of antiplatelet agents for unpublished studies.

49. American Diabetes Association. Aspirin therapy in diabetes. *Diabetes Care* 1997;20:1772–1773.

50. The BARI Investigators. Seven-year outcome in the Bypass Angioplasty Revascularization Investigation (BARI) by treatment and diabetic status. *J Am Coll Cardiol* 2000;35:1122–1129

51. Hasdai D, Granger CB, Srivatsa S, et al. Diabetes mellitus and outcome after primary coronary angioplasty for acute myocardial infarction: lessons from the GUSTO-IIb angioplasty study. *J Am Coll Cardiol* 2000;35:1502–1512.

52. Kleiman NS, Lincoff AM, Kereiakes DJ, et al. Diabetes mellitus, glycoprotein IIb/IIIa blockade, and heparin: evidence for a complex interaction in a multicenter trial. EPILOG Investigators. *Circulation* 1998;97:1912–1920.

53. Marso SP, Lincoff AM, Ellis SG, et al. Optimizing the percutaneous interventional outcomes for patients with diabetes mellitus: results of the EPISTENT (Evaluation of platelet IIb/IIIa inhibitor for stenting trial) diabetic substudy. *Circulation* 1999;100:2477–2484.

54. The EPISTENT Investigators. Randomised placebo-controlled and balloon-angioplasty-controlled trial to assess safety of coronary stenting with use of platelet glycoprotein- IIb/IIIa blockade. The EPISTENT Investigators. Evaluation of platelet IIb/IIIa inhibitor for stenting. *Lancet* 1998;352: 87–92.

55. Topol EJ, Mark DB, Lincoff AM, et al. Outcomes at 1 year and economic implications of platelet glycoprotein IIb/IIIa blockade in patients undergoing coronary stenting: results from a multicentre randomised trial. EPISTENT Investigators. Evaluation of Platelet IIb/IIIa Inhibitor for Stenting (published erratum appears in Lancet 2000 Mar 25;355:1104). *Lancet* 1999;354: 2019–2024.

56. The EPIC Investigation. Use of a monoclonal antibody directed against the platelet glycoprotein IIb/IIIa receptor in high-risk coronary angioplasty. *N Engl J Med* 1994;330:956–961.

57. Bhatt DL, Marso SP, Lincoff AM, Wolski KE, Ellis SG, Topol EJ. Abciximab reduces mortality in diabetics following percutaneous coronary intervention. *J Am Coll Cardiol* 2000;35:922–928.

Ronald Sigal
Assistant Professor of Medicine
University of Ottawa
Ottawa
Canada

Janine Malcolm
Fellow, Endocrinology and Metabolism
Ottawa Hospital
Ottawa
Canada

Competing interests: RS has been reimbursed by Bristol Myers Squibb, manufacturer of atorvastatin, for attending conferences. He has received speaker's fees from Eli Lilly (manufacturer of insulin and proglitazone), Novo Nordisk (manufacturer of insulin and repaglinide), GlaxoSmithkline (manufacturer of rosiglitazone), and Bayer (manufacturer of cerivastatin, aspirin, and home glucose testing devices). JM, none declared.

TABLE 1 Primary prevention of cardiovascular events in people with diabetes: evidence from systematic reviews and randomised trials (see text, pp 20, 23–25).

Study	Interventions	Study type	Duration (years)	Outcome	Events / Sample size (%)*		NNT	95% CI for NNT
					Intervention	Control		
Antihypertensive medication								
Cochrane meta-analysis: diabetes and hypertension[18]	Various	SR	5	CVD mortality and morbidity	121/647 (19%)	188/708 (27%)	13	9 to 28
UKPDS Hypertension Study[29,30]	"Tight" target BP (≤ 150/ ≤ 85) with captopril or atenolol v "less tight" target (≤ 180/ ≤ 105)	RCT	8.4	AMI (fatal or non-fatal) Stroke Peripheral vascular events	107/758 (14%) 38/758 (5.0%) 8/758 (1.1%)	83/390 (21%) 34/390 (8.7%) 8/390 (2.1%)	14 27 –	9 to 35 18 to 116 –
HOT[31]	Felodipine and ACE-inhibitor, or β blocker, with 3 distinct target BPs	RCT	3.8	AMI (fatal or non-fatal), stroke (fatal or non-fatal) or other cardiovascular death	22/499 (4.4%) Target diastolic BP 80 mmHg	45/501 (9.0%) Target diastolic BP 90 mmHg	22	16 to 57
FACET[28]	Fosinopril v amlodipine	RCT	2.9	AMI, stroke, or admission to hospital for angina	14/189 (7.4%) Fosinopril	27/191 (14%) Amlodipine	15	10 to 199
ABCD[27]	Enalapril v nisoldipine	RCT	5	AMI (fatal or non-fatal)	5/235 (2.1%) Enalapril	25/235 (11%) Nisoldipine	12	10 to 19
Syst-Eur[19]	Nitrendipine; enalapril ± hydrochlorothiazide (20 mmHg BP lowering) v placebo	RCT	2	MI, CHF, or sudden cardiac death	13/252 (5%)	31/240 (13%)	13	10 to 31

TABLE 1 continued

Lipid-lowering

AFCAPS/TexCAPS[32]	Lovastatin	RCT	5	MI, unstable angina, or sudden cardiac death	4/84 (4.8%)	6/71 (8.5%)	27	NS
SENDCAP[34]	Bezafibrate	RCT	3	MI or new ischaemic changes on ECG	5/64 (7.8%)	16/64 (25%)	6	5 to 20
Helsinki[33]	Gemfibrozil	RCT	5	MI or cardiac death	2/59 (3.4%)	8/76 (10.5%)	14	NS

Blood glucose control

DCCT[41,42]	Intensive insulin therapy in Type 1 diabetes	RCT	6.5	Major macrovascular events‡	23/711 (3.2%)	40/730 (5.5%)	45	28 to 728
UKPDS[39]	Intensive therapy with insulin and/or sulphyoaylurea v conventional therapy	RCT	5	MI (fatal or non-fatal)	387/2729 (14.2%)	186/1138 (16.3%)	46	NS
UKPDS[40]	Intensive therapy with metformin v conventional therapy	RCT	5	MI (fatal or non-fatal)	39/342 (11%)	73/411 (18%)	16	10 to 71

Aspirin

Physicians' Health Study[46]	Aspirin	RCT	5	MI (fatal or non-fatal)	11/275 (4.0%)	26/258 (10%)	16	12 to 47
ETDRS (mixed primary & secondary prevention)[47]	Aspirin	RCT	5	MI (fatal or non-fatal)	289/1856 (15.6%)	336/1855 (18.1%)	39	21 to 716

*Diabetic patients only. ‡Combined MI (fatal or non-fatal), sudden cardiac death, revascularisation procedure, angina with coronary artery disease confirmed by angiography or by noninvasive testing, stroke, lower limb amputation, peripheral arterial events requiring revascularisation, claudication with angiographic evidence of peripheral vascular disease. AMI, acute myocardial infarction; CHF, chronic heart failure; CVD, cardiovascular disease; MI, myocardial infarction; NNT, number needed to treat; RCT, randomised controlled trials; SR, systematic review.

TABLE 2 Secondary prevention of cardiovascular events in people with diabetes: evidence from systematic reviews and randomised trials (see text, pp 21, 24).

Study	Interventions	Study Type	Duration (years)	Outcome	Events / Sample size (%)* Intervention	Events / Sample size (%)* Control	NNT	95% CI for NNT
Antihypertensive medication								
Cochrane review: long-term secondary prevention[18]	Various antihypertensive medications	SR	≥ 1	CVD mortality and morbidity	130/316 (41%)	157/338 (46%)	19	NS
Cochrane review: short-term secondary prevention[18]	Various antihypertensive medications	SR	< 1	CVD mortality and morbidity	8/245 (3.3%)	21/288 (7.3%)	25	17 to 1145
Lipid-lowering								
4S[35]	Simvastatin	RCT	5.4	CHD death or non-fatal MI	24/105 (23%)	44/97 (45%)	5	3 to 10
CARE[36]	Pravastatin	RCT	5	Coronary disease death, non-fatal MI, or revascularisation	81/282 (29%)	112/304 (37%)	12	7 to 194
LIPID[37]	Pravastatin	RCT	6.1	CHD death or non-fatal MI	76/396 (19%)	88/386 (23%)	28	NS
Veterans[38]	Gemfibrozil	RCT	5.1	CHD death or non-fatal MI	88/309 (29%)	116/318 (37%)	13	7 to 144

TABLE 2 continued

Blood glucose control

DIGAMI[44,45]	Insulin infusion followed by intensive insulin therapy v usual care	RCT	3.4	Overall mortality	102/306 (33%)	138/314 (44%)	9	6 to 33
Aspirin								
Antiplatelet trialists[48]	Aspirin v placebo	SR	Median 2 years	CVD mortality and morbidity	415/2248 (19%)	502/2254 (22%)	26	17 to 66
Revascularization								
GUSTO IIb[51]	PTCA v alteplase	RCT	2	Death, nonfatal reinfarction or disabling stroke	PTCA 11/99 (11%)	Alteplase 13/78 (16%)	18	NS
BARI[50]	CABG v PTCA	RCT	7.7	Death or non-fatal q wave MI	CABG 60/173 (35%)	PTCA 85/170 (50%)	7	4 to 21
Glycoprotein IIb/IIIa blockers								
EPIC[56]/EPILOG[52]/EPISTENT[53-55]	Abciximab v control	Pooled	1	Overall death rate	26/540 (4.8%)	21/844 (2.5%)	43	23 to 422
EPIC[56]/EPILOG[52]/EPISTENT[53-55]	Abciximab v control	Pooled	1	Death or non-fatal MI	185/540 (34%)	246/844 (29%)	20	9 to 1423

*Diabetic patients only. CABG, coronary artery bypass grafting; CHD, coronary heart disease; CVD, cardiovascular disease; MI, myocardial infarction; NNT, number needed to treat; PTCA, percutaneous transluminal coronary angioplasty; RCT, randomised controlled trials; SR, systematic review.

TABLE 3 Mixed primary and secondary prevention of cardiovascular events in people with diabetes (see text, pp 21, 23, 25, 27–29).

Interventions	Study type	Duration (years)	Outcome	Events/sample size (%) (diabetic people only)		NNT	95% CI for NNT
				Intervention	Control		
Antihypertensive medication							
ACE Inhibitors v diuretics or calcium channel blockers[24]	Meta-analysis	2.8 to 6.2	CVD death, MI, CHF, angina, or stroke.	ACE inhibitor 158/733	Diuretics or calcium channel blockers 266/789	6	4 to 8
Diuretics v placebo[22]	Meta-analysis	2.2 to 4.8	Any coronary event, any stroke, sudden death, or death from embolism.	Diuretics 151/1000	Placebo 189/1000	26	Unavailable
Ramipril 10 mg daily versus placebo[23]	RCT	4.5	MI, stroke, or CVD. Overall mortality	277/1808 (15%) 196/1808 (11%)	351/1769 (20%) 240/1769 (14%)	22 32	14 to 43 19 to 98

ACE; angiotensin converting enzyme; CHF, congestive heart failure; CVD, cadiovascular disease; MI, myocardial infarction.

Search date January 2001

Margaret Thorogood, Melvyn Hillsdon and Carolyn Summerbell

INTERVENTIONS

Key Messages

Smoking

- Systematic reviews of RCTs have found that simple, one off, advice from a physician during a routine consultation is associated with 2% of smokers quitting smoking and not relapsing for 1 year. Additional encouragement or support may increase (by a further 3%) the effectiveness of the advice. Individual advice from a psychologist achieves a similar quit rate (3%), and advice from trained nurse counsellors, or from trained counsellors who are neither doctors nor nurses, increases quit rates compared with minimal intervention.

- One systematic review of RCTs and one subsequent RCT have found that nicotine replacement is an effective additional component of cessation strategies in smokers who smoke at least 10 cigarettes daily. We found no clear evidence that any method of delivery of nicotine is more effective than others. We found limited evidence from three RCTs with follow up of 2–6 years that the additional benefit of nicotine replacement therapy on quit rates reduces with time.

- One systematic review of RCTs found no evidence that acupuncture increased rates of smoking cessation at 12 months.

- One systematic review of RCTs found very limited evidence that exercise might increase smoking cessation.

- One systematic review of antidepressants used as part of a smoking cessation programme has found that buproprion increases quit rates. Moclobemide and anxiolytics did not significantly increase quit rates.

- Two systematic reviews have found that, in pregnant women, antismoking interventions increase abstinence rates and reduce the risk of low birthweight babies. Interventions without nicotine replacement were as effective as nicotine replacement in men and healthy non-pregnant women.

- One systematic review and two subsequent RCTs have found that antismoking advice improves smoking cessation in people at higher risk of smoking related disease.

- One systematic review has found that training health professionals to give antismoking advice increases the frequency of antismoking interventions being offered, but found no good evidence that the effectiveness of the interventions is increased.

Physical activity and diet

- We found weak evidence from systematic reviews and subsequent RCTs that counselling sedentary people increases physical activity compared with no intervention. Limited evidence from RCTs suggests that consultation with an exercise specialist versus a physician may increase physical activity at 1 year.

- One RCT found that, in women over 80 years, exercise advice delivered in the home by physiotherapists increased physical activity and reduced their risk of falling.

- Systematic reviews have found that advice on cholesterol lowering diet (that is, advice to lower fat intake or increase the ratio of polyunsaturated to saturated fatty acid) leads to a small reduction in blood cholesterol concentrations in the long term (6 months or more).

- Systematic reviews and one RCT have found that salt restriction significantly reduces blood pressure in people with hypertension, and found limited evidence that salt restriction was effective in preventing hypertension. The RCT found limited evidence that advice on restricting salt intake was less effective than advice on weight reduction in preventing hypertension.

- Systematic reviews found that a combination of advice on diet and exercise supported by behaviour therapy was probably more effective than either diet or exercise advice alone in the treatment of obesity, and might lead to sustained weight loss.

DEFINITION	Cigarette smoking, diet, and level of physical activity are important in the aetiology of many chronic diseases. Individual change in behaviour has the potential to decrease the burden of chronic disease, particularly cardiovascular disease.
INCIDENCE/ PREVALENCE	In the developed world, the decline in smoking has slowed and the prevalence of regular smoking is increasing in young people. A sedentary lifestyle is becoming increasingly common and the prevalence of obesity is increasing rapidly.
AIMS	To encourage individuals to reduce or abandon unhealthy behaviours and to take up healthy behaviours; to support the maintenance of these changes in the long term.
OUTCOMES	Ideally the outcomes considered would be clinical, and would relate to the underlying conditions (longevity, quality of life, rate of stroke, or myocardial infarction). However, most studies report proxy outcomes, such as the proportion of people changing behaviour (e.g. stopping smoking) in a specified period.
METHODS	*Clinical Evidence* search and appraisal January 2001.

QUESTION   **Which interventions reduce cigarette smoking?**

OPTION   **COUNSELLING**

Systematic reviews of RCTs have found that simple, one off advice from a physician during a routine consultation is associated with 2% of smokers quitting smoking and not relapsing for 1 year. Additional encouragement or support may increase (by a further 3%) the effectiveness of the advice. Individual advice from a psychologist achieves a similar quit rate (3%), and advice from trained nurse counsellors, or from trained counsellors who are neither doctors nor nurses, increases quit rates compared with minimal intervention.

Benefits: We found four systematic reviews.[1-4] The first (search date not stated, 17 RCTs, 14 438 smokers) evaluated simple advice from physicians. The advice was typically of less than 5 minutes duration. It found that 1.9% of smokers (95% CI 0.1% to 2.8%) stopped smoking as a direct result of the advice and did not relapse for at least 1 year.[1] Rates of cessation in the control groups ranged from 1.1% to 14.1%, and in the intervention groups from 1.5% to 14.5%. The results were similar when the analysis was confined to the six trials in which cessation was confirmed by biochemical markers. Ten RCTs assessed the effect of additional support, such as additional visits and encouragement or demonstrations of exhaled carbon monoxide in the person's breath. There was a high degree of heterogeneity (with rates of cessation ranging from −0.5% to +29%), but the overall estimate of smokers quitting for 1 year was 5% (95% CI 1% to 8%). Five trials of individual sessions with a psychologist found that the number of smokers quitting at 1 year as a result of advice was 2.8% (95% CI 1.3% to 4.2%). The second systematic review (search date 1998, 11 RCTs) of interventions provided by counsellors trained in smoking cessation (other than doctors and nurses) used a broad definition of counselling including all contacts with a smoker that lasted at least 10 minutes. Six of the RCTs had follow up for at least 1 year, whereas the rest had a minimum follow up of 6 months. The review found that counselling increased the rate of quitting (263/1381 [14%] quit with counselling v 194/1899 [10%] with control; OR of quitting 1.55, 95% CI 1.27 to 1.90).[2] The third review (search date 1999, 19 RCTs, 4 with follow up for < 1 year) considered the effectiveness of smoking interventions delivered by a nurse. It found that advice from a nurse increased the rate of quitting (621/4689 [13.2%] quit with advice v 402/3223 [12.5%] with control; OR 1.43, 95% CI 1.24 to 1.6).[3] The final systematic review (search date 1995) identified 23 trials of smoking advice in general practice.[4] In 20 of the trials, a general practitioner gave advice, although nurses or counsellors were also involved in four of these trials. In three trials, the advice was given solely by a nurse or health visitor. Smoking cessation was measured for between 6 months and 2 years. There was significant heterogeneity because of the inclusion of two trials (both involving only general practitioners) with notably larger effects. When these two trials were excluded, the review found that advice significantly increased the odds of smoking cessation (935/9361 [9.7%] quit with advice v 513/7952 [6.8%] with control; OR 1.32, 95% CI 1.18 to 1.48). The review found that (by indirect comparisons) intensive advice was more effective than brief advice (616/7651 [8%] quit with brief advice v 391/6486 [6%] with control; OR for quitting after brief advice 1.27, 95% CI 1.11 to 1.45; with intensive advice 319/2070 [15.4%] quit v 122/1106 [11.0%]; OR after intensive advice 1.46, 95% CI 1.18 to 1.80). Fifty smokers would need to be given brief advice (or 25 smokers given intensive advice) for one additional person to quit for at least 6 months.[4]

Harms: We found no evidence of harm.

Comment: The effects of advice may be considered disappointingly small, but a year on year reduction of 2% in the number of smokers would represent a significant public health gain (see smoking cessation under primary prevention, p 135).

| OPTION | NICOTINE REPLACEMENT |

One systematic review and one subsequent RCT have found that nicotine replacement is an effective component of cessation strategies in smokers who smoke at least 10 cigarettes a day. Fifteen such smokers would have to be treated with nicotine replacement to produce one extra non-smoker at 12 months, but this overestimates effectiveness, because relapse will continue after 12 months. Higher dose (4 mg) gum is more effective than lower dose (2 mg) gum in very dependent smokers. We

found no clear evidence that any one method of delivery of nicotine is more effective, or evidence of further benefit after 8 weeks' treatment with patches. Long term relapse may occur in people who quit, but the review found that the rate of relapse was not greater in those who quit with the aid of nicotine replacement. Abstinence after 1 week is a strong predictor of 12 month abstinence.

Benefits: **Abstinence at 12 months:** We found one systematic review and one subsequent RCT.[5,6] The systematic review (search date 2000) identified 48 trials of nicotine gum, 30 trials of nicotine transdermal patches, four of nicotine intranasal spray, four of inhaled nicotine, and two of sublingual tablet.[5] All forms of nicotine replacement were more effective than placebo. When the abstinence rates for all trials were pooled according to the longest duration of follow up available, the odds of abstinence were increased by 71% (95% CI 60% to 82%) with nicotine replacement compared with placebo. Seventeen per cent of smokers allocated to nicotine replacement successfully quit, compared with 10% in the control group. The review found no significant difference in benefit between different forms of nicotine replacement (OR for abstinence 1.63 for nicotine gum v 2.27 for nicotine nasal spray). In trials that directly compared 4 mg with 2 mg nicotine gum, the higher dose improved abstinence in highly dependent smokers (pooled OR of abstinence 2.67, 95% CI 1.69 to 4.22). Pooled analysis of six trials, which compared high dose versus standard dose patches, found that high dose may slightly increase abstinence (OR 1.21, 95% CI 1.03 to 1.42). The review found no evidence of a difference in effectiveness for 16 hour patches versus 24 hour patches, and no difference in effect in trials where the dose was tapered compared with those where the patches were withdrawn abruptly. Use of the patch for 8 weeks was as effective as longer use, and there was very weak evidence in favour of nicotine replacement in relapsed smokers. The subsequent RCT (3585 people) found that abstinence at 1 week was a strong predictor of 12 month abstinence (25% of those abstinent at 1 week were abstinent at 12 months v 2.7% of those not abstinent at 1 week).[6] One meta-analysis of relapse rates in nicotine replacement trials found that nicotine replacement increased abstinence at 12 months, but that the addition of nicotine replacement did not significantly affect relapse rates between 6 weeks and 12 months.[7] **Longer term abstinence:** We found three RCTs,[8-10] which found that nicotine replacement does not affect long term abstinence. In one RCT, which compared nicotine spray versus placebo, 47 people abstinent at 1 year were followed for up to a further 2 years and 5 months, after which there was still a significant, although smaller, difference in abstinence (in longer term 15.4% abstinent with nicotine spray v 9.3% with placebo; NNT for 1 extra person to abstain 7 at 1 year v 11 at 3.5 years).[8] The second RCT compared 5 months of nicotine patches plus nicotine spray versus the same patches plus a placebo spray. It found no significant difference between treatments after 6 years (16.2% abstinent with nicotine spray v 8.5% with placebo spray, P = 0.08).[9] The third trial compared patches delivering different nicotine doses versus placebo patches. The trial followed everyone that quit at 6 weeks for a further 4 to 5 years, and found no significant difference in relapse between the groups. Overall, 73% of people who quit at 6 weeks relapsed.[10]

Harms: Nicotine gum has been associated with hiccups, gastrointestinal disturbances, jaw pain, and orodental problems. Nicotine transdermal patches have been associated with skin sensitivity and irritation. Nicotine inhalers and nasal spray have been associated with local irritation at the site of administration. Nicotine sublingual tablets have been reported to cause hiccups, burning, and smarting sensations in the mouth, sore throat, coughing, dry lips, and mouth ulcers.[11]

Comment: Nicotine replacement may not represent an "easy cure" for nicotine addiction, but it does improve the cessation rate. The evidence suggests that the majority of smokers attempting cessation fail at any one attempt, or relapse over the next 5 years. Multiple attempts may be needed.

OPTION   ACUPUNCTURE

One systematic review found no evidence that acupuncture increases rates of smoking cessation at 12 months.

Benefits: We found one systematic review (search date 1999, 18 RCTs, 3772 people) comparing acupuncture with sham acupuncture, other treatment, or no treatment. Only five trials (2535 people) reported abstinence after at least 12 months.[12] The review found that acupuncture versus control treatment produced no significant reduction in smoking cessation at 12 months (OR 1.02, 95% CI 0.72 to 1.43).

Harms: None were documented.

Comment: None.

OPTION   PHYSICAL EXERCISE

One systematic review of RCTs found limited evidence that exercise might increase smoking cessation.

Benefits: We found one systematic review (search date 1999, 8 RCTs)[13] of exercise compared with control interventions. Four small RCTs in the review reported point prevalence of non-smoking at 12 months and found no significant benefit from exercise, but these studies were insufficiently powered to exclude a clinically important effect. One RCT (281 women) found that three exercise sessions a week for 12 weeks plus a cognitive behaviour programme (see glossary, p 53) improved continuous abstinence from smoking at 12 months compared with the behaviour programme alone (16/134 [12%] with exercise v 8/147 [5%] with control; ARR +6.5%, 95% CI –19% to +0.0%; RR 2.2, 95% CI 0.98 to 4.5).[14]

Harms: None were documented.

Comment: None.

OPTION ANTIDEPRESSANT AND ANXIOLYTIC TREATMENT

Systematic reviews have found that quit rates are significantly increased by buproprion, but not by moclobemide or anxiolytics.

Benefits: **Antidepressants:** We found one systematic review of antidepressants (search date 2000, 12 RCTs).[15] Eight of the RCTs (3230 people) reported 12 month cessation rates. It found that buproprion 300 mg daily increased cessation at 12 months compared with control treatment (4 RCTs; AR quitting 21% with buproprion v 8% with control; OR 2.73, 95% CI 1.90 to 3.94; NNT 8).[15] Another RCT in the review found that combined buproprion plus a nicotine patch was more efficacious than a patch alone (OR 2.65, 95% CI 1.58 to 4.45), but not more effective than buproprion alone. In two included trials (1 with 6 month and 1 with 12 month follow up), nortriptyline improved long term (6–12 month) abstinence rates compared with placebo (OR 2.83, 95% CI 1.59 to 5.03). One RCT of moclobemide found no significant difference in abstinence at 12 months. **Anxiolytics:** We found one systematic review of anxiolytics (search date 2000, 6 RCTs).[16] Four of the RCTs (626 people) reporting 12 month cessation rates found no significant increase in abstinence with anxiolytics versus control treatment.[16]

Harms: Headache, insomnia, and dry mouth were reported in people using buproprion.[15] Nortriptyline can cause sedation and urinary retention, and can be dangerous in overdose. The largest RCT found that discontinuation rates caused by adverse events were 3.8% with placebo, 6.6% for nicotine replacement therapy, 11.9% for buproprion, and 11.4% for buproprion plus nicotine replacement therapy.[17] Anxiolytics may cause dependence and withdrawal problems, tolerance, paradoxical effects, and impair driving ability.

Comment: None.

QUESTION Are smoking cessation interventions more effective in people at high risk of smoking related disease?

OPTION IN PREGNANT WOMEN

Two systematic reviews of RCTs have found that the effect of antismoking interventions in pregnant women increases abstinence rates and decreases the risk of giving birth to low birthweight babies. The increase in abstinence with non-nicotine replacement interventions was similar to the increase found in trials of nicotine replacement in men and non-pregnant women. One RCT found no evidence that nicotine patches increased quit rates in pregnant women compared with placebo, although birthweight was greater in babies born to mothers given active patches.

Benefits: We found two systematic reviews[1,18] and one additional RCT.[19] The most recent review (search date 1999, 34 RCTs) assessed smoking cessation interventions in pregnancy. It found that smoking cessation programmes improved abstinence (OR of abstinence in late pregnancy with antismoking programmes v no programmes 0.53, 95% 0.47 to 0.60).[18] The findings were similar if the analysis was restricted to trials in which abstinence was confirmed by means other than self reporting. The review also found that antismoking programmes reduced the risk of low birthweight babies, but found no evidence of an effect on the rates of very low birthweight babies or perinatal mortality, although the power to detect such effects was low (OR for low birthweight babies 0.80, 95% CI 0.69 to 0.99). The review calculated that of 100 smokers attending a first antenatal visit, 10 stopped spontaneously and a further six to seven stopped as the result of a smoking cessation programme. Five included trials examined the effects of interventions to prevent relapse in 800 women who had quit smoking. Collectively, these trials found no evidence that the interventions reduced relapse rate.[18] One earlier systematic review (search date not stated, 10 RCTs, 4815 pregnant women) of antismoking interventions[1] included one trial of physician advice, one trial of advice by a health educator, one trial of group sessions, and seven trials of behaviour therapy based on self help manuals. Cessation rates among trials ranged from 1.9–16.7% in the control groups and from 7.1–36.1% in the intervention groups. The review found that antismoking interventions significantly increased the rate of quitting (ARI with intervention v no intervention 7.6%, 95% CI 4.3% to 10.8%).[1] The additional RCT found that nicotine patches did not significantly alter quit rates in pregnant women compared with placebo. However, active patches were associated with greater birthweight in babies born to treated mothers (mean difference in birthweight with nicotine v placebo 186 g, 95% CI 35 g to 336 g).[19]

Harms: None documented.

Comment: The recent review found that some women quit smoking before their first antenatal visit, and the majority of these will remain abstinent.[18]

OPTION **IN PEOPLE AT HIGH RISK OF DISEASE**

One systematic review of RCTs and two subsequent RCTs have found that antismoking advice improves smoking cessation in people at high risk of smoking related disease.

Benefits: We found no trials in which the same intervention was used in high and low risk people. We found one systematic review (search date not stated, 4 RCTs, 13 208 healthy men at high risk of heart disease)[1] and two subsequent RCTs.[20,21] The review found that antismoking advice improved smoking cessation rates compared with control interventions (ARI of smoking cessation 21%, 95% CI 10% to 31%; NNT 5, 95% CI 4 to 10).[1] One early trial (223 men), which was included in the review, used non-random allocation after myocardial infarction. The intervention group was given intensive advice by the therapeutic team while in the coronary care unit. The trial found that the self reported cessation rate at 1 year or more was higher in the intervention group than the control group (63% quit in the intervention group v 28% in the control group; ARI of quitting 36%, 95% CI 23% to 48%).[22] The first subsequent RCT compared postal advice on smoking cessation versus no intervention in men aged 30–45 years with either a history of asbestos exposure, or forced expiratory volume in 1 second (FEV_1) in the lowest quartile for their age. Postal advice increased the self reported sustained cessation rate at 1 year compared with no intervention (5.6% with postal advice v 3.5%; $P < 0.05$; NNT 48).[20] The second RCT (100 people) compared minimal advice versus a 6 month programme of bedside counselling plus seven brief telephone counselling sessions after myocardial infarction. It found that the more intensive programme increased reported abstinence at 12 months compared with minimal counselling (AR of abstinence 55% with programme v 34% with minimal advice, $P = 0.05$).[21]

Harms: None were documented.

Comment: There was heterogeneity in the four trials included in the review, partly because of a less intense intervention in one trial and the recording of a change from cigarettes to other forms of tobacco as success in another. One of the included trials was weakened by use of self reported smoking cessation as an outcome and non-random allocation to the intervention.[22]

QUESTION   **Does training of professionals increase the effectiveness of smoking cessation interventions?**

One systematic review has found that training professionals increases the frequency of antismoking interventions being offered, but found no good evidence that antismoking interventions are more effective if the health professionals delivering the interventions received training.

Benefits: We found one systematic review (search date 2000, 9 RCTs),[23] which included eight RCTs of training medical practitioners and one RCT of training dental practitioners to give antismoking advice. All the trials took place in the USA. The training was provided on a group basis, and variously included lectures, videotapes, role plays, and discussion. The importance of setting quit dates and offering follow up was emphasised in most of the training programmes. The review found no good evidence that training professionals leads to higher quit rates in people receiving antismoking interventions from those professionals, although training increased the frequency with which such interventions were offered. Three of the trials used prompts and reminders to practitioners to deploy smoking cessation techniques, and found that prompts increased the frequency of health professional interventions.[23]

Harms: None were documented.

Comment: The results of the systematic review should be interpreted with caution because there were variations in the way the analysis allowed for the unit of randomisation.

QUESTION   **Which interventions increase physical activity in sedentary people?**

OPTION   **COUNSELLING**

We found weak evidence from systematic reviews and subsequent RCTs that sedentary people can be encouraged to increase their physical activity. Interventions that encourage moderate rather than vigorous

Cardiovascular disorders

exercise, and do not require attendance at a special facility, may be more successful. Increases in walking in previously sedentary women can be sustained over at least 10 years. Brief advice from a physician is probably not effective in increasing physical activity. We found limited evidence from RCTs that primary care consultation with an exercise specialist may increase physical activity at 1 year compared with no advice.

Benefits: We found two systematic reviews[24,25] and seven subsequent RCTs.[26-32] The first review (search date 1996, 11 RCTs based in the USA, 1699 people) assessed single factor physical activity promotion.[24] Seven trials evaluated advice to undertake exercise from home (mainly walking, but including jogging and swimming), and six evaluated advice to undertake facility based exercise (including jogging and walking on sports tracks, endurance exercise, games, swimming, and exercise to music classes). An increase in activity in the intervention groups was seen in trials in which home based moderate exercise was encouraged and regular brief follow up of participants was provided. In most of the trials, participants were self selected volunteers, so the effects of the interventions may have been exaggerated. The second systematic review (search date not stated, 3 RCTs, 420 people) compared "lifestyle" physical activity interventions with either standard exercise treatment or a control group.[25] Lifestyle interventions were defined as those concerned with the daily accumulation of moderate or vigorous exercise as part of everyday life. The first RCT (60 adults, 65–85 years old) found significantly more self reported physical activity in the lifestyle group than a standard exercise group. The second RCT (235 people, 35–60 years old) found no significant difference in physical activity between the groups. The third RCT (125 women, 23–54 years old) of encouraging walking found no significant difference in walking levels at 30 months' follow up between people receiving an 8 week behavioural intervention and those receiving a 5 minute telephone call and written information about the benefits of exercise, although both groups increased walking. Six of the additional trials involved primary care delivered interventions.[26-28,30-32] The two trials, in which advice was delivered by an exercise specialist rather than a physician, found significant improvement in self reported physical activity at long term (> 6 months) follow up compared with controls.[30,31] Short term improvement was found in two further trials, but not maintained at 9 months or 1 year.[27,28] One quasi-randomised trial (776 people in a primary care setting) tested the effect of brief physician advice plus a mailed leaflet on physical activity. It found short term improvement in self-reported activity with the intervention versus control, although after 12 months no significant difference was maintained.[29] One RCT (229 women) of encouraging women to increase walking found significantly increased walking in the intervention group. Ten year follow up of 86% of the original women in the trial found that women who had been encouraged to walk reported significantly more walking (median estimated calorie expenditure from self reported amount of walking 1344 kcal/week in women given encouragement *v* 924 kcal/week in women not encouraged to walk, P = 0.01).[33]

Harms: None of the reviews, or the trials, reported any incidences of harm from taking up exercise.

Comment: Self reporting of effects by people in a trial, especially where blinding to interventions is not possible (as is the case with advice or encouragement), is a potential source of bias. Several trials are in progress, including one in the UK, in which people in primary care have been randomised to two different methods of encouragement to increase walking, or to a no intervention arm. One ongoing multisite trial in the USA has randomised 874 people to one of three experimental counselling interventions.[34]

QUESTION What are effects of exercise advice in high risk people?

OPTION IN WOMEN AGED OVER 80 YEARS

One RCT found exercise advice increased physical activity in women aged over 80 years and decreased the risk of falling.

Benefits: We found no systematic review. One RCT (233 women > 80 years old, conducted in New Zealand) compared four visits from a physiotherapist who advised a course of 30 minutes of home based exercises three times a week that was appropriate for the individual, versus a similar number of social visits.[35] After 1 year, women who had received physiotherapist visits were significantly more active than women in the control group, and 42% were still completing the recommended exercise programme at least three times a week. The mean annual rate of falls in the intervention group was 0.87 compared with 1.34 in the control group, a difference of 0.47 falls a year (95% CI 0.04 to 0.90).

Harms: No additional harms in the intervention group were reported.

Comment: None.

QUESTION What are the effects on blood cholesterol of dietary advice to reduce fat, increase polyunsaturated fats, and decrease saturated fats?

OPTION COUNSELLING

Systematic reviews have found that advice on eating a cholesterol lowering diet (that is, advice to reduce fat intake or increase the polyunsaturated to saturated fatty acid ratio in the diet) leads to a small reduction in blood cholesterol concentrations in the long term (6 months or more). We found evidence of a dose response, in that dietary advice recommending more stringent reduction in fat and cholesterol intake lowered blood cholesterol more than less stringent advice. We found no evidence to support the effectiveness of such advice in primary care.

Benefits: **Effects on blood cholesterol:** We found three systematic reviews[11,36,37] and one subsequent RCT, which reported biochemical rather than clinical end points.[38] None of these systematic reviews included evidence after 1996. One review (search date 1993) identified five trials of cholesterol lowering dietary advice (principally advice from nutritionists or specially trained counsellors) with follow up for 9–18 months.[36] It found a reduction in blood cholesterol concentration in the intervention group of 0.22 mmol/litre

(95% CI 0.05 to 0.39 mmol/l) compared with the control group. However, there was significant heterogeneity (P < 0.02), with two outlying studies — one showing no effect and one showing a larger effect. This review excluded trials in people at high risk of heart disease. Another systematic review (search date 1996) identified 13 trials of more than 6 months' duration and included people at high risk of heart disease.[11] It found that dietary advice reduced blood cholesterol (mean reduction in blood cholesterol concentration with advice 4.5%, 95% CI 3.9% to 5.1%; given a mean baseline cholesterol of 6.3 mmol/litre, mean absolute reduction about 0.3 mmol/l). The third systematic review (search date 1995, 1 trial,[39] 76 people) found no significant difference between brief versus intensive advice from a general practitioner and dietician on blood cholesterol at 1 year.[37] The subsequent RCT (186 men and women at high risk of coronary heart disease) compared advice on healthy eating versus no intervention. At 1 year, it found no significant differences between groups in total and low density lipoprotein cholesterol concentrations for either sex, even though the reported percentage of energy from fat consumed by both women and men in the advice group decreased significantly compared with that reported by the women and men in the control group.[38] These results may reflect bias caused by self-reporting of dietary intake. **Effects on clinical outcomes:** We found two systematic reviews, which reported on morbidity and mortality.[11,40] The first (search date 1996) compared 13 separate and single dietary interventions.[11] It found no significant effect of dietary interventions on total mortality (OR 0.93, 95% CI 0.84 to 1.03) or coronary heart disease mortality (OR 0.93, 95% CI 0.82 to 1.06), but found a reduction in non-fatal myocardial infarction (OR 0.77, 95% CI 0.67 to 0.90). The second review (search date 1999, 27 studies including 40 intervention arms, 30 901 person years) found dietary advice to reduce or modify dietary fat versus no dietary advice had no significant effect on total mortality (HR 0.98, 95% CI 0.86 to 1.12) or cardiovascular disease mortality (HR 0.98, 95% CI 0.77 to 1.07), but significantly reduced cardiovascular disease events (HR 0.84, 95% CI 0.72 to 0.99).[40] RCTs in which people were followed for more than 2 years showed significant reductions in the rate of cardiovascular disease events. The relative protection from cardiovascular disease events was similar in both high and low risk groups, but was significant only in high risk groups.

Harms: We found no evidence about harms.

Comment: The finding of a 0.2–0.3 mmol/litre reduction in blood cholesterol in the two systematic reviews accords with the findings of a meta-analysis of the plasma lipid response to changes in dietary fat and cholesterol.[41] The analysis included data from 244 published studies (trial duration 1 day to 6 years), and concluded that adherence to dietary recommendations (30% energy from fat, < 10% saturated fat, and < 300 mg cholesterol per day) compared with average US dietary intake would reduce blood cholesterol by about 5%.

Cardiovascular disorders

| QUESTION | Does dietary advice to reduce sodium intake lead to a sustained fall in blood pressure? |

Systematic reviews and RCTs have found that salt restriction reduces blood pressure in people with normal blood pressure, and in people with hypertension. The effect was more pronounced in older people. We found no evidence of effects on morbidity and mortality.

Benefits: We found three systematic reviews[36,42,43] and one additional RCT[44] about the long term effects of advice to restrict salt. The first systematic review (search date 1993, 5 trials with follow up for 9–18 months) compared dietary advice (mainly from nutritionists or specially trained counsellors) with control treatment. It found that the advice slightly reduced systolic blood pressure (change in blood pressure: –1.9 mm Hg systolic, 95% CI –3.0 to –0.8 mm Hg), but not diastolic blood pressure (–1.2 mm Hg, 95% CI –2.6 to +0.2 mm Hg).[36] The second review (8 RCTs in adults over 44 years with and without hypertension) found no clearly significant systolic blood pressure changes after at least 6 months' follow up with advice on salt restriction versus no dietary advice either in people with hypertension (–2.9 mm Hg, 95% CI –5.8 to 0.0 mm Hg) or in people without hypertension (–1.3 mm Hg, 95% CI –2.7 to +0.1 mm Hg). Small but significant changes in mean diastolic blood pressure were found in people with hypertension (+2.1 mm Hg, 95% CI –4.0 to –0.1 mm Hg) but not in people without hypertension (–0.8 mm Hg, 95% CI –1.8 to +0.2 mm Hg).[42] The definitions of hypertension varied between the trials. The third review (search date 1996, 30 RCTs) found that in people aged over 44 years defined as having hypertension, a reduction in sodium intake of 100 mmol a day resulted in a decrease of 6.3 mm Hg in systolic blood pressure and 2.2 mm Hg in diastolic pressure.[43] For younger people with hypertension, the systolic fall was 2.4 mm Hg and the diastolic fall was negligible. Three RCTs of salt restriction followed people without hypertension for over 12 months, and found conflicting results. One RCT (181 people) found that advice to restrict salt was less effective in preventing hypertension in overweight people than advice on weight reduction at 7 years.[45] One RCT (585 people) found that advice to restrict salt was as effective as advice to reduce weight for reducing blood pressure in overweight people with hypertension at 15–36 months.[44]

Harms: None reported.

Comment: None.

| QUESTION | What are the effects of lifestyle interventions to achieve sustained weight loss? |

Systematic reviews and subsequent RCTs have found that a combination of advice on diet and exercise, supported by behaviour therapy, is probably more effective in achieving weight loss than either diet or exercise advice alone. A low energy, low fat diet is the most effective

lifestyle intervention for weight loss. RCTs have found no significant differences in weight loss between interventions to promote physical activity. Weight regain is likely, but weight loss of 2–6 kg may be sustained over at least 2 years.

Benefits: We found three systematic reviews,[46-48] and 12 additional RCTs.[49-60] One systematic review (search date 1995) identified 99 studies, including some that tested either dietary or physical activity interventions with or without a behaviour intervention component. The combination of diet and exercise in conjunction with behavioural therapy produced greater weight loss than diet alone. However, this finding was based on the results of one RCT in which a mean weight loss of 3.8 kg at 1 year was observed in a group receiving diet guidelines and behaviour intervention compared with a significantly different mean loss of 7.9 kg in a group receiving the same intervention plus a programme of walking.[46] The second systematic review of the detection, prevention, and treatment of obesity (search date 1999, 11 RCTs and additional prospective cohort studies) included eight RCTs comparing dietary prescriptions with exercise, counselling, or behavioural therapy for the treatment of obesity, and three RCTs comparing dietary counselling alone with no intervention. In both comparisons, initial weight loss was followed by gradual weight regain once treatment had stopped (mean difference in weight change at least 2 years after baseline: 2–6 kg for dietary prescription trials, and 2–4 kg for dietary counselling trials).[47] The third systematic review of RCTs and observational studies found similar results; it found that a combination of diet and exercise, supported by behaviour therapy, was more effective than any one or two of these individual interventions.[48] One additional RCT compared advice on an energy restricted diet to advice on a fat restricted diet.[53] Weight loss was greater on an energy restricted diet than on the fat restricted diet at 6 months (−11.2 kg v −6.1 kg, $P < 0.001$) and at 18 months (−7.5 kg v −1.8 kg, $P < 0.001$). Seven RCTs focused on physical activity.[49-51,55-57,60] The heterogeneity of interventions makes pooling of data inappropriate, but no major differences were found between the various behaviour therapies and exercise regimes. One RCT[52] found behavioural choice treatment (see glossary, p 53) versus standard behaviour therapy (see glossary, p 54) resulted in greater weight loss at 12 months (−10.1 kg v −4.3 kg, $P < 0.01$). One RCT (166 people) compared standard behaviour therapy plus support from friends with standard behaviour therapy without support. It found no additional weight loss at 16 months with social support from friends (−4.7 kg v −3.0 kg, $P < 0.3$).[54] A further RCT (62 women) found that 1 year weight loss was greater in women following a standard versus a modified cognitive behaviour programme (−3.6 kg v 2.0 kg, $P = 0.02$).[59]

Harms: The systematic reviews and RCTs provided no evidence about harms resulting from diet or exercise for weight loss.

Comment: None.

Cardiovascular disorders

One systematic review and additional RCTs have found that most types of maintenance strategy result in smaller weight gains or greater weight losses compared with no contact. Strategies that involve personal contact with a therapist, family support, walking training programmes, multiple interventions, or are weight focused appear most effective.

Benefits: We found one systematic review[46] and six additional RCTs.[61-66] The systematic review (search date 1995, 21 studies) compared different types and combinations of interventions. It found that increased contact with a therapist in the long term produced smaller weight gain or greater weight loss, and that additional self help peer groups, self management techniques, or involvement of the family or spouse may increase weight loss. The largest weight loss was seen in programmes using multiple strategies. Two additional small RCTs (102 people[61] and 100 people in two trials[65]) assessed simple strategies without face to face contact with a therapist. Frequent phone contacts, optional food provision, continued self monitoring, urge control, or relapse prevention did not reduce the rate of weight regain. One small RCT (117 people) found that phone contacts plus house visits did reduce the rate of weight regain compared with no intervention (3.65 kg v 6.42 kg, P = 0.048).[62] One RCT (82 women) compared two walking programmes (4.2 MJ/week or 8.4 MJ/week) plus diet counselling versus diet counselling alone following a 12 week intensive weight reduction programme.[66] Both walking programmes reduced weight regain at 1 year (reduction in weight gain compared with dietary counselling alone 2.7 kg, 95% CI 0.2 kg to 5.2 kg with low intensity programme and 2.6 kg, 95% CI 0.0 kg to 5.1 kg with high intensity programme). At 2 years, weight regain was not significantly different between high intensity programme and control, but was reduced in the low intensity group (reduction in weight gain 3.5 kg, 95% CI 0.2 kg to 6.8 kg with low intensity programme and 0.2 kg, 95% CI –3.1 kg to +3.6 kg). One additional small RCT (67 people) found that people on a weight focused programme maintained weight loss better than those on an exercise focused programme (0.8 kg v 4.4 kg, P < 0.01).[63] One 5 year RCT (489 menopausal women) compared behavioural intervention in two phases aimed at lifestyle changes in diet and physical activity with lifestyle assessment. People in the intervention group were encouraged to lose weight during the first 6 months (phase I), and thereafter maintain this weight loss for a further 12 months (phase II). The intervention resulted in weight loss compared to control during the first 6 months (–8.9 lb v –0.8 lb, P < 0.05), most of which was sustained over phase II (–6.7 lb v +0.6 lb, P < 0.05).[64]

Harms: We found no direct evidence that interventions designed to maintain weight loss are harmful.

Comment: Weight regain is common. The resource implication of providing long term maintenance of any weight loss may be a barrier to the routine implementation of maintenance programmes.

QUESTION   **What are the effects of lifestyle advice to prevent weight gain?**

One small RCT found that low intensity education increased weight loss. An extension of this RCT found no significant effect on weight gain from a mailed newsletter with or without a linked financial incentive.

Benefits: We found three systematic reviews,[46,47,67] which included the same two RCTs.[68,69] The second RCT was an extension of the first. The first RCT (219 people) compared low intensity education with a financial incentive to maintain weight versus an untreated control group. It found significantly greater average weight loss in the intervention group than in the control group (−2.1 lb *v* −0.3 lb, P = 0.03).[68] The second RCT (228 men and 998 women) compared a monthly newsletter versus the newsletter plus a lottery incentive versus no contact. There was no significance difference in weight gain after 3 years between the groups (1.6 kg *v* 1.5 kg *v* 1.8 kg).[60]

Harms: None reported.

Comment: None.

QUESTION   **What are the effects of training professionals in promoting reduction of body weight?**

One systematic review of poor quality RCTs found little evidence on the sustained effect of interventions to improve health professionals' management of obesity. One subsequent small RCT found limited evidence that training for primary care doctors in nutrition counselling plus a support programme reduced body weight of the people in their care over 1 year.

Benefits: We found one systematic review (search date 1998, 12 RCTs, 5 with follow up > 1 year)[70] and one subsequent RCT.[71] The studies in the review were heterogeneous and poor quality. The subsequent RCT (45 people) compared nutrition counselling training plus a support programme for primary care doctors versus usual care.[71] The nutrition supported intervention compared with usual care increased weight loss at 1 year (additional weight loss 2.3 kg, P < 0.001).

Harms: None reported.

Comment: The doctors were randomly allocated to treatment but the analysis of results was based on the people in the care of those doctors. No allowance was made for cluster bias. This increases the likelihood that the additional weight loss could have occurred by chance.

GLOSSARY

Behavioural choice treatment A cognitive behavioural intervention based on a decision making model of women's food choice. This relates situation specific eating behaviour to outcomes and goals using decision theory. The outcomes and goals governing food choice extend beyond food related factors to include self esteem and social acceptance.

Cognitive behaviour programme Traditional cognitive behavioural topics (e.g. self-monitoring, stimulus control, coping with cravings and high risk situations, stress management, and relaxation techniques) along with topics of particular importance to women (e.g. healthy eating, weight management, mood management, and managing work and family).

Standard behaviour therapy A behavioural weight management programme that incorporates moderate calorie restriction to promote weight loss.

REFERENCES

1. Law M, Tang JL. An analysis of the effectiveness of interventions intended to help people stop smoking. *Arch Intern Med* 1995;155:1933–1941. Search date not specified but before 1995; primary sources Medline and Index Medicus; dates not given, but selected trials range from 1967 to 1993.

2. Lancaster T, Stead LF. Individual behavioural counselling for smoking cessation. In: The Cochrane Library, Issue 4, 2000. Oxford: Update Software. Search date October 1998; primary sources Cochrane Tobacco Addiction Group Trials Register to October 1998.

3. Rice VH, Stead LF. Nursing interventions for smoking cessation. In: The Cochrane Library, Issue 1, 2000. Oxford: Update Software. Search date May 1999; primary sources Cochrane Tobacco Addiction Group Trials Register to May 1999, and Cinahl 1983 to May 1999.

4. Ashenden R, Silagy C, Weller D. A systematic review of the effectiveness of promoting lifestyle change in general practice. *Family Practice* 1997; 14:160–176. Search date May 1995; primary sources Medline, Psychlit, Sociofile, Cinahl, Embase, and Drug; all searched from the year of their inception up to May 1995.

5. Silagy C, Mant D, Fowler G, Lancaster T. Nicotine replacement therapy for smoking cessation. In: The Cochrane Library, Issue 4, 2000. Oxford: Update Software. Search date April 2000; primary sources Cochrane Tobacco Addiction Group Trials Register.

6. Tonneson P, Paoletti P, Gustavsson G, et al. Higher dose nicotine patches increase one year smoking cessation rates: results from the European CEASE trial. *Eur Respir J* 1999;13:238–246.

7. Stapleton J. Cigarette smoking prevalence, cessation and relapse. *Stat Methods Med Res* 1998;7:187–203. Search date and primary sources not given.

8. Stapleton JA, Sutherland G, Russell MA. How much does relapse after one year erode effectiveness of smoking cessation treatments? Long term follow up of a randomised trial of nicotine nasal spray. *BMJ* 1998;316:830–831.

9. Blondal T, Gudmundsson J, Olafsdottir I, et al. Nicotine nasal spray with nicotine patch for smoking cessation: randomised trial with six years follow up. *BMJ* 1999;318:285–289.

10. Daughton DM, Fortmann SP, Glover ED, et al. The smoking cessation efficacy of varying doses of nicotine patch delivery systems 4 to 5 years post-quit day. *Prev Med* 1999;28:113–118.

11. Ebrahim S, Davey Smith G. *Health promotion in older people for the prevention of coronary heart disease and stroke.* Health promotion effectiveness reviews series, No 1. London: Health Education Authority, 1996. Search date December 1994; primary sources Medline, hand searches of reference lists, and citation search on BIDS for Eastern European trials.

12. White AR, Rampes H, Ernst E. Acupuncture for smoking cessation. In: The Cochrane Library, Issue 4, 2000. Oxford: Update Software. Search date 1999; primary sources Cochrane Tobacco Addiction Group Register, Medline, Psychlit, Dissertation Abstracts, Health Planning and Administration, SocialSciSearch, Smoking and Health, Embase, Biological Abstracts and Drug.

13. Ussher MH, Taylor AH, West R, McEwen A. Does exercise aid smoking cessation? *Addiction* 2000; 95:199–208.

14. Marcus BH, Albrecht AE, King TK, et al. The efficacy of exercise as an aid for smoking cessation in women. *Arch Intern Med* 1999;159: 1229–1234.

15. Hughes JR, Stead LF, Lancaster T. Antidepressants for smoking cessation. In: The Cochrane Library, Issue 4, 2000. Oxford Update Software. Search date July 2000; primary sources Cochrane Tobacco Addiction Group trials register.

16. Hughes JR, Stead LF, Lancaster T. Anxiolytics for smoking cessation. In: The Cochrane Library, Issue 4, 2000. Oxford Update Software. Search date July 2000; primary sources Cochrane Tobacco Addiction Group trials register.

17. Jorenby DE, Leischow SJ, Nides MA, et al. A controlled trial of sustained-release buproprion. A nicotine patch, or both for smoking cessation. *N Engl J Med* 1999;340:685–691.

18. Lumley J, Oliver S, Waters E. Interventions for promoting smoking cessation during pregnancy. In: The Cochrane Library, Issue 4, 2000. Oxford: Update Software. Search date October 1998; primary sources Cochrane Tobacco Addiction Group Trials Register to October 1998.

19. Wisborg K, Henriksen TB, Jespersen LB, Secher NJ. Nicotine patches for pregnant smokers: A randomized controlled study. *Obstet Gynecol* 2000;96:967–971.

20. Humerfelt S, Eide GE, Kvale G, et al. Effectiveness of postal smoking cessation advice: a randomized controlled trial in young men with reduced FEV$_1$ and asbestos exposure. *Eur Respir J* 1998;11: 284–290.

21. Dornelas EA, Sampson RA, Gray JF, Waters D, Thompson PD. A randomized controlled trial of smoking cessation counselling after myocardial infarction. *Prev Med* 2000;30:261–268.

22. Burt A, Thornley P, Illingworth D, et al. Stopping smoking after myocardial infarction. *Lancet* 1974; 1:304–306.

23. Lancaster T, Silagy C, Fowler G, Spiers I. Training health professionals in smoking cessation. In: The Cochrane Library, Issue 4, 2000. Oxford: Update Software. Search date 2000; primary sources Specialised Register of the Cochrane Tobacco Addiction Group.

24. Hillsdon M, Thorogood M. A systematic review of physical activity promotion strategies. *Br J Sports Med* 1996;30:84–89. Search date 1996; primary sources Medline, Excerpta Medica, Sport, SCISearch 1966 to 1996, and hand search of reference lists.

25. Dunn AL, Anderson RE, Jakicic JM. Lifestyle physical activity interventions. History, short- and long-term effects and recommendations. *Am J Prev Med* 1998;15:398–412. Search date not given; primary sources Medline, Current Contents, Biological Abstracts, The Johns Hopkins Medical Institutions Catalog, Sport Discus, and Grateful Med.

26. Goldstein MG, Pinto BM, Marcus BH, et al. Physician-based physical activity counseling for middle-aged and older adults: a randomised trial. *Ann Behaviour Med* 1999;1:40–47.

27. Harland J, White M, Drinkwater C, et al. The Newcastle exercise project: a randomised controlled trial of methods to promote physical activity in primary care. *BMJ* 1999;319:828–832.

28. Taylor, A, Doust, J, Webborn, N. Randomised controlled trial to examine the effects of a GP exercise referral programme in Hailsham, East Sussex, on modifiable coronary heart disease risk factors. *J Epidemiol Community Health* 1998;52: 595–601.

29. Bull F, Jamorozik K. Advice on exercise from a family physician can help sedentary patients to become active. *Am J Prev Med* 1998;15:85–94.

30. Stevens W, Hillsdon M, Thorogood M, McArdle D. Cost-effectiveness of a primary care based physical activity intervention in 45–74 year old men and women; a randomised controlled trial. *Br J Sports Med* 1998;32:236–241.

31. Halbert JA, Silagy CA, Finucane PM, Withers RT, Hamdorf PA. Physical activity and cardiovascular risk factors: effect of advice from an exercise specialist in Australian general practice. *Med J Aust* 2000;173:84–87.

32. Norris SL, Grothaus LC, Buchner DM, Pratt M. Effectiveness of physician-based assessment and counseling for exercise in a staff model HMO. *Prev Med* 2000;30:513–523.

33. Pereira MA, Kriska AN, Day RD, et al. A randomized walking trial in postmenopausal women. *Arch Intern Med* 1998;158:1695–1701.

34. King A, Sallis JF, Dunn AL, et al. Overview of the activity counselling trial (ACT) intervention for promoting physical activity in primary health care settings. *Med Sci Sports Exerc* 1998;30: 1086–1096.

35. Campbell AJ, Robertson MC, Gardner MM, et al. Randomised controlled trial of a general practice programme of home based exercise to prevent falls in elderly women. *BMJ* 1997;315: 1065–1069.

36. Brunner E, White I, Thorogood M, et al. Can dietary interventions change diet and cardiovascular risk factors? A meta-analysis of randomised controlled trials. *Am J Public Health* 1997;87:1415–1422. Search date July 1993; primary sources computer and manual searches of databases and journals. No further details given.

37. Tang JL, Armitage JM, Lancaster T, et al. Systematic review of dietary intervention trials to lower blood total cholesterol in free living subjects. *BMJ* 1998;316:1213–1220. Search date 1996; primary sources Medline, Human Nutrition, Embase, and Allied and Alternative Health 1966 to 1995; hand search of *Am J Clin Nutr*, and reference list checks.

38. Stefanick ML, Mackey S, Sheehan M, et al. Effects of diet and exercise in men and postmenopausal women with low levels of HDL cholesterol and high levels of LDL cholesterol. *N Engl J Med* 1998;339:12–20.

39. Tomson Y, Johannesson M, Aberg H. The costs and effects of two different lipid intervention programmes in primary health care. *J Intern Med* 1995;237:13–17.

40. Hooper L, Summerbell C, Higgins J, et al. Dietary advice, modification or supplementation aimed at lipid lowering for prevention of cardiovascular disease in patients with and without ischaemic heart disease. In: The Cochrane Library, Issue 4, 2000. Oxford: Update Software. Search date 1999, primary sources Cochrane Library, Medline, Embase, CAB Abstracts, CVRCT registry, related Cochrane groups' trial registers, trials known to experts in the field, and biographies.

41. Howell WH, McNamara DJ, Tosca MA, et al. Plasma lipid and lipoprotein responses to dietary fat and cholesterol: a meta-analysis. *Am J Clin Nutr* 1997;65:1747–1764. Search date 1994; primary source Medline 1966 to February 1994, hand search of selected review publications and bibliographies.

42. Ebrahim S, Davey Smith G. Lowering blood pressure: a systematic review of sustained effects of non-pharmacological interventions. *J Public Health* 1998;2:441–448. Search date April 1998; primary sources Medline and hand searches of reference lists.

43. Fodor JG, Whitmore B, Leenen F, Larochelle P. Recommendations on dietary salt. *Can Med Assoc J* 1999;160(suppl 9):29–34. Search date 1996; primary sources Medline, hand searches of reference lists, personal files, and contact with experts.

44. Whelton PK, Appel LJ, Espeland MA, et al. Sodium reduction and weight loss in the treatment of hypertension in older persons. A randomized controlled Trial of Nonpharmacologic Interventions in the Elderly (TONE). *JAMA* 1998;279:839–846.

45. He J, Whelton PK, Appel LJ, et al. Long-term effects of weight loss and dietary sodium reduction on incidence of hypertension. *Hypertension* 2000;35:544–549.

46. Glenny A-M, O'Meara S, Melville A, Shelton T, Wilson C. The treatment and prevention of obesity: a systematic review of the literature. *Int J Obesity* 1887;21;715–737. Published in full as NHS CRD report 1997, No10. *Systematic review of interventions in the treatment and prevention of obesity.* http://ww.york.ac.uk/inst/crd/obesity.htm. Search date 1995; primary sources Medline; Embase; DHSS data; Current Research in UK; Science citation index; Social science citation index; Conference Proceedings index; SIGLE; Dissertation Abstracts; Sport; Drug Info; AMED (Allied and alternative medicine; ASSI (abstracts and indexes); CAB; NTIS (national technical information dB); Directory of Published Proceedings (Interdoc); Purchasing Innovations database; Health promotion database; S.S.R.U.; DARE (CRD, database of systematic reviews); NEED (CRD, database of health economic reviews); all databases searched from starting date to the end of 1995.

47. Douketis JD, Feightner JW, Attia J, Feldman WF. Periodic health examination, 1999 update. Detection, prevention and treatment of obesity. Canadian Task Force on Preventive Health Care. *Can Med Assoc J* 1999;160:513–525. Search date 1999; primary sources Medline (1996 to April 1998); Current Contents (1966 to 1999); and hand search of references.

48. The National Heart, Lung, and Blood Institute. Clinical guidelines on the identification, evaluation, and treatment of overweight and obesity in adults. Bethesda Maryland: National Institutes of Health, 1998; website http://www.nhlbi.nih.gov/nhlbi/guidelns/ob_home.htm

49. Wing RR, Polley BA, Venditti E, et al. Lifestyle intervention in overweight individuals with a family history of diabetes. *Diabetes Care* 1998;21: 350–359.

50. Anderson RE, Wadden TA, Barlett SJ, et al. Effects of lifestyle activity v structured aerobic exercise in obese women. *JAMA* 1999;281:335–340.

51. Jakicic JM, Winters C, Lang W, Wing RR. Effects of intermittent exercise and use of home exercise

equipment on adherence, weight loss, and fitness in overweight women. *JAMA* 1999;282: 1554–1560.

52. Sbrocco T, Nedegaard RC, Stone JM, Lewis EL. Behavioural choice treatment promotes continuing weight loss. *J Consult Clin Psychol* 1999;67: 260–266.

53. Harvey-Berino J. Calorie restriction is more effective for obesity treatment than dietary fat restriction. *Ann Behav Med* 1999;21:35–39.

54. Wing RR, Jeffery RW. Benefits of recruiting participants with friends and increasing social support for weight loss and maintenance. *J Consult Clin Psychol* 1999;67:132–138.

55. Jeffery RW, Wing RR, Thorson C, Burton LR. Use of personal trainers and financial incentives to increase exercise in a behavioural weight loss program. *J Consult Clin Psychol* 1998;66: 777–783.

56. Craighead LW, Blum MD. Supervised exercise in behavioural treatment for moderate obesity. *Behav Ther* 1989;20:49–59.

57. Donnelly JE, Jacobsen DJ, Heelan KS, Seip R, Smith S. The effects of 18 months of intermittent vs. continuous exercise on aerobic capacity, body weight and composition, and metabolic fitness in previously sedentary, moderately obese females. *Int J Obesity* 2000;24:566,–572.

58. Kunz K, Kreimel K, Gurdet C, Lenhart P, Wirth B, Irsigler, K. Comparison of behaviour modification and conventional dietary advice in a long-term weight reduction programme for obese women [abstract]. *Diabetologia* 1982;23:181.

59. Rapoport L, Clark M, Wardle J. Evaluation of a modified cognitive-behavioural programme for weight management. *Int J Obesity* 2000;24: 1726–1737.

60. Wing R, Epstein LH, Paternostro-Bayles M, et al. Exercise in a behavioural weight control program for obese patients with type 2 (non insulin dependent) diabetes. *Diabetologica* 1988;31: 902–909.

61. Bonato DP, Boland FJ. A comparison of specific strategies for long-term maintenance following a behavioural treatment program for obese women. *Int J Eat Disord* 1986;5:949–958.

62. Hillebrand TH, Wirth A. Evaluation of an outpatient care program for obese patients after an inpatient treatment. *Prav Rehab* 1996;8:83–87.

63. Leermakers EA, Perri MG, Shigaki CL, Fuller PR. Effects of exercise-focused versus weight-focused maintenance programs on the management of obesity. *Addict Behav* 1999;24:219–227.

64. Simkin-Silverman LR, Wing RR, Boraz MA, Meilan EN, Kuller LH. Maintenance of cardiovascular risk factor changes among middle-aged women in a lifestyle intervention trial. *Women's Health: Research on Gender, Behaviour, and Policy* 1998; 4:255–271.

65. Wing RR, Jeffery RW, Hellerstedt WL, Burton LR. Effect of frequent phone contacts and optional food provision on maintenance of weight loss. *Ann Behav Med* 1996;18:172–176.

66. Fogelholm M, Kukkonen-Harjula K, Nenonen A, Pasanen M. Effects of walking training on weight maintenance after a very-low-energy diet in premenopausal obese women: a randomized controlled trial. *Arch Intern Med* 2000;160: 2177–2184.

67. Hardeman W, Griffin S, Johnston M, et al. Interventions to prevent weight gain: a systematic review of psychological models and behaviour change methods. *Int J Obesity* 2000;4:131–143. Search date not stated; primary sources Medline, Embase, Psychlit, The Cochrane Library, Current Contents, ERIC, HealthStar, Social Science Citation Index, and hand searches of reference lists.

68. Forster JL, Jeffery RW, Schmid TL, Kramer FM. Preventing weight gain in adults: a pound of prevention. *Health Psychol* 1988;7:515–525.

69. Jeffery RW, French SA. Preventing weight gain in adults: the pound of prevention study. *Am J Public Health* 1999;89:747–751.

70. Harvey EL, Glenny A, Kirk SFL, Summerbell CD. Improving health professionals' management and the organisation of care for overweight and obese people. In: The Cochrane Library, Issue 4, 2000. Oxford: Update Software. Search date January 1998; primary sources specialised registers of the Cochrane Effective Practice and Organisation of Care Group May 1997; The Cochrane Depression, Anxiety and Neurosis Group August 1997; The Cochrane Diabetes Group August 1997; The Cochrane Controlled Trials Register September 1997; Medline 1966 to January 1998; Embase 1988 to December 1997; Cinahl 1982 to November 1997; Psychlit 1974 to December 1997; Sigle 1980 to November 1997; Sociofile 1974 to October 1997; Dissertation Abstracts 1861 to January 1998; Conference Papers Index 1973 to January 1998; Resource Database in Continuing Medical Education; hand searches of seven key journals; and contacts with experts in the field.

71. Ockene IS, Hebert JR, Ockene JK, et al. Effect of physician-delivered nutrition counseling training and an office-support program on saturated fat intake, weight, and serum lipid measurements in a hyperlipidemic population: Worcester area trial for counseling in hyperlipidemia (WATCH). *Arch Intern Med* 1999;159:725–731.

Margaret Thorogood
Reader in Public Health and Preventative Medicine

Melvyn Hillsdon
Lecturer in Health Promotion

London School of Hygiene and Tropical Medicine, University of London, UK

Carolyn Summerbell
Reader in Human Nutrition
School of Health, University of Teesside, Middlesborough, UK

Competing interests: None declared.

Search date December 2000

William H Herman

QUESTIONS

INTERVENTIONS

Beneficial

Trade off between benefits and harms

Key Messages

- We found strong evidence from one systematic review and three large subsequent RCTs that intensive compared with conventional treatment reduces the development and progression of microvascular and neuropathic complications in both type 1 and type 2 diabetes. A second systematic review of RCTs has found that intensive treatment is associated with a small reduction in cardiovascular risk.

- We found no evidence that intensive treatment causes adverse cardiovascular outcomes. RCTs have found that intensive treatment is associated with hypoglycaemia and weight gain without adverse impact on neuropsychological function or quality of life.

- Large RCTs have found that diabetic complications increase with HbA1c concentrations above the non-diabetic range.

DEFINITION Diabetes mellitus is a group of disorders characterised by hyperglycaemia (definitions vary slightly, one current US definition is fasting plasma glucose $\geq$ 7.0 mmol/l or $\geq$ 11.1 mmol/l 2 hours after a 75 g oral glucose load, on two or more occasions). Intensive treatment is designed to achieve blood glucose values as close to the non-diabetic range as possible. The components of such treatment are education, counselling, monitoring, self management, and pharmacological treatment with insulin or oral antidiabetic agents to achieve specific glycaemic goals.

INCIDENCE/ PREVALENCE Diabetes is diagnosed in around 5% of adults aged 20 years or older in the USA.[1] A further 2.7% have undiagnosed diabetes on the basis of fasting glucose. The prevalence is similar in men and women, but diabetes is more common in some ethnic groups. The prevalence in people aged 40–74 years has increased over the past decade.

AETIOLOGY/ RISK FACTORS Diabetes results from deficient insulin secretion, decreased insulin action, or both. Many processes can be involved, from autoimmune destruction of the β cells of the pancreas to incompletely understood abnormalities that result in resistance to insulin action. Genetic factors are involved in both mechanisms. In type 1 diabetes there is an absolute deficiency of insulin. In type 2 diabetes, insulin resistance and an inability of the pancreas to compensate are involved. Hyperglycaemia without clinical symptoms but sufficient to cause tissue damage can be present for many years before diagnosis.

PROGNOSIS Severe hyperglycaemia causes numerous symptoms, including polyuria, polydipsia, weight loss, and blurred vision. Acute, life threatening consequences of diabetes are hyperglycaemia with ketoacidosis or the non-ketotic hyperosmolar syndrome. There is increased susceptibility to certain infections. Long term complications of diabetes include retinopathy (with potential loss of vision), nephropathy (leading to renal failure), peripheral neuropathy (increased risk of foot ulcers, amputation, and Charcot joints), autonomic neuropathy (cardiovascular, gastrointestinal, and genitourinary dysfunction), and greatly increased risk of atheroma affecting large vessels (macrovascular complications of stroke, myocardial infarction, or peripheral vascular disease). The physical, emotional, and social impact of diabetes and demands of intensive treatment can also create problems for people with diabetes and their families. One systematic review (search date 1998) of observational studies in people with type 2 diabetes found a positive association between increased blood glucose concentration and mortality.[2] It found no minimum threshold level.

AIMS To slow development and progression of the microvascular, neuropathic, and cardiovascular complications of diabetes, while minimising adverse effects of treatment (hypoglycaemia and weight gain) and maximising quality of life.

OUTCOMES Quality of life; short term burden of treatment; long term clinical complications; risks and benefits of treatment. Both the development of complications in people who have previously been free of them, and the progression of complications, are used as outcomes. Scales of severity are used to detect disease progression (e.g. 19

step scales of diabetic retinopathy; normoalbuminuria, microalbuminuria, and albuminuria for nephropathy; absence or presence of clinical neuropathy).

METHODS *Clinical Evidence* search and appraisal December 2000.

QUESTION   **What are the effects of intensive versus conventional glycaemic control?**

One systematic review and three subsequent RCTs in people with type 1 and type 2 diabetes have found that intensive treatment compared with conventional treatment reduces development and progression of microvascular and neuropathic complications. A second systematic review in people with type 1 diabetes, and two additional RCTs in people with type 2 diabetes, have found no evidence that intensive treatment increases adverse cardiovascular outcomes. Intensive treatment reduced the number of macrovascular events but had no significant effect on the number of people who developed macrovascular disease. Intensive treatment is associated with hypoglycaemia and weight gain, but does not seem to affect neuropsychological function or quality of life adversely.

Benefits: **Microvascular and neuropathic complications:** We found one systematic review (search date 1991, 16 small RCTs of type 1 diabetes)[3] and three subsequent long term RCTs (see table 1, p 64),[4-6] which found the relative risks of retinopathy, nephropathy, and neuropathy were all significantly reduced by intensive treatment versus conventional treatment. In one subsequent RCT (1441 people with type 1 diabetes) about half had no retinopathy and half had mild retinopathy at baseline.[4] At 6.5 years, intensive treatment significantly reduced the progression of retinopathy and neuropathy. After a further 4 years, the benefit was maintained, regardless of whether people stayed in the groups to which they were initially randomised.[7] The difference in the median HbA1c concentration for people initially randomised to intensive or conventional care narrowed. The proportion of people with worsening retinopathy and nephropathy was also significantly lower for those who had received intensive treatment. However, another subsequent RCT[6] compared a conventional dietary treatment policy with two different intensive treatment policies based on sulfonylurea and insulin (3867 people with newly diagnosed type 2 diabetes; age 25–65 years; fasting plasma glucose 6.1–15.0 mmol/l after 3 months' dietary therapy; no symptoms of hyperglycaemia; follow up 10 years). HbA1c rose steadily in both groups. Intensive treatment was associated with a significant reduction in any diabetes related end point (40.9 *v* 46.0 events/1000 person years; RRR 12%, 95% CI 1% to 21%), but no significant effect on diabetes related deaths (10.4 *v* 11.5 deaths/1000 person years; RRR +10%, 95% CI −11% to +27%) or all cause mortality (17.9 *v* 18.9 deaths/1000 person years; RRR +6%, 95% CI −10% to +20%). Secondary analysis found that intensive treatment was associated with a significant reduction in microvascular end points (8.6 *v* 11.4/1000 person years; RRR 25%, 95% CI 7% to 40%) compared with conventional treatment (see table 1, p 64).[6] **Cardiovascular outcomes:** We found one systematic review[8] and two additional RCTs.[5,6] The systematic review (6 RCTs, 1731 people with type 1 diabetes followed for 2–8 years) found that intensive insulin treatment versus conventional treatment decreased the number of macrovascular events (OR 0.55, 95% CI 0.35 to 0.88), but had no significant effect on the number of people developing macrovascular disease (OR 0.72, 95% CI 0.44 to 1.17) or on macrovascular mortality (OR 0.91, 95% CI 0.31 to 2.65). The additional RCTs included people with type 2 diabetes.[5,6] In the first RCT the number of major cerebrovascular, cardiovascular, and peripheral vascular events in the intensive treatment group was half that of the conventional treatment group (0.6 v 1.3 events/100 person years), but the event rate in this small trial was low and the results were not significant.[5] In the second RCT, intensive treatment versus conventional treatment was associated with a non-significant reduction in the risk of myocardial infarction (AR 387/2729 [14%] with intensive treatment v 186/1138 [16%] with conventional treatment; RRR +13%, 95% CI −2% to +27%), a non-significant increase in the risk of stroke (AR 148/2729 [5.4%] v 55/1138 [4.8%]; RRI +12%, 95% CI −17% to +51%), and a non-significant reduction in the risk of amputation or death from peripheral vascular disease (AR 29/2729 [1.1%] v 18/1138 [1.6%]; RRR +33%, 95% CI −20% to +63%).[6]

Harms: **Hypoglycaemia:** We found one systematic review[9] and three additional RCTs.[5,6,10] The systematic review (search date 1996, 14 RCTs with at least 6 months' follow up and monitoring of HbA1c, 2067 people with type 1 diabetes followed for 0.5–7.5 years) found that the median incidence of severe hypoglycaemia was 7.9 episodes/100 person years among intensively treated people and 4.6 episodes/100 person years among conventionally treated people (OR 3.0, 95% CI 2.5 to 3.6). The risk of severe hypoglycaemia was associated with the degree of HbA1c lowering in the intensive treatment groups (P = 0.005). The three additional RCTs included people with type 2 diabetes with lower baseline rates of hypoglycaemia. In the first RCT (110 people), there was no significant difference in rates of hypoglycaemia between groups.[5] In the second RCT (3867 people), the rates of major hypoglycaemic episodes per year were 0.7% with conventional treatment, 1.0% with chlorpropamide, 1.4% with glibenclamide, and 1.8% with insulin. People in the intensive treatment group had significantly more hypoglycaemic episodes than those in the conventional group (P < 0.0001).[6] In the third RCT (1704 overweight people) major hypoglycaemic episodes occurred in 0.6% of overweight people in the metformin treated group.[10] **Weight gain:** Four RCTs found more weight increase with intensive treatment than with standard treatment.[4-6,11] One RCT found weight remained stable in people with type 1 diabetes in the conventional treatment group, but body mass index increased by 5.8% in the intensive treatment group (95% CI not presented, P < 0.01).[11] In the second RCT (1441 people with type 2 diabetes), intensive treatment was associated with increased risk of developing a body weight more than 120% above the ideal (12.7 cases per 100 person years with intensive treatment v 9.3 cases per 100 person years with conventional treatment; RR 1.33). At 5 years, people treated intensively gained 4.6 kg more than people treated conventionally (CI not presented for weight data).[4] In the third RCT, the increase in body mass index from baseline to 6 years was not significant in either group (intensive treatment group 20.5 to 21.2 kg/m^2, conventional treatment group 20.3 to 21.9 kg/m²).[5] In the fourth RCT, weight gain at 10 years was significantly higher in people with type 2 diabetes in the intensive treatment group compared with people in the conventional treatment group (mean 2.9 kg, $P < 0.001$), and people assigned insulin had a greater gain in weight (4.0 kg) than those assigned chlorpropamide (2.6 kg) or glibenclamide (1.7 kg).[6] We found one systematic review (search date 1996, 10 RCTs)[12] and one subsequent RCT[10] comparing metformin and sulfonylurea. Meta-analysis in the review found that sulfonylurea was associated with an increase in weight from baseline and metformin with a decrease (difference 2.9 kg, 95% CI 1.1 to 4.4 kg). In the subsequent RCT, overweight participants randomly assigned to intensive blood glucose control with metformin had a similar change in body weight to the conventional treatment group, and less increase in mean body weight than people receiving intensive treatment with sulfonylureas or insulin.[10] **Neuropsychological impairment:** We found no systematic review on neuropsychological impairment, but found two RCTs.[13-16] One RCT (102 people) compared intensified with standard treatment in people with type 1 diabetes. It found no cognitive impairment associated with hypoglycaemia after 3 years.[13,14] The second RCT found that intensive treatment did not affect neuropsychological performance.[15] People who had repeated episodes of hypoglycaemia did not perform differently from people who did not have repeated episodes.[16] **Quality of life:** We found three RCTs, which reported quality of life in people undergoing intensive versus conventional treatment.[17-19] Together, they suggest that quality of life is lowered by complications, but is not lowered directly by intensive versus conventional treatment. The first RCT (1441 people) found that intensive treatment did not reduce quality of life in people with type 1 diabetes.[17] Severe hypoglycaemia was not consistently associated with a subsequent increase in distress caused by symptoms or decline in the quality of life. In the primary prevention intensive treatment group, however, repeated severe hypoglycaemia (three or more events resulting in coma or seizure) tended to increase the risk of distress caused by symptoms. The second RCT (77 adolescents with type 1 diabetes) found after 1 year that behavioural intervention plus intensive diabetes management versus intensive diabetes management alone significantly improved quality of life, diabetes and medical self-efficacy, and HbA1c (7.5% v 8.5%, $P = 0.001$).[18] The behavioural intervention included six small group sessions and monthly follow up aimed at social problem solving, cognitive behaviour modification, and conflict resolution. The third RCT of intensive versus conventional treatment of type 2 diabetes assessed quality of life in two large cross sectional samples at 8 and 11 years after randomisation (disease specific measures in 2431 people and generic measures in 3104 people), and also in a small cohort (diabetes specific quality of life measures in 374 people 6 months after randomisation and annually thereafter for 6 years).[19] The cross sectional studies found no significant effect of intensive versus conventional treatment on scores for mood, cognitive mistakes, symptoms, work satisfaction, or general health. The longitudinal study also found no significant difference in quality of life scores other than a small increase in the number of symptoms in people allocated to conventional than to intensive treatment. In the cross sectional studies, people who had macrovascular or microvascular complications in the last year had lower quality of life than people without complications. People treated with insulin who had two or more hypoglycaemic episodes during the previous year reported more tension, more overall mood disturbance, and less work satisfaction than those with no hypoglycaemic attacks (after adjusting for age, time from randomisation, systolic blood pressure, HbA1c, and sex). It was unclear whether frequent hypoglycaemic episodes affected quality of life, or whether people with certain personality traits or symptoms simply reported increased numbers of hypoglycaemic attacks.

Comment: None.

QUESTION   **What is the optimum target blood glucose?**

Large RCTs in people with type 1 and type 2 diabetes have found that risk of development or progression of complications increases progressively as HbA1c increases above the non-diabetic range.

Benefits: We found no systematic review but found two large RCTs.[4,6] The first RCT (1441 people with type 1 diabetes) found that lower HbA1c was associated with a lower risk of complications.[4,20] The second RCT (3867 people with type 2 diabetes) found that, as concentrations of HbA1c were reduced, the risk of complications fell but the risk of hypoglycaemia increased.[6,19] A further analysis of the second RCT (3642 people who had HbA1c measured 3 months after the diagnosis of diabetes and who had complete data whether or not they were randomised in the trial) found that each 1% reduction in mean HbA1c was associated with reduced risk of any diabetes-related microvascular or macrovascular event (RR 0.79, 95% CI 0.76 to 0.83), diabetes related death (RR 0.79, 95% CI 0.73 to 0.85), all cause mortality (RR 0.86, 95% CI 0.81 to 0.91), microvascular complications (RR 0.63, 95% CI 0.59 to 0.67), and myocardial infarction (RR 0.86, 95% CI 0.79 to 0.92).[21] These prospective observational data suggest that there is no lower glycaemic threshold for the risk of complications; the better the glycaemic control, the lower the risk of complications. They also suggest that the rate of increase of risk for microvascular disease with hyperglycaemia is greater than that for macrovascular disease.

Harms: Both RCTs found that hypoglycaemia was increased by intensive treatment.[19,20]

Comment: It is difficult to weigh the benefit of reduced complications against the harm of increased hypoglycaemia. The balance between benefits and harms of intensive treatment in type 1 diabetes may be less favourable in children under 13 years or in older adults, and in people with repeated severe hypoglycaemia or unawareness of hypoglycaemia. Similarly, the balance between benefits and harms of intensive treatment in type 2 diabetes may be less favourable in people over 65 years or in those with longstanding diabetes. The benefit of intensive treatment is limited by the complications of advanced diabetes (such as blindness, end stage renal disease or cardiovascular disease), major comorbidity, and reduced life expectancy. The risk of intensive treatment is increased by a history of severe hypoglycaemia or unawareness of hypoglycaemia, advanced autonomic neuropathy, or cardiovascular disease, and impaired ability to detect or treat hypoglycaemia (such as altered mental state, immobility, or lack of social support). For people likely to have limited benefit or increased risk with intensive treatment, it may be more appropriate to negotiate less intensive goals for glycaemic management that reflect the person's self determined goals of care and willingness to make lifestyle modifications.

REFERENCES

1. Harris MI, Flegal KM, Cowie CC, et al. Prevalence of diabetes, impaired fasting glucose, and impaired glucose tolerance in US adults: the third national health and nutrition examination survey, 1988–1994. *Diabetes Care* 1998;2:518–524.
2. Groeneveld Y, Petri H, Hermans J, et al. Relationship between blood glucose level and mortality in type 2 diabetes mellitus: a systematic review. *Diabet Med* 1999;16:2–13. Search date 1998; primary source Medline 1996 to 1998.
3. Wang PH, Lau J, Chalmers TC. Meta-analysis of effects of intensive blood glucose control on late complications of type I diabetes. *Lancet* 1993; 341:1306–1309. Search date 1991; primary sources Medline 1966 to December 1991.
4. The Diabetes Control and Complications Trial Research Group. The effect of intensive treatment of diabetes on the development and progression of long-term complications in insulin-dependent diabetes mellitus. *N Engl J Med* 1993;329:977–986.
5. Ohkubo Y, Kishikawa H, Arake E, et al. Intensive insulin therapy prevents the progression of diabetic microvascular complications in Japanese patients with non-insulin-dependent diabetes mellitus: a randomized prospective 6-year study. *Diabetes Res Clin Pract* 1995;28:103–117.
6. UK Prospective Diabetes Study Group. Intensive blood-glucose control with sulphonylureas or insulin compared with conventional treatment and risk of complications in patients with type 2 diabetes. *Lancet* 1998;352:837–853.
7. The DCCT/Epidemiology of Diabetes Interventions and Complications Research Group. Retinopathy and nephropathy in patients with type 1 diabetes four years after a trial of intensive therapy. *N Engl J Med* 2000;342:381–389.
8. Lawson ML, Gerstein HC, Tsui E, et al. Effect of intensive therapy on early macrovascular disease in young individuals with type 1 diabetes. *Diabetes Care* 1999;22:B35–B39. Search date 1996; primary sources Medline, Citation Index, reference lists, and personal files.
9. Egger M, Smith GD, Stettler C, et al. Risk of adverse effects of intensified treatment in insulin-dependent diabetes mellitus: a meta-analysis. *Diabet Med* 1997;14:919–928. Search date not given; primary sources Medline, reference lists, and specialist journals.
10. UK Prospective Diabetes Study Group. Effect of intensive blood-glucose control with metformin on complications in overweight patients with type 2 diabetes. *Lancet* 1998;352:854–865.
11. Reichard P, Berglund B, Britz A, et al. Intensified conventional insulin treatment retards the microvascular complications of insulin-dependent

diabetes mellitus (IDDM): the Stockholm diabetes intervention study (SDIS) after 5 years. *J Intern Med* 1991;30:101–108.
12. Johansen K. Efficacy of metformin in the treatment of NIDDM. *Diabetes Care* 1999;22:33–37. Search date January 1996; primary sources current list of medical literature 1957 to 1959; Index Medicus 1959 to 1965; Medline 1966 to January 1966; Embase 1989 to January 1996, and hand searched references.
13. Reichard P, Nilsson BY, Rosenqvist U. The effect of long-term intensified insulin treatment on the development of microvascular complications of diabetes mellitus. *N Engl J Med* 1993;29: 304–309.
14. Reichard P, Berglund A, Britz A, et al. Hypoglycaemic episodes during intensified insulin treatment: increased frequency but no effect on cognitive function. *J Intern Med* 1991;229:9–16.
15. The Diabetes Control and Complications Trial Research Group. Effects of intensive diabetes therapy on neuropsychological function in adults in the diabetes control and complications trial. *Ann Intern Med* 1996;124:379–388.
16. Austin EJ, Deary IJ. Effects of repeated hypoglycaemia on cognitive function. A psychometrically validated reanalysis of the diabetes control and complications trial data. *Diabetes Care* 1999;22:1273–1277.
17. The Diabetes Control and Complications Trial Research Group. Influence of intensive diabetes treatment on quality-of-life outcomes in the diabetes control and complications trial. *Diabetes Care* 1996;19:195–203.
18. Grey M, Boland EA, Davidson M, Li J, Tamborlane W. Coping skills training for youth with diabetes mellitus has long-lasting effects on metabolic control and quality of life. *J Pediatr* 2000;137: 107–113.
19. UK Prospective Diabetes Study Group. Quality of life in type 2 diabetic patients is affected by complications but not by intensive policies to improve blood glucose or blood pressure control (UKPDS 37). *Diabetes Care* 1999;22:1125–1136.
20. The Diabetes Control and Complications Trial Research Group. The absence of a glycaemic threshold for the development of long-term complications: the perspective of the diabetes control and complications trial. *Diabetes* 1996; 45:1289–1298.
21. Stratton IM, Adler AI, Neil HAW, et al on behalf of the UK Prospective Diabetes Study Group. Association of glycaemia with macrovascular and microvascular complications of type 2 diabetes (UKPDS 35): prospective observational study. *BMJ* 2000;321:450–412.

William H Herman

Professor of Internal Medicine and Epidemiology
University of Michigan Medical Center, Ann Arbor, Michigan, USA

Competing interests: None declared.

TABLE 1 Risk (odds ratio) for development or progression of microvascular, nephropathic, and neuropathic complications with intensive versus conventional treatment. Odds ratio, number needed to treat, and confidence intervals were all calculated from data in papers (see text, p 59).

	Systematic Review[3]	DCCT[4]	Kumamoto[5]	UKPDS[6]
Studies	16 RCTs	RCT	RCT	RCT
Number of participants	–	1441	110	3867
Type of diabetes	Type 1	Type 1	Type 2	Type 2*
Follow up	8 to 60 months	6.5 years	6 years	10 years
Change in HbA1c	1.4%	2.0%	2.0%	0.9%
Progression of retinopathy				
OR (95% CI)	0.49 (0.28 to 0.85)	0.39 (0.28 to 0.55)	0.25 (0.09 to 0.65)	0.66 (0.48 to 0.92)
NNT (95% CI) over duration of study	–	5 (4 to 7)	4 (3 to 11)	10 (6 to 50)
Development of retinopathy				
OR (95% CI)	–	0.22 (0.14 to 0.36)	–	–
NNT (95% CI) over duration of study	–	6 (5 to 7)	–	–
Development or progression of nephropathy				
OR (95% CI)	0.34 (0.20 to 0.58)	0.50 (0.39 to 0.63)	0.26 (0.09 to 0.76)	0.54 (0.25 to 1.18)
NNT (95% CI) over duration of study	–	7 (6 to 11)	5 (4 to 19)	–
Development or progression of neuropathy				
OR (95% CI)	–	0.36 (0.24 to 0.54)	–	0.42 (0.23 to 0.78)
NNT (95% CI) over duration of study	–	13 (11 to 18)	–	5 (3 to 16)

*All participants had fasting plasma glucose > 6.0 mmol/L on two occasions: 93% had fasting plasma glucose ≥ 7.0 mmol/L (American Diabetic Association criterion) and 86% had fasting plasma glucose ≥ 7.8 mmol/L (WHO criterion). CI, confidence interval; NNT, number needed to treat; OR, odd ratio.

INTERVENTIONS

Key Messages

Non-drug treatments

- We found conflicting evidence about multidisciplinary care. One systematic review has found that multidisciplinary approaches to nutrition, patient counselling, and education reduce hospital admissions, may improve quality of life, and enhance patient knowledge. However, the review excluded one large RCT that found that multidisciplinary follow up increased re-admission rates.

- RCTs have found that prescribed exercise training improves functional capacity and quality of life, and reduces the rate of adverse cardiac events.

Drug and invasive treatments

- Two systematic reviews and recent RCTs have found that angiotensin converting enzyme (ACE) inhibitors reduce mortality, admission to hospital for heart failure, and ischaemic events in people with heart failure. Relative benefits are similar in different groups of people, but absolute benefits are greater in people with severe heart failure.

- One systematic review and one recent RCT found no evidence of a difference between angiotensin II receptor blockers and ACE inhibitors in their effects on mortality, or on functional capacity and symptoms.

- RCTs have found that positive inotropic drugs improve symptoms but do not reduce mortality. Many of the non-digoxin positive inotropic drugs may increase mortality. Only digoxin has been found to improve morbidity in people already receiving diuretics and ACE inhibitors.

- Systematic reviews found strong evidence that adding a β blocker to ACE inhibitors decreases the rate of death and admission to hospital. The reviews found less robust evidence that β blockers improve exercise capacity and reduce mortality.

- We found no evidence supporting the use of calcium channel blockers in heart failure.

- One RCT has found that, in people with severe heart failure, adding an aldosterone receptor antagonist to ACE inhibitor treatment reduces mortality compared with ACE inhibitors alone.

- Systematic reviews have found weak evidence suggesting that amiodarone may reduce mortality in people with heart failure.

- Evidence extrapolated from one systematic review in people treated after a myocardial infarction suggests that non-amiodarone antiarrhythmic drugs may increase mortality in people with heart failure.

- One systematic review has found good evidence that an implantable cardiac defibrillator (ICD) reduces mortality in people with heart failure who have experienced a cardiac arrest. The review found conflicting evidence for prophylactic implantation of ICDs in people at high risk of arrhythmia.

- We found no RCTs of anticoagulation in people with heart failure. We found conflicting evidence from two large retrospective cohort studies.

- We found no RCTs of antiplatelet agents versus placebo in people with heart failure. Retrospective analyses have included too few events to establish or exclude a clinically important effect of antiplatelet agents in people with heart failure.

- RCTs have found good evidence that, in people with asymptomatic left ventricular systolic dysfunction, ACE inhibitors delay the onset of symptomatic heart failure and reduce cardiovascular events.

DEFINITION   Heart failure occurs when abnormality of cardiac function causes failure of the heart to pump blood at a rate sufficient for metabolic requirements, or maintains cardiac output only with a raised filling pressure. It is characterised clinically by breathlessness, effort intolerance, fluid retention, and poor survival. It can be caused by systolic or diastolic dysfunction and is associated with neurohormonal changes.[1] Left ventricular systolic dysfunction (LVSD) is defined as a left ventricular ejection fraction (LVEF) below 0.40. It can be symptomatic or asymptomatic. Defining and diagnosing diastolic heart failure can be difficult. Recently proposed criteria include: (1) clinical evidence of heart failure; (2) normal or mildly abnormal left ventricular systolic function; and (3) evidence of abnormal left ventricular relaxation, filling, diastolic distensibility, or diastolic stiffness.[2] The clinical utility of these criteria is limited by difficulty in standardising assessment of the last criterion.

INCIDENCE/ PREVALENCE   Both the incidence and prevalence of heart failure increase with age. Under 65 years of age the incidence is 1/1000 men a year and 0.4/1000 women a year. Over 65 years, incidence is 11/1000 men a year and 5/1000 women a year. Under 65 years the prevalence of heart failure is 1/1000 men and 1/1000 women; over 65 years the prevalence is 40/1000 men and 30/1000 women.[3] The prevalence of asymptomatic LVSD is 3% in the general population.[4-6] The mean age of people with asymptomatic LVSD is lower than that for symptomatic individuals. Both heart failure and asymptomatic LVSD are more common in men.[4-6] The prevalence of diastolic heart failure in the community is unknown. The prevalence of heart failure with preserved systolic function in people in hospital with clinical heart failure varies from 13% to 74%.[7,8] Less than 15% of people with heart failure under 65 years have normal systolic function, whereas the prevalence is about 40% in people over 65 years.[7]

AETIOLOGY/ RISK FACTORS Coronary artery disease is the most common cause of heart failure.[3] Other common causes include hypertension and idiopathic dilated congestive cardiomyopathy. After adjustment for hypertension, the presence of left ventricular hypertrophy remains a risk factor for the development of heart failure. Other risk factors include cigarette smoking, hyperlipidaemia, and diabetes mellitus.[4] The common causes of left ventricular diastolic dysfunction are coronary artery disease and systemic hypertension. Other causes are hypertrophic cardiomyopathy, restrictive or infiltrative cardiomyopathies, and valvular heart disease.[8]

PROGNOSIS The prognosis of heart failure is poor, with 5 year mortality ranging from 26–75%.[3] Up to 16% of people are re-admitted with heart failure within 6 months of first admission. In the USA it is the leading cause of hospital admission among people over 65 years old.[3] In people with heart failure, a new myocardial infarction increases the risk of death (RR 7.8, 95% CI 6.9 to 8.8); 34% of all deaths in people with heart failure are preceded by a major ischaemic event.[9] Sudden death, mainly caused by ventricular arrhythmias, is responsible for 25–50% of all deaths, and is the most common cause of death in people with heart failure.[10] The presence of asymptomatic LVSD increases an individual's risk of having a cardiovascular event. One large prevention trial found that, for a 5% reduction in ejection fraction, the risk ratio for mortality was 1.20 (95% CI 1.13 to 1.29), for hospital admission for heart failure it was 1.28 (95% CI 1.18 to 1.38), and for development of heart failure it was 1.20 (95% CI 1.13 to 1.26).[4] The annual mortality of patients with diastolic heart failure varies in observational studies (1.3–17.5%).[7] Reasons for this variation include age, the presence of coronary artery disease, and variation in the partition value used to define abnormal ventricular systolic function. The annual mortality for left ventricular diastolic dysfunction is lower than found in patients with systolic dysfunction.[11]

AIMS To relieve symptoms; to improve quality of life; to reduce morbidity and mortality, with minimum adverse effects.

OUTCOMES Functional capacity (assessed by the New York Heart Association [NYHA] functional classification or more objectively by using standardised exercise testing or the 6 minute walk test);[12] quality of life (assessed with questionnaires);[13] mortality; adverse effects of treatment. Proxy measures of clinical outcome (e.g. LVEF, hospital re-admission rates) are used here only when clinical outcomes are unavailable.

METHODS *Clinical Evidence* search and appraisal October 2000.

Heart failure

| QUESTION | What are the effects of non-drug treatments? |

| OPTION | MULTIDISCIPLINARY INTERVENTIONS |

We found conflicting evidence. One systematic review has found that multidisciplinary approaches to nutrition, patient counselling, and education reduce hospital admissions, may improve quality of life, and enhance patient knowledge. However, the review excluded a large RCT, which found that multidisciplinary follow up increased re-admission rates.

Benefits:
We found one systematic review (search date 1998, 7 RCTs, 1164 people with heart failure), which compared treatment for 1–6 months in a multidisciplinary programme versus conventional care alone.[14] The multidisciplinary programme included non-drug treatments such as nutrition advice, counselling, patient education, and exercise training. Six of the RCTs (666 people) were chosen for analysis in the systematic review. The RCTs found that multidisciplinary programmes reduced hospital use, and improved quality of life, functional capacity, patient satisfaction, and compliance with diet and medication compared with conventional care. The four RCTs (543 people) that reported hospital re-admissions over 1–6 months found significant reductions with the intervention (89/286 [31%] with intervention v 116/257 [45%] with control; ARR 14%, 95% CI 6% to 21%; RRR 31%, 95% CI 13% to 47%; NNT 7, 95% CI 5 to 17). The seventh RCT was excluded from analysis in the systematic review but it is not clear how this study differs from those included, apart from its findings. The seventh study included 504 men with heart failure who received conventional follow up or an intensive follow up with their primary care physician and a nurse. This RCT found an increased hospital re-admission rate over 6 months in the intervention group compared with controls (130/249 [52%] for intervention v 106/255 [42%] for control; ARI 11%, 95% CI 2% to 19%; RRI 26%, 95% CI 5% to 46%). Combination of the results of this study with the others found that the intervention had no definite effect compared with control (219/535 [41%] for intervention v 222/512 [43%] for control; ARR +2.4%, 95% CI −3.6% to +8.2%; RRR +5.6%, 95% CI −8% to +19%).

Harms:
We found no reports of harm associated with multidisciplinary management.[14]

Comment:
Studies were small, involved highly selected patient populations, and were usually performed in academic centres so results may not generalise to smaller community centres. The systematic review excluded, without *a priori* exclusion criteria, a seventh RCT that found different effects. Interventions varied among studies, and relative merits of each strategy are unknown. Studies generally lasted less than 6 months, and it is not known how well people adhere to treatment over the longer term. Larger studies are needed to define the effects on mortality and morbidity of longer term multidisciplinary interventions.

OPTION   **EXERCISE**

RCTs have found that prescribed exercise training improves functional capacity and quality of life. One recent RCT has also found that exercise significantly reduces adverse cardiac events.

Benefits: We found one non-systematic review,[15] two systematic reviews,[16,17] one overview of RCTs from a collaborative group,[18] and one subsequent RCT[19] of exercise training in people with heart failure. The reviews and overview identified 20 small RCTs, which reported only proxy outcomes (maximum exercise time [see glossary, p 82], oxygen uptake, various biochemical measures, and unvalidated symptom scores) in a small number of people over a few weeks. No significant adverse effects were found. The subsequent RCT (99 people with heart failure, 88 men) compared 12 months of exercise training versus a control group with no exercise.[19] After 12 months, exercise compared with control improved quality of life (P < 0.001), fatal or non-fatal cardiac events (17/50 [34%] with training v 37/49 [76%] with control; ARR 42%, 95% CI 20% to 58%; RRR 55%, 95% CI 27% to 77%; NNT 2), mortality (9/50 [18%] v 20/49 [41%]; RRR 56%, 95% CI 13% to 80%; NNT 4), and hospital re-admission for heart failure (5/50 [10%] v 14/49 [29%]; ARR 19%, 95% CI 3% to 25%; RRR 65%, 95% CI 12% to 88%; NNT 5).[19]

Harms: The reviews and overview reported no important adverse effects associated with prescribed exercise training.[15,16,18]

Comment: The studies were small, involved highly selected patient populations, and were performed in well resourced academic centres. The results may not generalise to smaller community centres. The specific form of exercise training varied among studies and the relative merits of each strategy are unknown. The studies generally lasted less than 1 year and long term effects are unknown. Larger studies over a longer period are needed.

QUESTION   **What are the effects of drug treatments in heart failure?**

OPTION   **ANGIOTENSIN CONVERTING ENZYME (ACE) INHIBITORS**

Two systematic reviews and recent RCTs have found that ACE inhibitors reduce mortality, admission to hospital for heart failure, and ischaemic events in people with heart failure. Relative benefits are similar in different groups of people, but absolute benefits are greater in people with severe heart failure.

Benefits: We found two systematic reviews of ACE inhibitors versus placebo in heart failure.[20,21] The first systematic review (search date 1994, 32 RCTs, duration 3–42 months, 7105 people, NYHA class II or worse [see glossary, p 82])[20] found that ACE inhibitors versus placebo reduced mortality (611/3870 [16%] with ACE inhibitors v 709/3235 [22%] with placebo; ARR 6%, 95% CI 4% to 8%; OR 0.77, 95% CI 0.67 to 0.88; NNT 16). Relative reductions in mortality were similar in different subgroups (stratified by age, sex, cause of heart failure, and NYHA class). The second systematic overview (search date not stated, 5 RCTs, 12 763 people with left ventricular dysfunction or heart failure, mean duration 35 months) analysed results from individuals in long term and large RCTs that compared ACE inhibitors versus placebo.[21] Three RCTs were in people for 1 year after myocardial infarction. In these three post infarction trials (5966 people), ACE inhibitor versus placebo significantly reduced mortality (702/2995 [23.4%] v 866/2971 [29.1%]; OR 0.74, 95% CI 0.66 to 0.83), re-admission for heart failure (355/2995 [11.9%] v 460/2971 [15.5%]; OR 0.73, 95% CI 0.63 to 0.85), and reinfarction (324/2995 [10.8%] v 391/2971 [13.2%]; OR 0.80, 95% CI 0.69 to 0.94]). For all five trials, ACE inhibitors versus placebo reduced mortality (1467/6391 [23.0%] v 1710/6372 [26.8%]; OR 0.80, 95% CI 0.74 to 0.87), reinfarction (571/6391 [8.9%] v 703/6372 [11.0%]; OR 0.79, 95% CI 0.70 to 0.89), and re-admission for heart failure (876/6391 [13.7%] v 1202/6372 [18.9%]; OR 0.67, 95% CI 0.61 to 0.74). The benefits began soon after the start of therapy, persisted long term, were independent of age, sex, and baseline use of diuretics, aspirin, and β blockers. Although there was a trend towards greater relative reduction in mortality or re-admission for heart failure in people with lower ejection fractions, benefit was apparent over the range examined. **Other ischaemic events:** Individual RCTs that studied high risk groups found that ACE inhibitors significantly reduced some ischaemic event rates. One RCT in people with left ventricular dysfunction found that, compared with placebo, ACE inhibitors reduced myocardial infarction (combined fatal or non-fatal myocardial infarction: 9.9% v 12.3%; RRR 23%, 95% CI 2% to 39%), hospital admission for angina (15% v 19%; RRR 27%, 95% CI 12% to 40%), and the combined end point of cardiac death, non-fatal myocardial infarction, or hospital admission for angina (43% v 51%; RRR 23%, 95% CI 14% to 32%).[9] Effects on hospital re-admissions were observed shortly after starting ACE inhibitor treatment, although effects on ischaemic events were not apparent for at least 6 months and peaked at 36 months. **Dosage:** We found one large RCT (3164 people with NYHA class II-IV heart failure), which compared low dose lisinopril (2.5 mg or 5.0 mg daily) versus high dose lisinopril (32.5 mg or 35 mg daily).[22] It found no significant difference in mortality (717/1596 [44.9%] with low dose v 666/1568 [42.5%] with high dose; ARR 8%, 95% CI not given; hazard ratio 0.92, 95% CI 0.80 to 1.03; P = 0.128), but found that high dose lisinopril reduced the combined outcome of death or hospital admission for any reason (1338 events with low dose [83.8%] v 1250 events with high dose [79.7%]; ARR 12%; hazard ratio 0.88, 95% CI 0.82–0.96; P = 0.002) and reduced admissions for heart failure (1576 admissions with low dose v 1199 admissions with high dose; ARR 24%; P = 0.002). **Comparison of different ACE inhibitors:** The first systematic review found similar benefits with different ACE inhibitors.[20]

Harms: We found no systematic review. The main adverse effects documented in large trials were cough, hypotension, hyperkalaemia, and renal dysfunction. Compared with placebo, ACE inhibitors increased the incidence of cough (37% v 31%; ARI 7%, 95% CI 3% to 11%; RRI 23%, 95% CI 11% to 35%; NNH 14), dizziness or fainting (57%

v 50%; ARI 7%, 95% CI 3% to 11%; RRI 14%, 95% CI 6% to 21%; NNH 14), increased creatinine concentrations above 177 µmol/litre (10.7% v 7.7%; ARI 3%, 95% CI 0.6% to 6%; RRI 38%, 95% CI 9% to 67%; NNH 34), and increased potassium concentrations above 5.5 mmol/litre (ARs 6.4% v 2.5%; ARI 4%, 95% CI 2% to 7%; RRI 156%, 95% CI 92% to 220%; NNH 26).[23] Angioedema was not found to be more common with ACE inhibitors than placebo (3.8% taking enalapril v 4.1% taking placebo; ARI +0.3%, 95% CI −1.4% to +1.5%).[23] The trial comparing low and high doses of lisinopril found that most adverse effects were more common with high dose (no P value reported; dizziness: 12% with low dose v 19% with high dose; hypotension: 7% with low dose v 11% with high dose; worsening renal function: 7% with low dose v 10% with high dose; significant change in serum potassium concentration: 7% with low dose v 7% with high dose), although there was no difference in withdrawal rates between groups (17% discontinued with high dose v 18% with low dose). The trial found that cough was less commonly experienced with high dose compared with low dose lisinopril (cough: 13% with low dose v 11% with high dose).

Comment: The relative beneficial effects of ACE inhibitors were similar in different subgroups of people with heart failure. Most RCTs evaluated left ventricular function by assessing LVEF, but some studies defined heart failure clinically, without measurement of left ventricular function in people at high risk of developing heart failure (soon after myocardial infarction). It is unclear whether there are additional benefits from adding ACE inhibitor therapy to people with heart failure who are already taking antiplatelet therapy, and of adding antiplatelet therapy to people with heart failure who are already taking an ACE inhibitor (see antiplatelet agents, p 79).

OPTION   ANGIOTENSIN II RECEPTOR BLOCKERS

One RCT has found that angiotensin II receptor antagonists improve symptom indices compared with placebo. RCTs found no evidence that angiotensin II receptor blockers altered functional capacity or symptoms compared with ACE inhibitors, but the trials were too small to rule out clinically important differences. We found moderate evidence from one RCT that angiotensin II receptor blockers are as effective as ACE inhibitors in reducing all cause mortality.

Benefits: **Versus placebo:** We found one overview[24] and one additional RCT.[18] The overview (3 RCTs, all 12 weeks' duration, 890 people with heart failure NYHA class II and III) found that losartan versus placebo significantly reduced mortality (11/616 [1.8%] with losartan v 13/274 [4.7%] with placebo; OR 0.34, 95% CI 0.14 to 0.80).[24] The RCT (844 people with heart failure NYHA class II and III) compared 12 weeks of candesartan cilexetil (4 mg daily, 208 people v 8 mg daily, 212 people v 16 mg daily, 213 people) versus placebo (211 people).[25] It found that 16 mg candesartan cilexetil daily versus placebo improved exercise time in a standardised symptom limited bicycle ergonometry exercise (47.2 v 30.8 seconds, P = 0.0463). All doses of candesartan cilexetil compared with placebo significantly improved the dyspnoea fatigue index (see glossary, p 82) score (P < 0.001). **Versus ACE inhibitors:**

We found one overview (3 RCTs, 1004 people)[24] and one subsequent RCT.[26] Two of the RCTs in the overview (116 people, NYHA class II and III, duration 8 weeks; and 166 people, NYHA class III and IV, duration 12 weeks) compared losartan versus enalapril. The third RCT in the overview (722 people, NYHA class II and III, duration 48 weeks) compared losartan versus captopril. The overview combined the results of these RCTs and found no significant reduction in mortality for losartan versus ACE inhibitors (25/538 [4.6%] with losartan v 34/466 [7.3%] with ACE inhibitors; OR 0.60, 95% CI 0.34 to 1.04). The subsequent RCT (3152 people, aged $\geq$ 60 years, NYHA class II–IV, LVEF $\leq$ 40%) found losartan (titrated to 50 mg once daily) versus captopril (titrated to 50 mg three times daily) produced no significant differences in mortality after a median of 555 days (280/1578 [17.7%] with losartan v 250/1574 [15.9%] with captopril; HR 1.13, 95% CI 0.95 to 1.35; P = 0.16). There was also no significant difference in sudden death or resuscitated cardiac arrest (142/1578 [9.0%] v 115/1574 [7.3%]; HR 1.25, 95% CI 0.98 to 1.60; P = 0.08).[26] Significantly fewer patients in the losartan group discontinued study treatment because of adverse effects (9.7% v 14.7%; P < 0.001), including cough (0.3% v 2.7%).

Harms: We found no systematic review. The RCT comparing different doses of candesartan cilexetil versus placebo found no evidence of a difference among groups for serious adverse events (placebo 4.7%; 4 mg 1.4%; 8 mg 5.7%; 16 mg 5.6%) or withdrawal because of adverse events (placebo 4.3%; 4 mg 1.9%; 8 mg 4.7%; 16 mg 5.6%).[25]

Comment: The overview of losartan was company sponsored and included all clinical studies in their evaluation programme.[24] None of the trials of an angiotensin II receptor blocker compared with an ACE inhibitor have been designed with mortality as the primary end point. In people who are truly intolerant of an ACE inhibitor the evidence supports the use of an angiotensin II receptor blocker with the expectation, at the very least, of symptomatic improvement of the heart failure. Pilot studies have examined the efficacy, tolerability, and safety of combining angiotensin II receptor blockers and ACE inhibitors in people with symptomatic heart failure.[27,28] Larger studies are in progress.

OPTION	POSITIVE INOTROPIC AGENTS

We found no evidence that positive inotropic drugs other than digoxin reduce mortality and morbidity in people with heart failure, and most RCTs found that they increased mortality. One well designed RCT found that digoxin decreased the rate of hospital admissions and cointervention for worsening heart failure in people already receiving diuretics and ACE inhibitors, although it found no evidence of an effect on mortality.

Benefits: **Digoxin:** We found one systematic review (search date 1992, 13 RCTs, duration 3–24 weeks, 1138 people with heart failure and sinus rhythm)[29] and one recent large RCT.[30] The systematic review found that six of the 13 RCTs enrolled people without assessment of ventricular function and may have included some people with mild or no heart failure. Other limitations of the older trials included crossover designs and small sample sizes. In people who were in sinus rhythm with heart failure, the systematic review found fewer people with clinical worsening of heart failure (52/628 [8.3%] with digoxin v 131/631 [20.8%] with placebo; ARR 12.5%, 95% CI 9.5% to 14.7%; RRR 60%, 95% CI 46% to 71%) but did not find a definite effect on mortality (16/628 [2.5%] with digoxin v 15/631 [2.4%] with placebo; ARR −0.2%, 95% CI −2.6% to +1.1%; RRR −7%, 95% CI −113% to +47%). The subsequent large RCT randomised 6800 people (88% male, mean age 64 years, NYHA class I–III, 94% already taking ACE inhibitors, 82% taking diuretics) to blinded additional treatment with either digoxin or placebo for a mean of 37 months.[30] Digoxin did not reduce all cause mortality compared with placebo (1181/3397 [34.8%] with digoxin v 1194/3403 [35.1%] with placebo; ARR +0.3%, 95% CI −2.0% to +2.6%; RRR 0.9%, 95% CI −6% to +7%). The number of people admitted to hospital for worsening heart failure was substantially reduced in the digoxin group over 37 months (910/3397 [27%] for digoxin v 1180/3403 [35%] for placebo; ARR 8%, 95% CI 6% to 10%; RRR 23%, 95% CI 17% to 28%; NNT 13) as was the combined outcome of death or hospital admission caused by worsening heart failure (1041/3397 [31%] for digoxin v 1291/3403 [38%] for placebo; ARR 7.3%, 95% CI 5.1% to 9.4%; RRR 19%, 95% CI 13% to 25%; NNT 14). **Other inotropic agents:** Non-digitalis inotropic agents have been evaluated in RCTs, including up to 3600 people. Some of these studies found improved functional capacity and quality of life but not consistently across all studies. We found no evidence that positive inotropic agents decrease mortality; most RCTs found increased risk of death (see harms below).

Harms: We found no systematic review. **Digoxin:** The RCT (6800 people) found that more participants had suspected digoxin toxicity in the digoxin group versus placebo (11.9% v 7.9%; ARI 4%, 95% CI 2.4% to 5.8%; RRI 50%, 95% CI 30% to 73%; NNH 25).[30] The trial found no evidence that digoxin increased the risk of ventricular fibrillation or tachycardia compared with placebo (37/3397 [1.1%] with digoxin v 27/3403 [0.8%] with placebo; ARI +0.3%, 95% CI −0.1% to +1.0%; RRI 37%, 95% CI −16% to +124%). Digoxin compared with placebo increased rates of supraventricular arrhythmia (2.5% with digoxin v 1.2% with placebo; ARI 1.3%, 95% CI 0.5% to 2.4%; RRI 108%, 95% CI 44% to 199%; NNH 77) and second or third degree atrioventricular block (1.2% v 0.4%; ARI 0.8%, 95% CI 0.2% to 1.8%; RRI 193%, 95% CI 61% to 434%; NNH 126). **Other inotropic agents:** RCTs found that non-digitalis positive inotropic agents increase mortality compared with placebo.[10] One RCT (1088 people with heart failure) found milrinone versus placebo increased mortality over 6 months (168/561 [30%] v 127/527 [24%] for placebo; ARI 6%, 95% CI 0.5% to 12%; RRI 24%, 95% CI 2% to 49%; NNH 17).[31] Another RCT (3833 people with heart failure) found increased mortality with 60 mg vesnarinone a day versus placebo for 9 months (292/1275 [23%] for 60 mg vesnarinone v 242/1280 [19%] for placebo; ARI 4%, 95% CI 1% to 8%; RRI 21%, 95% CI 4% to 40%; NNH 25).[10]

Comment: None.

Heart failure

OPTION	β BLOCKERS

We found strong evidence from systematic reviews of RCTs that adding β blockers to standard treatment with ACE inhibitors in people with moderate heart failure reduces the rate of death or hospital admission. The reviews found less robust evidence that β blockers improve exercise capacity.

Benefits: We found one recent systematic review[32] and two subsequent large RCTs[29,30] of the effects of β blockers in heart failure. The systematic review (search date not stated, 18 RCTs of β blockers versus placebo, 1.5–44 months, 3023 people with heart failure) obtained details of outcomes directly from trial investigators.[32] The participants had idiopathic dilated cardiomyopathy (1718 people) or ischaemic heart disease (1513 people). Trials in people after an acute myocardial infarction were excluded. Most participants had NYHA class II or III symptoms. The systematic review found strong evidence that β blockers reduced the combined outcome of death or admission to hospital (239/1486 [16%] on β blockers v 293/1155 [25%] on placebo; ARR 9%, 95% CI 7% to 12%; RRR 37%, 95% CI 26% to 46%; NNT 11). The result was robust to the addition of neutral results from further trials. The review also found that addition of β blockers reduced total mortality compared with placebo (130/1718 [8%] for β blockers v 156/1305 [12%] for placebo; ARR 4%, 95% CI 2% to 6%; RRR 37%, 95% CI 21% to 50%; NNT 23) and improved NYHA class. These results were less robust (the conclusion could be altered by addition or removal of only one moderate sized study). The two subsequent RCTs[33,34] found stronger evidence of reduced mortality from the additional use of β blockers compared with placebo in heart failure. The first RCT (2647 people, NYHA class III–IV) compared additional bisoprolol versus placebo.[33] The RCT was stopped early because of significant reduction in the bisoprolol group after 1.3 years in all cause mortality (156/1327 [11.8%] for bisoprolol v 228/1320 [17.3%] for placebo; ARR 5.5%, 95% CI 3.0% to 7.6%; RRR 32%, 95% CI 18% to 44%; NNT 18) and sudden deaths (48/1327 [3.6%] for bisoprolol v 83/1320 [6.3%] for placebo; ARR 2.7%, 95% CI 1.2% to 3.7%; RRR 42%, 95% CI 19% to 60%; NNT 37). The second RCT (3991 people, NYHA class II–IV) compared additional controlled release metoprolol versus placebo.[34] It was stopped early because of significant reduction in the metoprolol group of mortality after 1 year (145/1990 [7.3%] for metoprolol v 217/2001 [10.8%] for placebo; ARR 3.6%, 95% CI 1.9% to 4.9%; RRR 33%, 95% CI 18% to 45%; NNT 28), sudden death and deaths from worsening heart failure.

Harms: Fears that β blockers may cause excessive problems with worsening heart failure, bradyarrhythmias, or hypotension have not been confirmed. In one RCT, the overall drug discontinuation rate for adverse reactions was 7.8% in the placebo group and 5.7% in the carvedilol group.[32] The findings from the RCT of metoprolol were similar, with the study drug discontinued in 13.9% of the controlled release metoprolol group and in 15.3% of the placebo group (RR 0.91, 95% CI 0.78 to 1.06).[34]

Comment: Good evidence was found for the use of β blockers in people with moderate symptoms (NYHA class II–III) receiving standard treatment, including ACE inhibitors. The value of β blockers needs clarification in NYHA class IV, in heart failure with preserved ejection fraction, in asymptomatic LVSD, and in heart failure after an acute myocardial infarction. The RCTs of β blockers have consistently found a mortality benefit, but it is not clear whether or not the benefit is a class effect. One recent small RCT (150 people) of metoprolol versus carvedilol found some differences in surrogate outcomes, but both drugs produced similar improvements in symptoms, submaximal exercise tolerance, and quality of life.[35] An RCT is comparing the effect of metoprolol versus carvedilol on survival.[35]

OPTION   CALCIUM CHANNEL BLOCKERS

We found no evidence that calcium channel blockers are of benefit in people with heart failure.

Benefits: **After myocardial infarction:** See calcium channel blockers under acute myocardial infarction, p 94. **Other heart failure:** We found one non-systematic review (3 RCTs, 1790 people with heart failure)[10] and one subsequent RCT.[10] One RCT (1153 people, NYHA class III–IV, LVEF < 0.30, using diuretics digoxin and ACE inhibitors) found that amlodipine versus placebo had no significant effect on the primary combined end point of all cause mortality and hospital admission for cardiovascular events over 14 months (222/571 [39%] for amlodipine v 246/582 [42%] for placebo; ARR +3.4%, 95% CI –2.3% to +8.8%; RRR 8%, 95% CI –6% to +21%).[36] Subgroup analysis of people with primary cardiomyopathy found a reduction in mortality (45/209 [22%] for amlodipine v 74/212 [35%] for placebo; ARR 13%, 95% CI 5% to 20%; RRR 38%, 95% CI 15% to 57%; NNT 7). There was no significant difference in the group with heart failure caused by coronary artery disease. The subsequent RCT (186 people, idiopathic dilated cardiomyopathy, NYHA class I–III) compared diltiazem versus placebo.[10] It found no evidence of a difference in survival with diltiazem versus placebo in those who did not have a heart transplant, although people on diltiazem had improved cardiac function, exercise capacity, and subjective quality of life. A third RCT (451 people with mild heart failure, NYHA class II–III) compared felodipine versus placebo.[10] No significant adverse or beneficial effect was found.

Harms: Calcium channel blockers have been found to exacerbate symptoms of heart failure or increase mortality in people with pulmonary congestion after myocardial infarct or ejection fraction less than 0.40 (see calcium channel blockers under acute myocardial infarction, p 94).[10]

Comment: Many of the RCTs were underpowered and had wide confidence intervals. An RCT is in progress to test the hypothesis that amlodipine decreases mortality in people with primary dilated cardiomyopathy.

| OPTION | ALDOSTERONE RECEPTOR ANTAGONISTS |

One recent large RCT of people with severe heart failure (on usual treatment including ACE inhibitor) has found that adding an aldosterone receptor antagonist (spironolactone) further decreases mortality.

Benefits: We found no systematic review. We found one RCT of spirono-lactone (25 mg daily) versus placebo in 1663 people with heart failure (NYHA class III–IV, LVEF < 0.35, all taking ACE inhibitors and loop diuretics, and most taking digoxin).[37] The trial was stopped early because of a significant reduction in the primary end point of all cause mortality for spironolactone versus placebo after 2 years (mortality 284/822 [35%] for spironolactone v 386/841 [46%] for placebo; ARR 11%, 95% CI 7% to 16%; RRR 25%, 95% CI 15% to 34%; NNT 9).

Harms: The trial found no evidence that spironolactone in combination with an ACE inhibitor may result in an increased incidence of clinically significant hyperkalaemia. Gynaecomastia or breast pain was reported in 10% of men given spironolactone and 1% of men given placebo.[37]

Comment: The RCT was large and well designed. As only NYHA functional class III–IV patients were randomised into the study, these data cannot necessarily be generalised to people with milder heart failure.

| OPTION | ANTIARRHYTHMIC DRUG TREATMENT |

Systematic reviews found weak evidence that amiodarone reduces total mortality in people with heart failure. Other antiarrhythmic agents may increase mortality in people with heart failure.

Benefits: **Amiodarone:** We found two systematic reviews of the effects of amiodarone versus placebo in heart failure.[38,39] The most recent review (10 RCTs, 4766 people) included people with a wide range of conditions (symptomatic and asymptomatic heart failure, ventricular arrhythmia, recent myocardial infarction, and recent cardiac arrest).[38] Eight of these studies reported the number of deaths. The review found that treatment with amiodarone over 3–24 months reduced the risk of death from any cause compared with placebo or conventional treatment (436/2262 [19%] for amiodarone v 507/2263 [22%] for control; ARR 3%, 95% CI 0.8% to 5.3%; RRR 14%, 95% CI 4% to 24%; NNT 32). This review did not perform any subgroup analyses to reveal the effect of amiodarone on people with heart failure. The earlier systematic review found eight RCTs (5101 people after myocardial infarction) of prophylactic amiodarone versus placebo or usual care and five RCTs (1452 people with heart failure).[39] Mean follow up was 16 months. Analysis of data from all 13 RCTs found a lower total mortality with amiodarone than control (10.9% v 12.3% dead per year). The effect was significant with some methods of calculation (fixed effects model: OR 0.87, 95% CI 0.78 to 0.99) but not with others (random effects model: OR 0.85, 95% CI 0.71 to 1.02). The effect of amiodarone was significantly greater in RCTs that compared amiodarone versus usual care than in placebo controlled RCTs. Deaths classified as arrhythmic death or sudden death were significantly reduced by

Cardiovascular disorders

amiodarone compared with placebo (OR 0.71, 95% CI 0.59 to 0.85). Subgroup analysis found a significant effect of amiodarone in the five heart failure RCTs (19.9% deaths per year v 24.3% in the placebo group; OR 0.83, 95% CI 0.70 to 0.99). **Other antiarrhythmics:** Apart from β blockers, other antiarrhythmic drugs seem to increase mortality in people at high risk (see antiarrhythmics under secondary prevention of ischaemic cardiac events, p 168).

Harms: **Amiodarone:** Amiodarone was not found to increase the non-arrhythmic death rate (OR 1.02, 95% CI 0.87 to 1.19).[39] In placebo controlled RCTs, after 2 years 41% of people in the amiodarone group and 27% in the placebo group had permanently discontinued study medication.[34] In 10 RCTs of amiodarone versus placebo, amiodarone increased the odds of reporting adverse drug reactions compared with placebo (OR 2.22, 95% CI 1.83 to 2.68). Nausea was the most common adverse effect. Hypothyroidism was the most common serious adverse effect (7.0% of amiodarone treated group versus 1.1% of controls). Hyperthyroidism (1.4% v 0.5%), peripheral neuropathy (0.5% v 0.2%), lung infiltrates (1.6% v 0.5%), bradycardia (2.4% v 0.8%), and liver dysfunction (1.0% v 0.4%) were all more common in the amiodarone group.[39] **Other antiarrhythmics:** These agents (particularly class I antiarrhythmics) may increase mortality (see antiarrhythmics under secondary prevention of ischaemic cardiac events, p 168).

Comment: **Amiodarone:** RCTs of amiodarone versus usual treatment found larger effects than placebo controlled trials.[39] These findings suggest bias; unblinded follow up may be associated with reduced usual care or improved adherence with amiodarone. Further studies are required to assess the effects of amiodarone treatment on mortality and morbidity in people with heart failure.

OPTION **IMPLANTABLE CARDIAC DEFIBRILLATORS**

Three RCTs have found good evidence that the ICD reduces mortality in people with heart failure who have experienced a cardiac arrest. The review found conflicting evidence for prophylactic implantation of ICDs in people at risk of arrhythmia.

Benefits: We found no systematic review. We found three RCTs examining the effects of ICDs in people with left ventricular dysfunction.[40-42] The first RCT (1016 people resuscitated after ventricular arrhythmia plus either syncope or other serious cardiac symptom plus left ventricular ejection fraction ≤ 0.40) compared an ICD versus an antiarrhythmic drug (mainly amiodarone).[40] ICDs versus an antiarrhythmic drug improved survival at 1, 2, and 3 years (1 year survival: 89.3% with ICD v 82.3% with antiarrhythmic; 2 year survival 81.6% v 73.7%; 3 year survival 75.4% v 64.1%). The second RCT included 196 people with NYHA class I–III heart failure and previous myocardial infarction, a left ventricular ejection fraction ≤ 0.35, a documented episode of asymptomatic unsustained ventricular tachycardia, and inducible non-suppressible ventricular tachyarrhythmia on electrophysiologic study.[41] Ninety five people received an implantable defibrillator and 101 received conventional medical treatment. The trial found that ICDs compared with conventional treatment reduced mortality over a mean of 27 months (deaths: 15/95 [16%] with ICD [11 from cardiac cause] v 39/101 [39%] with conventional therapy [27 from cardiac cause]; HR 0.46, 95% CI 0.26 to 0.82). The third RCT included 1055 people aged under 80 years who were scheduled for coronary artery bypass surgery, had a left ventricular ejection less than 0.36, and had electrocardiographic abnormalities. It found that ICD (446 people) at the time of bypass surgery versus no ICD (454 people) produced no significant difference in mortality over a mean of 32 months (deaths: 101/446 [23%] with ICD [71 from cardiac causes] v 95/454 [21%] with control [72 from cardiac causes]; HR 1.07, 95% CI 0.81 to 1.42; P = 0.64).[42]

Harms: The three RCTs found that the main adverse effects of ICDs were infection (about 5%), pneumothorax (about 2%), bleeding requiring further operation (about 1%), serious haematomas (about 3%), cardiac perforation (about 0.2%), problems with defibrillator lead (about 7%), and malfunction of defibrillator generator (about 3%).[40-42]

Comment: The RCTs were all in people with previous ventricular arrhythmias. It is uncertain whether asymptomatic ventricular arrhythmia is in itself a predictor of sudden death in people with moderate or severe heart failure.[43] The role of ICDs in other groups of people with heart failure awaits evaluation. Several RCTs of prophylactic ICD treatment are ongoing in people with heart failure and in survivors of acute myocardial infarction.[44]

OPTION ANTICOAGULATION

We found no RCTs of anticoagulation in people with heart failure. We found conflicting evidence from two large retrospective cohort studies.

Benefits: We found no RCTs of anticoagulation in people with heart failure. We found conflicting evidence from two large retrospective cohort studies.[45,46] The first retrospective analysis (2 RCTs) assessed the effect of anticoagulants used at the discretion of individual investigators on the incidence of stroke, peripheral arterial embolism, and pulmonary embolism.[45] One RCT (642 men with chronic heart failure) compared hydralazine and isosorbide dinitrate versus prazosin versus placebo. The other RCT (804 men with chronic heart failure) compared enalapril plus isosorbide dinitrate versus hydralazine plus isosorbide dinitrate. All people were given digoxin and diuretics. The retrospective analysis found that without treatment the incidence of all thromboembolic events was low (2.7 per 100 patient years in the first RCT, 2.1 per 100 patient years in the second RCT) and that anticoagulation did not reduce the incidence of thromboembolic events (2.9 per 100 patient years in the first RCT, 4.8 per 100 patient years in the second RCT). In this group of people, atrial fibrillation was not found to be associated with a higher risk of thromboembolic events. The second retrospective analysis included two large RCTs, which compared enalapril versus placebo in 2569 people with symptomatic and asymptomatic left ventricular dysfunction.[46] The analysis found that people treated with warfarin at baseline had significantly lower risk of death during follow up (hazards ratio adjusted for baseline differences 0.76, 95% CI 0.65 to 0.89). Warfarin use was associated with a reduction in the combined outcome of death plus hospitalisation for heart failure (adjusted HR 0.82, 95% CI 0.72 to 0.93). The benefit with warfarin use was not significantly influenced by the presence or absence of symptoms, randomisation to enalapril or placebo, gender, presence or absence of atrial fibrillation, age, ejection fraction, NYHA classification, or cause of heart failure. Warfarin reduced cardiac mortality, specifically deaths that were sudden, associated with heart failure, or associated with myocardial infarction.

Harms: Neither cohort study reported harms of anticoagulation.

Comment: Neither of the retrospective studies were designed to determine the incidence of thromboembolic events in heart failure or the effects of treatment. Neither study included information about the intensity of anticoagulation or warfarin use. We found several additional cohort studies, which showed a reduction in thromboembolic events with anticoagulation, but they all reported results for groups of people that were too small to provide useful data. An RCT is needed to compare anticoagulation versus no anticoagulation in people with heart failure.

OPTION   ANTIPLATELET AGENTS

We found no RCTs. Retrospective analyses have included two few events to establish or exclude a clinically important effect of antiplatelet agents in people with heart failure. In people not taking ACE inhibitors we found limited evidence from one retrospective cohort analysis that the incidence of thromboembolic events in people with heart failure was low and not significantly improved with antiplatelet therapy. It is unclear from limited evidence from two retrospective cohort analyses whether there are additional reductions in the incidence of thromboembolic events from adding ACE inhibitor therapy to antiplatelet therapy in people with heart failure. It is unclear whether adding antiplatelet therapy to ACE inhibitor treatment in people with heart failure is beneficial.

Benefits: **In people not taking ACE inhibitors:** We found no systematic review and no RCTs. We found one retrospective cohort analysis of one RCT in 642 men with heart failure.[45] The RCT compared hydralazine plus isosorbide dinitrate versus prazosin versus placebo in men receiving digoxin and diuretics. Aspirin, dipyridamole, or both, were used at the discretion of the investigators. The number of thromboembolic events was low in both groups (only 1 stroke and no pulmonary or peripheral emboli in 184 patient years of treatment with antiplatelet drugs v 21 strokes, 4 peripheral and 4 pulmonary emboli in 1068 patient years of treatment without antiplatelet drugs; 0.5 events per 100 patient years with antiplatelet agents v 2.0 events per 100 patient years without antiplatelet agents; P = 0.07). **In people taking ACE inhibitors:** We found no RCTs. We found two large retrospective cohort studies.[45,47] The first retrospective analysis (1 RCT) assessed the effect of antiplatelet agents used at the discretion of individual investigators on the incidence of stroke, peripheral arterial embolism, and pulmonary embolism.[45] The RCT (804 men with chronic heart failure) compared enalapril plus isosorbide dinitrate versus hydralazine plus isosorbide dinitrate. It found that the incidence of all thrombo-embolic events was low without antiplatelet treatment and, although antiplatelet agents reduced the thromboembolic rate, the difference was not significant (2.1 events per 100 patient years with no antiplatelet agent v 1.6 per 100 patient years with antiplatelet agents; P = 0.48). The second cohort analysis included two large RCTs, which compared enalapril versus placebo (2569 people with symptomatic and asymptomatic left ventricular dysfunction). It found that people treated with antiplatelet agents at baseline had a significantly lower risk of death (HR adjusted for baseline differences 0.82, 95% CI 0.73 to 0.92).[47] Subgroup analysis suggested that an effect of antiplatelet agents might be present in people who were randomised to placebo (mortality HR for antiplatelet treatment at baseline v no antiplatelet treatment at baseline 0.68, 95% CI 0.58 to 0.80), but not in people randomised to enalapril (mortality HR for antiplatelet treatment v no antiplatelet treatment 1.00, 95% CI 0.85 to 1.17).

Harms: Neither study reported harms of treatment.

Comment: Both retrospective studies have limitations common to studies with a retrospective cohort design. One study did not report on the proportions of people taking aspirin and other antiplatelet agents.[45] The other study noted that more than 95% of people took aspirin, but the dosage and consistency of antiplatelet use was not noted.[47] One retrospective overview (4 RCTs, 96 712 people, search date not stated) provided additional evidence about the effect of aspirin on the benefits of early ACE inhibitors in heart failure.[48] It found a similar reduction in 30 day mortality with ACE inhibitor versus control for those people not taking aspirin compared to those taking aspirin (no aspirin: OR 0.90, 95% CI 0.81 to 1.01; aspirin: OR 0.94, 95% CI 0.89 to 0.99). However, the analysis may not be valid because the group of people who did not receive aspirin were older and had a worse baseline prognosis than those taking aspirin. The effects of antiplatelet therapy in combination with ACE inhibitors in people with heart failure requires further research.

QUESTION What are the effects of ACE inhibitors in people at high risk of heart failure?

RCTs have found good evidence that ACE inhibitors can delay development of symptomatic heart failure and reduce the frequency of cardiovascular events in people with asymptomatic LVSD, and in people with other cardiovascular risk factors for heart failure.

Benefits: **In people with asymptomatic LVSD:** We found no systematic review but found two RCTs. One large RCT examined ACE inhibitors versus placebo over 40 months in people with asymptomatic LVSD (LVEF < 0.35).[49] It found no evidence that ACE inhibitors significantly decreased total mortality and cardiovascular mortality compared with placebo (all cause mortality: 313/2111 [14.8%] for ACE inhibitor v 334/2117 [15.8%] for placebo; ARR 0.9%, 95% CI −1.3% to +2.9%; RRR 6%, 95% CI −8% to +19%; cardiovascular mortality: 265/2111 [12.6%] for ACE inhibitor v 298/2117 [14.1%] for placebo; ARR +1.5%, 95% CI −0.6% to +3.3%; RRR 11%, 95% CI −4% to +24%). During the study, more people assigned to the placebo than to the enalapril group received digoxin, diuretics, or ACE inhibitor that were not part of the study protocol, which may have contributed to the lack of significant difference in mortality between the two groups. Compared with placebo, ACE inhibitors reduced symptomatic heart failure, reduced hospital admission for heart failure, and reduced fatal or non-fatal myocardial infarction (symptomatic heart failure: 438/2111 [21%] for ACE inhibitor v 640/2117 [30%] for placebo; ARR 9.5%, 95% CI 7% to 12%; RRR 31%, 95% CI 23% to 39%; NNT 11; admission for heart failure: 306/2111 [15%] for ACE inhibitor v 454/2117 [21%] for placebo; ARR 7%, 95% CI 5% to 9%; RRR 32%, 95% CI 23% to 41%; NNT 14; fatal or non-fatal myocardial infarction: 7.6% for ACE inhibitor v 9.6% for placebo; ARR 2%, 95% CI 0.4% to 3.4%; RRR 21%, 95% CI 4% to 35%).[9,49] A second trial in asymptomatic people after myocardial infarction with documented LVSD found that ACE inhibitors (captopril) reduced mortality and reduced risk of ischaemic events compared with placebo.[50] **In people with other risk factors:** We found one large RCT comparing ramipril 10 mg daily versus placebo in 9297 high risk people (people with vascular disease or diabetes plus one other cardiovascular risk factor) who were not known to have LVSD or heart failure, for a mean of 5 years.[51] It found that ramipril reduced the risk of heart failure (9.0% with ramipril v 11.5% with placebo, RR 0.77, 95% CI 0.67 to 0.87, P < 0.001). Ramipril also reduced the combined risk of myocardial infarction or stroke or cardiovascular death, reduced the risk of these outcomes separately, and reduced all cause mortality (see ACE inhibitors in people at high risk under secondary prevention of ischaemic cardiac events, p 167). During the trial, 496 people underwent echocardiography; 2.6% of these people were found to have ejection fraction less than 0.40. Retrospective review of charts found that left ventricular function had been documented in 5193 people; 8.1% had a reduced ejection fraction.

Harms: We found no systematic review. The first RCT over 40 months found that a high proportion of people in both groups reported adverse effects (76% in the enalapril group v 72% in the placebo group).[49] Dizziness or fainting (46% v 33%) and cough (34% v 27%) were reported more often in the enalapril group (no P value reported). The incidence of angioedema was the same (1.4%) in both groups. Study medication was permanently discontinued by 8% of the participants in the enalapril group versus 5% in the placebo group (no P value reported).

Comment: Asymptomatic LVSD is prognostically important, but we found no prospective studies that have assessed the usefulness of screening to detect its presence.

<hr>

QUESTION   **What are the effects of treatments for diastolic heart failure?**

We found no randomised controlled trials in people with diastolic heart failure.

Benefits: We found no systematic review or RCTs in people with diastolic heart failure.

Heart failure

Harms: We found no evidence on the harms of treatments for diastolic heart failure.

Comment: The causes of diastolic dysfunction vary among people with diastolic heart failure. Current treatment is empirical, based on the results of small clinical studies, and consists of treating the underlying cause and coexistent conditions with interventions optimised for individuals.[6,52,53] RCTs with clinically relevant outcome measures are needed to determine the benefits and harms of treatment in diastolic heart failure.

GLOSSARY

Dyspnoea fatigue index Measures impact of breathlessness on ability to carry out activities of daily living, with a scale from 0 to 12.

Exercise time This is the total time in seconds that a person is able to pedal in a standardised symptom limited bicycle ergonometry exercise test.

NYHA class Classification of severity by symptoms. Class I: no limitation of physical activity; ordinary physical activity does not cause undue fatigue or dysponea. Class II: slight limitation of physical activity; comfortable at rest, but ordinary physical activity results in fatigue or dysponea. Class III: limitation of physical activity; comfortable at rest, but less than ordinary activity causes fatigue or dysponea. Class IV: unable to carry on any physical activity without symptoms; symptoms are present even at rest; if any physical activity is undertaken, symptoms are increased.

REFERENCES

1. Poole-Wilson PA. History, definition, and classification of heart failure. In: Poole-Wilson PA, Colucci WS, Massie BM, Chatterjee K, Coats AJS, eds. *Heart failure. Scientific principles and clinical practice.* London: Churchill Livingston, 1997: 269–277.

2. Working Group Report. How to diagnose diastolic heart failure: European Study Group on Diastolic Heart Failure. *Eur Heart J* 1998;19:990–1003.

3. Cowie MR, Mosterd A, Wood DA, et al. The epidemiology of heart failure. *Eur Heart J* 1997; 18:208–225.

4. McKelvie RS, Benedict CR, Yusuf S. Prevention of congestive heart failure and management of asymptomatic left ventricular dysfunction. *BMJ* 1999;318:1400–1402.

5. Bröckel U, Hense HW, Museholl M, Döring A, Riegger GA, Schunkert H. Prevalence of left ventricular dysfunction in the general population [abstract]. *J Am Coll Cardiol* 1996;27(suppl A):25.

6. Mosterd A, deBruijne MC, Hoes A, Deckers JW, Hofman A, Grobbee DE. Usefulness of echocardiography in detecting left ventricular dysfunction in population-based studies (the Rotterdam study). *Am J Cardiol* 1997;79: 103–104.

7. Vasan RS, Benjamin EJ, Levy D. Congestive heart failure with normal left ventricular systolic function. *Arch Intern Med* 1996;156:146–157.

8. Davie AP, Francis CM, Caruana L, Sutherland GR, McMurray JV. The prevalence of left ventricular diastolic filling abnormalities in patients with suspected heart failure. *Eur Heart J* 1997;18: 981–984.

9. Yusuf S, Pepine CJ, Garces C, et al. Effect of enalapril on myocardial infarction and unstable angina in patients with low ejection fractions. *Lancet* 1992;340:1173–1178.

10. Gheorghiade M, Benatar D, Konstam MA, Stoukides CA, Bonow RO. Pharmacotherapy for systolic dysfunction: a review of randomized clinical trials. *Am J Cardiol* 1997;80(suppl 8B): 14–27H.

11. Gaasch WH. Diagnosis and treatment of heart failure based on LV systolic or diastolic dysfunction. *JAMA* 1994;271:1276–1280.

12. Bittner V, Weiner DH, Yusuf S, et al, for the SOLVD Investigators. Prediction of mortality and morbidity with a 6-minute walk test in patients with left ventricular dysfunction. *JAMA* 1993;270: 1702–1707.

13. Rogers WJ, Johnstone DE, Yusuf S, et al, for the SOLVD Investigators. Quality of life among 5 025 patients with left ventricular dysfunction randomized between placebo and enalapril. The studies of left ventricular dysfunction. *J Am Coll Cardiol* 1994;23:393–400.

14. Rich MW. Heart failure disease management: a critical review. *J Cardiac Fail* 1999;5:64–75. Search dates 1983 to 1998; primary sources Medline; references in published articles.

15. Miller TD, Balady GJ, Fletcher GF. Exercise and its role in the prevention and rehabilitation of cardiovascular disease. *Ann Behav Med* 1997;19: 220–229.

16. Dracup K, Baker DW, Dunbar SB, et al. Management of heart failure. II. Counseling, education and lifestyle modifications. *JAMA* 1994; 272:1442–1446. Search date 1993; primary sources Medline; Embase.

17. Piepoli MF, Flater M, Coats AJS. Overview of studies of exercise training in chronic heart failure: the need for a prospective randomized multi-centre European trial. *Eur Heart J* 1998;19: 830–841. Search date and primary sources not stated; computed-aided search performed.

18. European Heart Failure Training Group. Experience from controlled trials of physical training in chronic heart failure. Protocol and patient factors in effectiveness in the improvement in exercise tolerance. *Eur Heart J* 1998;19:466–475.

19. Belardinelli R, Georgiou D, Cianci G, Purcaro A. Randomized, controlled trial of long-term moderate exercise training in chronic heart failure. Effects on functional capacity, quality of life, and clinical outcomes. *Circulation* 1999;99: 1173–1182.

20. Garg R, Yusuf S, for the Collaborative Group on ACE Inhibitor Trials. Overview of randomized trials of angiotensin-converting enzyme inhibitors on mortality and morbidity in patients with heart failure. *JAMA* 1995;273:1450–1456. Search date 1994; primary sources Medline; correspondence with investigators and pharmaceutical firms.

21. Flather M, Yusuf S, Kober L, et al, for the ACE-Inhibitor Myocardial Infarction Collaborative Group. Long-term ACE-inhibitor therapy in patients with heart failure or left-ventricular dysfunction: a systematic overview of data from individual patients. *Lancet* 2000;355:1575–1581. Search date not stated; primary sources Medline; Ovid; and hand searches of reference lists and personal contact with researchers, colleagues and principal investigators of the trials identified.

22. Packer M, Poole-Wilson PA, Armstrong PW, et al, on behalf of the ATLAS Study Group. Comparative effects of low and high doses of the angiotensin-converting enzyme inhibitor, lisinopril, on morbidity and mortality in chronic heart failure. *Circulation* 1999;100:2312–2318.

23. SOLVD Investigators. Effect of enalapril on survival in patients with reduced left ventricular ejection fractions and congestive heart failure. *N Engl J Med* 1991;325:293–302.

24. Sharma D, Buyse M, Pitt B, Rucinska EJ, and the Losartan Heart Failure Mortality Meta-analysis Study Group. Meta-analysis of observed mortality data from all-controlled, double-blind, multiple-dose studies of losartan in heart failure. *Am J Cardiol* 2000;85:187–192.

25. Riegger GAJ, Bouzo H, Petr P, et al, for the Symptom, Tolerability, Response to Exercise Trial of Candesartan Cilexetil in Heart Failure (STRETCH) Investigators. Improvement in exercise tolerance and symptoms of congestive heart failure during treatment with candesartan cilexetil. *Circulation* 1999;100:2224–2230.

26. Pitt B, Poole-Wilson PA, Segal R, et al, on behalf of the ELITE II investigators. Effect of losartan compared with captopril on mortality in patients with symptomatic heart failure: randomised trial. *Lancet* 2000;355:1582–1587.

27. McKelvie R, Yusuf S, Pericak D, Lindgren E, Held P, for the RESOLVD Investigators. Comparison of candesartan, enalapril, and their combination in congestive heart failure: randomized evaluation of strategies for left ventricular dysfunction (RESOLVD pilot study). *Circulation* 1999;100:1056–1064.

28. Hamroff G, Katz SD, Mancini D, et al. Addition of angiotensin II receptor blockade to maximal angiotensin-converting enzyme inhibition improves exercise capacity in patients with severe congestive heart failure. *Circulation* 1999;99: 990–992.

29. Kraus F, Rudolph C, Rudolph W. Wirksamkeit von Digitalis bei Patienten mit chronischer Herzinsuffizienz und Sinusrhythmus. *Herz* 1993; 18:95–117. Search date 1992; primary source Medline.

30. Digitalis Investigation Group. The effect of digoxin on mortality and morbidity in patients with heart failure. *N Engl J Med* 1997;336:525–533.

31. Packer M, Carver JR, Rodeheffer RJ, et al, for the PROMISE Study Research Group. Effect of oral milrinone on mortality in severe chronic heart failure. *N Engl J Med* 1991;325:1468–1475.

32. Lechat P, Packer M, Chalon S, Cucherat M, Arab T, Boissel J-P. Clinical effects of β-adrenergic blockade in chronic heart failure. A meta-analysis of double-blind, placebo-controlled, randomized trials. *Circulation* 1998;98:1184–1191. Search date not stated; primary sources Medline; reference lists; colleagues; pharmaceutical industry.

33. CIBIS-II Investigators and Committees. The cardiac insufficiency bisoprolol study II (CIBIS-II): a randomised trial. *Lancet* 1999;353:9–13.

34. MERIT-HF Study Group. Effect of metoprolol CR/XL in chronic heart failure: metoprolol CR/XL randomised intervention trial in congestive heart failure. *Lancet* 1999;353:2001–2007.

35. Metra M, Giubbini R, Nodari S, Boldi E, Modena MG, Cas LD. Differential effects of β-blockers in patients with heart failure: a prospective, randomized, double-blind comparison of the long-term effects of metoprolol versus carvedilol. *Circulation* 2000;102:546–551.

36. Packer M, O'Connor CM, Ghali JK, et al, for the Prospective Randomized Amlodipine Survival Evaluation Study Group. Effect of amlodipine on morbidity and mortality in severe chronic heart failure. *N Engl J Med* 1996;335:1107–1114.

37. Pitt B, Zannad F, Remme WJ, et al, for the Randomized Aldactone Evaluation Study Investigators. The effects of spironolactone on morbidity and mortality in patients with severe heart failure. *N Engl J Med* 1999;341:709–717.

38. Piepoli M, Villani GQ, Ponikowski P, Wright A, Flather MD, Coats AJ. Overview and meta-analysis of randomised trials of amiodarone in chronic heart failure. *Int J Cardiol* 1998;66:1–10. Search date 1997; primary sources unspecified computerised literature database.

39. Amiodarone Trials Meta-Analysis Investigators. Effect of prophylactic amiodarone on mortality after acute myocardial infarction and in congestive heart failure: meta-analysis of individual data from 6500 patients in randomised trials. *Lancet* 1997; 350:1417–1424. Search date not stated; primary sources literature review, computerised literature review, and discussion with colleagues.

40. The Antiarrhythmic versus Implantable Defibrillators (AVID) Investigators. A comparison of antiarrhythmic-drug therapy with implantable defibrillators I patients resuscitated from near-fatal ventricular arrhythmias. *N Engl J Med* 1997;337: 1576–1583.

41. Moss AJ, Hall WJ, Cannom DS, et al. Improved survival with an implanted defibrillator in patients with coronary disease at high risk for ventricular arrhythmia. *N Engl J Med* 1996;335:1933–1940.

42. Bigger JT for The Coronary Artery Bypass Graft (CABG) Patch Trial Investigators. Prophylactic use of implanted cardiac defibrillators in patients at high risk for ventricular arrhythmias after coronary-artery bypass graft surgery. *N Engl J Med* 1997; 337:1569–1575.

43. Teerlink JR, Jalaluddin M, Anderson S, et al. Ambulatory ventricular arrhythmias in patients with heart failure do not specifically predict an increased risk of sudden death. *Circulation* 2000; 101:40–46.

44. Connolly SJ. Prophylactic antiarrhythmic therapy for the prevention of sudden death in high-risk patients: drugs and devices. *Eur Heart J* 1999(suppl C):31–35.

45. Dunkman WB, Johnson GR, Carson PE, Bhat G, Farrell L et al, for the V-HeFT Cooperative Studies Group. Incidence of thromboembolic events in congestive heart failure. *Circulation* 1993;87: 94–101.

46. Al-Khadra AS, Salem DN, Rand WM, et al. Warfarin anticoagulation and survival: A cohort analysis from the studies of left ventricular dysfunction. *J Am Coll Cardiol* 1998;31:749–753.

Heart failure

47. Al-Khadra AS, Salem DN, Rand WM, Udelson JE, Smith JJ, et al. Antiplatelet agents and survival: A cohort analysis from the studies of left ventricular dysfunction (SOLVD) Trial. *J Am Coll Cardiol* 1998; 31:419–425.

48. Latini R, Tognoni G, Maggioni AP, Baigent C, Braunwald E, et al, on behalf of the Angiotensin-converting Enzyme Inhibitor Myocardial Infarction Collaborative Group. Clinical effects of early angiotensin-converting enzyme inhibitor treatment for acute myocardial infarction are similar in the presence and absence of aspirin. Systematic overview of individual data from 96 712 randomized patients. *J Am Coll Cardiol* 2000;35: 1801–1807.

49. SOLVD Investigators. Effect of enalapril on mortality and the development of heart failure in asymptomatic patients with reduced left ventricular ejection fractions. *N Engl J Med* 1992; 327:685–691.

50. Rutherford JD, Pfeffer MA, Moyé LA, et al. Effects of captopril on ischaemic events after myocardial infarction. *Circulation* 1994;90: 1731–1738.

51. The Heart Outcome Prevention Evaluation Study Investigators. Effects of an angiotensin-converting-enzyme inhibitor, ramipril, on cardiovascular events in high-risk patients. *N Engl J Med* 2000; 342:145–153.

52. The Task Force of the Working Group on Heart Failure of the European Society of Cardiology: The treatment of heart failure. *Eur Heart J* 1997;18: 736–753.

53. Tendera M. Ageing and heart failure: the place of ACE inhibitors in heart failure with preserved systolic function. *Eur Heart J* 2000;2(suppl I):I8–I14.

Robert McKelvie
Associate Professor of Medicine
McMaster University
Hamilton
Ontario
Canada

Competing interests: None declared.

Search date November 2000 (Acute myocardial infarction).
Search date December 2000 (Cardiogenic shock).

Shamir Mehta, Philip Urban and Edoardo De Benedetti

QUESTIONS

INTERVENTIONS

Key Messages

Improving outcomes in acute myocardial infarction (AMI)

- Good evidence from systematic reviews supports the following interventions in people presenting with symptoms of AMI:
  - Aspirin (at least 160 mg chewed and swallowed immediately and continued daily for at least a few years and perhaps lifelong).
  - Thrombolytic treatment (streptokinase ± intravenous/subcutaneous heparin or tissue plasminogen activator [tPA] + intravenous heparin) in people with ST elevation on their presenting electrocardiogram (ECG).
  - β Blocker (started intravenously within hours of infarction and continued orally for several years) in people without contraindications.
  - Angiotensin converting enzyme (ACE) inhibitor (started within 24 hours of infarction and continued daily) for about a month in people at low risk of death, and for several months in people with heart failure at any time during hospital admission or with a left ventricular ejection fraction less than 40%.

- Nitrates (shown to be safe for symptomatic relief in this setting, but to have at most a modest effect on mortality).
- In high risk people who present early (< 4 hours after onset of symptoms) and have ST elevation, primary percutaneous transluminal coronary angioplasty (PTCA) is more effective than thrombolytic treatment provided it can be performed quickly (< 90 mins after hospital arrival) by an experienced operator and staff in a high volume centre.

■ Systematic reviews found no evidence of mortality benefit from calcium channel blockers during or after AMI; there is potential for increased mortality in people with heart failure.

Cardiogenic shock after AMI

■ Two RCTs have found that early invasive cardiac revascularisation versus initial medical treatment alone improves survival in people with cardiogenic shock after AMI.

■ One RCT found no significant reduction in mortality with thrombolysis in people with cardiogenic shock after AMI.

■ One abstract from an RCT found no reduction in mortality with intra-aortic balloon counterpulsation in people with cardiogenic shock after AMI.

■ In cardiogenic shock after AMI we found no evidence from RCTs about the effects of positive inotropes, vasodilators, pulmonary artery catheterisation, ventricular assistance devices, cardiac transplantation, or early cardiac surgery.

DEFINITION   **AMI:** The sudden occlusion of a coronary artery leading to myocardial death. **Cardiogenic shock:** Defined clinically as a poor cardiac output plus evidence of tissue hypoxia that is not improved by correction of reduced intravascular volume.[1] When a pulmonary artery catheter is used, cardiogenic shock may be defined as a cardiac index (see glossary, p 99) below 2.2 litres/minute/m^2 despite an elevated pulmonary capillary wedge pressure (≥ 15 mm Hg).[1-3]

INCIDENCE/   **AMI:** One of the most common causes of mortality in both
PREVALENCE developed and developing nations. In 1990, ischaemic heart disease was the leading cause of death worldwide, accounting for about 6.3 million deaths. The age standardised incidence varies among and within countries.[4] Each year, about 900 000 people in the USA experience an AMI and about 225 000 of them die. About half of these people die within 1 hour of symptoms and before reaching a hospital emergency room.[5] Event rates increase with age for both sexes and are higher in men than in women, and in poorer than richer people at all ages. The incidence of death from AMI has fallen in many Western countries over the past 20 years. **Cardiogenic shock:** Cardiogenic shock occurs in about 7% of people admitted to hospital with AMI.[6] Of these, about half have established cardiogenic shock at the time of admission to hospital, and most of the others develop it during the first 24–48 hours of their admission.[7]

AETIOLOGY/ RISK FACTORS

AMI: The immediate mechanism of AMI is rupture of an atheromatous plaque causing thrombosis and occlusion of coronary arteries and myocardial death. Factors that may convert a stable plaque into an unstable plaque (the "active plaque") have yet to be fully elucidated; however, shear stresses, inflammation, and autoimmunity have been proposed. The changing rates of coronary heart disease in different populations are only partly explained by changes in the standard risk factors for ischaemic heart disease (particularly fall in blood pressure and smoking). **Cardiogenic shock:** Cardiogenic shock after AMI usually follows a reduction in functional ventricular myocardium, and is caused by left ventricular infarction (79% of people with cardiogenic shock), more often than by right ventricular infarction (3% of people with cardiogenic shock).[8] Cardiogenic shock after AMI may also be caused by cardiac structural defects, such as mitral valve regurgitation due to papillary muscle dysfunction (7% of people with cardiogenic shock), ventricular septal rupture (4% of people with cardiogenic shock), or cardiac tamponade following free wall rupture (1% of people with cardiogenic shock). Major risk factors for cardiogenic shock after AMI are previous myocardial infarction, diabetes mellitus, advanced age, hypotension, tachycardia or bradycardia, congestive heart failure with Killip class II–III (see glossary, p 99), and low left ventricular ejection fraction (ejection fraction < 35%).[7,8]

PROGNOSIS

AMI: AMI may lead to a host of mechanical and electrical complications, including death, ventricular dysfunction, congestive heart failure, fatal and non-fatal arrhythmias, valvular dysfunction, myocardial rupture, and cardiogenic shock. **Cardiogenic shock:** Mortality rates for people in hospital with cardiogenic shock after AMI vary between 50–80%.[2,3,6,7] Most deaths occur within 48 hours of the onset of shock (see figure 1, p 105). People surviving until discharge from hospital have a reasonable long term prognosis (88% survival at 1 year).[10]

AIMS

To relieve pain; to restore blood supply to heart muscle; to reduce incidence of complications (such as congestive heart failure, myocardial rupture, valvular dysfunction, fatal and non-fatal arrhythmia); to prevent recurrent ischaemia and infarction; and to decrease mortality.

OUTCOMES

Efficacy outcomes: Rates of major cardiovascular events, including death, recurrent AMI, refractory ischaemia, and stroke. **Safety outcomes:** Rates of major bleeding and intracranial haemorrhage.

METHODS

AMI: *Clinical Evidence* search and appraisal November 2000. **Cardiogenic shock:** *Clinical Evidence* search and appraisal December 2000.

| QUESTION | Which treatments improve outcomes in acute myocardial infarction (AMI)? |

Shamir Mehta

| OPTION | ASPIRIN |

One systematic review has found that, in people with AMI, aspirin reduces mortality (1 life saved per 40 people treated during the acute phase), reinfarction (1 fewer non-fatal reinfarction per 100 people treated), and stroke (1 fewer non-fatal stroke per 300 people treated). The evidence suggests an optimal dose of aspirin of 160–325 mg acutely, followed by long term treatment with at least 75 mg/day indefinitely.

Benefits: **Aspirin versus placebo:** We found one systematic review (search date 1990, 9 RCTs, 18 773 people), which compared antiplatelet agents versus placebo soon after the onset of AMI and for a period of at least 1 month afterwards.[11] The absolute and relative benefits found in the systematic review are shown in figure 2, p 106. The largest of the RCTs (17 187 people with suspected AMI) compared placebo versus aspirin (162.6 mg) chewed and swallowed on the day of AMI and continued daily for 1 month.[12] In subsequent long term follow up, the mortality benefit was maintained for up to 4 years.[13] In the systematic review, the most widely tested aspirin regimens were 75–325 mg/day.[11] Doses throughout this range seemed similarly effective, with no evidence that "higher" doses were more effective (500–1500 mg/day; odds reduction compared with placebo 21%, 95% CI 14% to 27%) than "medium" doses (160–325 mg/day; odds reduction 28%, 95% CI 22% to 33%) or "lower" doses (75–160 mg/day; odds reduction 26%, 95% CI 5% to 42%). There was insufficient evidence for efficacy of doses below 75 mg/day. One study found that administering a loading dose of 160–325 mg/day achieved a prompt antiplatelet effect.[14]

Harms: In the largest RCT, there was no significant increase in rates of cerebral haemorrhage or bleeds requiring transfusion (0.4% on aspirin and placebo).[12] There was a small absolute excess of "minor" bleeding (ARI 0.6%, 95% CI not provided; P < 0.01).

Comment: None.

| OPTION | THROMBOLYSIS |

Systematic reviews have found that prompt thrombolytic treatment (within 6 hrs and perhaps up to 12 hrs and longer after the onset of symptoms) reduces mortality in people with AMI and ST elevation or bundle branch block on their presenting ECG. Fifty six people would need treatment in the acute phase to prevent one additional death. Strokes, intracranial haemorrhage, and major bleeds are more common in people given thrombolysis, with one additional stroke for every 250 people treated and one additional major bleed for every 143 people treated. The reviews have found that intracranial haemorrhage is more common in people of advanced age and low body weight, those with hypertension on admission, and those given tPA rather than another thrombolytic agent.

Benefits: **Versus placebo:** We found one overview (9 large RCTs, 58 600 people with suspected AMI) comparing thrombolysis versus placebo.[15] Baseline ECGs showed ST segment elevation in 68% of people, and ST segment depression, T wave abnormalities, or no abnormality in the rest. Thrombolysis versus placebo reduced short term mortality (9.6% with thrombolysis v 11.5% with placebo; ARR 1.9%; RR 0.82, 95% CI 0.77 to 0.87; NNT 56). Greatest benefit was found in the large group of people presenting with ST elevation (RR 0.79) or bundle branch block (RR 0.75). Reduced rates of death were seen in people with all types of infarct, but the benefit was several times greater in those with anterior infarction (ARR 3.7%) compared with those with inferior infarction (ARR 0.8%) or infarctions in other zones (ARR 2.7%). Long term follow up of one of the RCTs found that the benefit of thrombolysis versus placebo on mortality persists at 12 years (36/107 [34%] dead with thrombolysis v 55/112 [49%] with placebo; ARR 15%, 95% CI 2.4% to 29%; RR 0.69, 95% CI 0.49 to 0.95; NNT 7).[16] **Timing of treatment:** The systematic review found that when the thrombolytic treatment was given, the greater the absolute benefit (see figure 3, p 107). For each hour of delay, the absolute risk reduction for death decreased by 0.16% (ARR for death if given within 6 hrs of symptoms 3%; ARR for death if given 7–12 hrs after onset of symptoms 2%).[17] Too few people in the systematic review received treatment more than 12 hours after the onset of symptoms to determine whether the benefits of thrombolytic treatment given after 12 hours would outweigh the risks. Extrapolation of the data (see figure 3, p 107) suggests that, at least for people with ST elevation, there may be some net benefit of treatment between 12 and 18 hours after symptom onset (ARR for death 1%). **Streptokinase versus tPA:** We found one non-systematic review[17] (3 large RCTs;[18-20] see table 1, p 102) comparing streptokinase versus tPA. The first RCT was unblinded and in people with ST elevation and symptoms of AMI for less than 6 hours. Participants were first randomised to intravenous tPA 100 mg over 3 hours or streptokinase 1.5 MU over 1 hour, and then further randomised to subcutaneous heparin 12 500 U twice daily beginning 12 hours later, or no heparin. It found that heparin added no significant benefit (AR of death in hospital 8.5% v 8.9% on no heparin; RRR 0.05, 95% CI –0.04 to +0.14).[18] In the second RCT, people with suspected AMI presenting within 24 hours of symptoms were randomised to receive either streptokinase 1.5 MU over 1 hour, tPA 0.6 MU/kg every 4 hours, or anisoylated plasminogen streptokinase activator complex (APSAC) 30 U every 3 minutes, and then further randomised to subcutaneous heparin 12 500 U starting at 7 hours and continued for 7 days, or no heparin. All received aspirin on admission. At 35 days, mortality was similar among the three regimens (streptokinase 10.6%, APSAC 10.5%, tPA 10.3%), and the addition of heparin provided no significant benefit (AR of death 10.3% v 10.6% on no heparin).[19] The third RCT was unblinded and in people with ST segment elevation presenting within 6 hours of symptom onset. Participants were randomised to one of four regimens: streptokinase 1.5 MU over 1 hour plus subcutaneous heparin 12 500 U twice daily starting 4 hours after thrombolytic treatment; streptokinase 1.5 MU over 1 hour plus intravenous heparin 5000 U bolus followed by 1000 U every hour; accelerated tPA 15 mg bolus then 0.75 mg/kg over 30 minutes followed by 0.50 mg/kg over 60 minutes, plus intravenous heparin 5000 U bolus then 1000 U every hour; or tPA 1.0 mg/kg over 60 minutes, 10% given as a bolus, plus streptokinase 1.0 MU over 60 minutes.[20] Meta-analysis of the three trials, weighted by sample size, found no significant difference in the combined outcome of any stroke or death (ARs 9.4% for streptokinase only regimens v 9.2% for tPA based regimens, including the combined tPA and streptokinase arm in the third trial; ARR for tPA v streptokinase 0.2%, 95% CI −0.2% to +0.5%; RRR 2.1%).[17]

Harms: **Stroke/intracerebral haemorrhage:** The risk of stroke was increased by thrombolytic treatment given in the acute phase (ARI compared with placebo 0.4%, 95% CI 0.2% to 0.5%; NNH 250).[15] In the third trial comparing different thrombolytic treatments, the overall incidence of intracerebral haemorrhage was 0.7% and of stroke 1.4%, of which 31% were severely disabling and 50% were intracerebral haemorrhages. The risk of haemorrhagic stroke was higher with tPA (AR 0.72%) than with streptokinase and subcutaneous heparin (AR 0.49%), or with streptokinase and intravenous heparin (AR 0.54%; P = 0.03 for tPA compared with combined streptokinase arms).[20] **Predictive factors for stroke/intracranial haemorrhage:** Multivariate analysis of data from a large database of people who experienced intracerebral haemorrhage after thrombolytic treatment identified four independent predictors of increased risk of intracerebral haemorrhage: age 65 years or older (OR 2.2, 95% CI 1.4 to 3.5); weight less than 70 kg (OR 2.1, 95% CI 1.3 to 3.2); hypertension on admission (OR 2.0, 95% CI 1.2 to 3.2); and use of tPA rather than another thrombolytic agent (OR 1.6, 95% CI 1.0 to 2.5). Absolute risk of intracranial haemorrhage was 0.26% on streptokinase in the absence of risk factors, and 0.96%, 1.32%, and 2.17% in people with one, two, or three risk factors.[21] Analysis of 592 strokes in 41 021 people from the trials found seven factors to be predictors of intracerebral haemorrhage: advanced age, lower weight, history of cerebrovascular disease, history of hypertension, higher systolic or diastolic pressure on presentation, and use of tPA rather than streptokinase.[22,23] **Major bleeding:** The risk of major bleeding was increased by thrombolytic treatment given in the acute phase (ARI compared with placebo 0.7%, 95% CI 0.6% to 0.9%; NNH 143).[15] Bleeding was most common in people undergoing procedures (coronary artery bypass grafting or PTCA). Spontaneous bleeds were observed most often in the gastrointestinal tract.[20]

Comment: The evidence suggests that it is far more important to administer prompt thrombolytic treatment than to debate which thrombolytic agent should be used. A strategy of rapid use of any thrombolytic in a broad population is likely to lead to the greatest impact on mortality. When the results of RCTs are taken together, tPA based regimens do not seem to confer a significant advantage in the combined outcome of any stroke and death (unrelated to stroke) over streptokinase. The legitimacy of combining the results of the three trials can be questioned, as the selection criteria and proto-cols differed in important aspects (see review for arguments to justify combining the results of these trials despite their apparent differences).[17]

OPTION β BLOCKERS

Systematic reviews have found that oral β blockers given within hours of infarction reduce both mortality and reinfarction in people with AMI. Adding β blockers to thrombolytic treatment confers additional benefit. Most benefit is obtained from long term use of β blockers.

Benefits:
Given within hours of infarction: We found two systematic reviews (search date 1997[24] and search date not stated[25]) and one overview[26] of early use of β blockers. The older reviews identified 27 RCTs and found that, within 1 week of treatment, β blockers significantly reduced the risk of death and major vascular events (RR for the combined outcome of death, non-fatal cardiac arrest, or non-fatal reinfarction 0.84, 1110 events v 1298 events; 95% CI not provided; P < 0.001). The largest of the RCTs (16 027 people with AMI) compared intravenous atenolol 5–10 mg given immediately followed by 100 mg orally given daily for 7 days versus standard treatment (no β blocker).[27] After 7 days, atenolol reduced vascular mortality compared with control (3.9% with atenolol v 4.6% with control; ARR 0.7%; RR 0.85, 95% CI 0.73 to 0.88; NNT 147). The RCT found more benefit in people with ECG evidence of AMI at entry (in people with ECG suggesting anterior infarction, inferior infarction, both, or bundle branch block, AR of death 5.33% on atenolol, 6.49% for controls; ARR 1.16%; NNT 86, 95% CI not provided). People older than 65 years and those with large infarcts had the most benefit.[27] The more recent systematic review (82 RCTs, 54 234 people)[24] separately analysed 51 short term RCTs (up to 6 wks after the onset of pain) and 31 long term RCTs. Most of the RCTs did not include thrombolysis. In the short term studies, seven RCTs reported no deaths and many reported only a few. Meta-analysis of the RCTs that reported at least one death found that β blockers versus placebo reduced mortality, but the reduction was not significant in the short term (ARR 0.4%; OR 0.96, 95% CI 0.85 to 1.08). In the longer term RCTs, β blockers versus placebo significantly reduced mortality over 6 months to 4 years (OR 0.77, 95% CI 0.69 to 0.85). About 84 people would need treatment for 1 year to avoid one death. No significant difference in effectiveness was found between different types of β blocker (based on cardio-selectivity or intrinsic sympathomimetic activity). Most evidence was obtained with propranolol, timolol, and metoprolol. **In people receiving thrombolytic treatment:** We found one RCT (1434 people with AMI), which compared early versus delayed metoprolol in people who had been given thrombolysis (tPA).[28] Early treatment began on day 1 (intravenous then oral) and delayed treatment on day 6 (oral). At 6 days, people receiving early treatment had significantly lower rates of reinfarction (AR 2.7% early v 5.1% delayed, 95% CI not provided; P = 0.02) and recurrent chest pain (AR 18.8% v 24.1%; P < 0.02). There were no early (6 days) or late (1 year) differences observed in mortality or left ventricular ejection

Cardiovascular disorders

fraction between the two groups. **Long term use:** See β blockers under secondary prevention of ischaemic cardiac events, p 166.

Harms: People with asthma or severe congestive cardiac failure were excluded from most trials. Many of the early trials tended to enrol people at low risk of death soon after AMI. In people given immediate rather than delayed β blockers following tPA, there was a non-significant increased frequency of heart failure during the initial admission to hospital (15.3% v 12.2%; P = 0.10).[28] The presence of first degree heart block and bundle branch block was associated with an increased frequency of adverse events.

Comment: β Blockers may reduce rates of cardiac rupture and ventricular fibrillation. This may explain why people older than 65 years and those with large infarcts benefited most, as they also have higher rates of these complications. The trials were mostly conducted in the prethrombolytic era. The trial comparing early versus delayed β blockade after thrombolysis was too small to rule out an effect on mortality of β blockers when added to thrombolysis.[28]

| OPTION | ANGIOTENSIN CONVERTING ENZYME (ACE) INHIBITORS |

One systematic review has found that ACE inhibitors used within 24 hours of onset of symptoms reduce mortality in people with AMI. The question of whether ACE inhibitors should be offered to everyone presenting with AMI or only to people with signs of heart failure remains unresolved.

Benefits: **In all people after an AMI:** We found one overview[29] and one systematic review[30] of ACE inhibitors versus placebo after myocardial infarction. The overview (4 large RCTs, 98 496 people) compared ACE inhibitors versus placebo given to all people irrespective of clinical heart failure or left ventricular dysfunction, within 36 hours of the onset of symptoms of AMI.[29] After 30 days, ACE inhibitors versus placebo reduced mortality (7.1% with ACE inhibitors v 7.6% with placebo; RR 0.93, 95% CI 0.89 to 0.98; NNT 200). Most of this benefit was in the first 7 days after AMI. The absolute benefit was larger in some high risk groups: people in Killip class II–III (see glossary, p 99) (clinically moderate to severe heart failure at first presentation; RR 0.91; NNT 71, 99% CI 36 to 10 000), people with heart rates greater than 100 beats a minute at entry (RR 0.86; NNT 44, 99% CI 25 to 185), and people with an anterior AMI (RR 0.87; NNT 94, 99% CI 56 to 303). ACE inhibitors also reduced the incidence of non-fatal cardiac failure (AR 14.6% v 15.2%, 95% CI not provided; P = 0.01). The systematic review (search date 1997, 15 RCTs, 15 104 people) found similar results.[30] **In selected people after an AMI:** A selective strategy was tested in three trials.[31-33] Treatment was restricted to people with clinical heart failure, objective evidence of left ventricular dysfunction, or both, and was started a few days after AMI (about 6000 people). These trials found consistently that long term treatment with ACE inhibitors in this selected population was associated with a significant reduction in mortality and reinfarction (RRRs from 1 trial:[29] for cardiovascular death 21%, 95% CI 5% to 35%; for development of severe heart failure 37%, 95% CI 20% to 50%; for congestive heart failure requiring admission to hospital 22%, 95% CI 4% to 37%; and for recurrent AMI 25%, 95% CI 5% to 40%).

Harms: The systematic review found an excess of persistent hypotension (AR 17.6% v 9.3%, 95% CI for difference not provided; P < 0.01) and renal dysfunction (AR 1.3% v 0.6%; P < 0.01) in people given ACE inhibitors.[29] The relative and absolute risks of these adverse effects were uniformly distributed across both the high and lower cardiovascular risk groups.

Comment: The largest benefits of ACE inhibitors in AMI are seen when treatment is started within 24 hours. The evidence does not answer the question of which people with an AMI should be offered ACE inhibitors, and for how long after AMI it remains beneficial to start treatment with an ACE inhibitor. We found one systematic review (search date not stated; based on individual data from about 100 000 people in RCTs of ACE inhibitors), which found that people receiving both aspirin and ACE inhibitors had the same relative risk reduction as those receiving ACE inhibitors alone (i.e. there was no evidence of a clinically relevant interaction between ACE inhibitors and aspirin).[34]

OPTION	NITRATES

RCTs performed before and during the thrombolytic era have found that intravenous nitrates are safe in the acute management of symptoms in people with AMI, but may reduce mortality only slightly.

Benefits: **Without thrombolysis:** We found one systematic review (search date not stated, 10 RCTs comparing intravenous glyceryl trinitrate or nitroprusside v placebo, 2000 people with AMI).[35] The trials were all conducted in the prethrombolytic era. Nitrates reduced the relative risk of death by 35% (95% CI 16% to 55%). The observed benefit of nitrates seemed to be mostly during the acute hospitalisation period, with modest or little long term survival benefit. **With aspirin/ thrombolysis:** During the thrombolytic era, two large RCTs compared nitrates given acutely versus placebo in 58 050 and 17 817 people with AMI (90% received aspirin and about 70% received thrombolytic treatment).[36,37] In one RCT, people received oral controlled release isosorbide mononitrate glyceryl trinitrate 30–60 mg/day.[36] In the other RCT, people received intravenous glyceryl trinitrate for 24 hours followed by transdermal glyceryl trinitrate 10 mg daily.[37] Neither trial found a significant improvement in survival, either in the total sample or in subgroups of people at different risks of death. Nitrates were a useful adjunctive treatment to help control symptoms in people with AMI.

Harms: The systematic review and the large trials found no significant harm associated with routine use of nitrates in people with AMI.[35-37]

Comment: The two large trials had features that may have caused them not to find a benefit even if one exists: a large proportion of people took nitrates outside the study; there was a high rate of concurrent use of other hypotensive agents; people were relatively low risk; and nitrates were not titrated to blood pressure and heart rate.[36,37]

Cardiovascular disorders

RCTs have found that calcium channel blockers given to people within the first few days of an AMI do not reduce deaths, and may increase deaths in people with reduced left ventricular function.

Benefits: **Dihydropyridine calcium channel blockers:** We found one non-systematic review (2 large RCTs)[38] comparing short acting nifedipine versus placebo in people treated within the first few days of AMI.[39,40] Neither found evidence of benefit and both found trends towards increased mortality on nifedipine. One trial was terminated prematurely because of lack of efficacy. It found a 33% increase in mortality on nifedipine that did not reach significance.[40] We found insufficient data on sustained release nifedipine, amlodipine, or felodipine in this setting. **Verapamil:** We found one systematic review (search date 1997, 7 RCTs, 6527 people),[41] which found that verapamil versus placebo in AMI had no significant effect on mortality (RR 0.86, 95% CI 0.71 to 1.04).

Harms: Two systematic reviews (search dates not stated) of trials of any kind of calcium channel blockers in people with AMI found a non-significant increase in mortality of about 4% and 6%.[42,43] One trial (2466 people with AMI) compared diltiazem 60 mg orally four times daily starting 3–15 days after AMI versus placebo.[44] Overall there was no effect on total mortality or reinfarction between the two groups, but subgroup analysis found a 41% increase in death or reinfarction in people with congestive heart failure (RRI 1.41, 95% CI 1.01 to 1.96).

Comment: None.

One systematic review has found that, in the short term, primary PTCA is at least as effective as (and possibly superior to) thrombolysis in the treatment of AMI, in terms of reducing mortality, reinfarction, and haemorrhagic stroke. However, the trials were conducted mainly in high volume, specialist centres. The effectiveness of PTCA compared with thrombolysis in less specialist centres remains to be defined.

Benefits: We found two systematic reviews[45,46] of primary PTCA versus primary thrombolysis in people with AMI. **Death and reinfarction:** The first systematic review (search date 1996, 10 RCTs, 2606 people) found that primary PTCA versus primary thrombolysis reduced mortality at 30 days after intervention (4.4% for primary PTCA v 6.5% for primary thrombolysis; ARR 2.1%; OR 0.66, 95% CI 0.46 to 0.94; NNT 48).[45] The effect was similar regardless of which thrombolysis regimen was used. There was significant reduction in the combined end point of death and reinfarction with PTCA (OR 0.58, 95% CI 0.44 to 0.76). The largest single RCT (1138 people, ST elevation on ECG within 12 hrs of symptom onset) found less favourable results. It compared primary PTCA versus accelerated tPA.[47] At 30 days, there was no significant difference in mortality between the two groups (AR 5.7% v 7.0%), but primary PTCA significantly reduced the primary end point of death, non-fatal

AMI, or non-fatal disabling stroke (AR 9.6% v 13.7% on tPA; OR 0.67, 95% CI 0.47 to 0.97). This effect was substantially attenuated by 6 months. One of the included studies has reported long term follow up; it found that primary PTCA versus primary thrombolysis improves mortality over 5 years (25/194 [13%] with angioplasty v 48/201 [24%] with streptokinase; RR 0.54, 95% CI 0.36 to 0.87).[48] The second systematic review (search date 1998, 10 RCTs, 2573 people) found overall similar results, with significant reductions in mortality and in reinfarction.[46]

Harms: **Stroke:** The review found that PTCA was associated with a significant reduction in the risk of all types of stroke (AR 0.7% v 2.0%) and haemorrhagic stroke (AR 0.1% v 1.1%).[45] In the largest trial, the collective rate of haemorrhagic stroke in people given thrombolysis was 1.1%, substantially higher than that observed in trials comparing thrombolysis with placebo.[47] This may have been because the trials summarised above were in older people and used tPA. However, the lower rates of haemorrhagic stroke with primary PTCA were consistent across almost all trials, and this may be the major advantage of PTCA over thrombolysis.

Comment: Although collectively the trials found an overall short term reduction in deaths with PTCA compared with thrombolysis, there were several pitfalls common to individual trials, most of which may have inflated the benefit of PTCA.[49] Trials comparing PTCA with thrombolysis could not be easily blinded, and ascertainment of end points that required some judgement, such as reinfarction or stroke, may have been influenced by the investigators' knowledge of the treatment allocation (only 1 trial had a blinded adjudication events committee). Also, people allocated to PTCA were discharged 1–2 days earlier than those allocated to thrombolysis, which favoured PTCA by reducing the time for detection of in-hospital events. In addition, the trials conducted before the largest trial[47] should be viewed as hypothesis generating, in that the composite outcome (death, reinfarction, and stroke) was not prospectively defined, and attention was only placed on these end points after there seemed to be some benefit on post hoc analysis. The results are also based on short term outcomes only and do not provide information on collective long term benefit. For example, in the largest trial the composite end point was significant at 30 days but with a wide degree of uncertainty, and this was substantially attenuated to a non-significant difference by 6 months.[47] The lower mortality and reinfarction rates reported with primary PTCA are promising but not conclusive, and the real benefits may well be smaller. Only in a minority of centres that perform a high volume of PTCA, and in the hands of experienced interventionists, may primary PTCA be clearly superior to thrombolytic treatment. Elsewhere, primary PTCA may be of greatest benefit in people with contraindications to thrombolysis, in people in cardiogenic shock, or in people where the mortality reduction with thrombolysis is modest and the risk of intracranial haemorrhage is increased, for example, elderly people.[50] The value of PTCA over thrombolysis in people presenting to hospital more than 12 hours after onset of chest pain remains to be tested.

Cardiovascular disorders

Philip Urban and Edoardo De Benedetti

OPTION **EARLY INVASIVE CARDIAC REVASCULARISATION**

Two RCTs have found that early invasive cardiac revascularisation versus initial medical treatment alone improves survival in people with cardiogenic shock after AMI.

Benefits: We found no systematic review. We found two RCTs comparing early invasive cardiac revascularisation (see glossary, p 99) versus initial medical therapy alone for people with cardiogenic shock within 48 hours of AMI (see comment below).[2,3,51] The first RCT (302 people) found a significant reduction in mortality at 6 and 12 months with early invasive cardiac revascularisation (see table 2, p 104).[2,51] The second RCT (55 people) found a non-significant reduction in mortality at both 30 days and at 12 months with early invasive cardiac revascularisation (see table 2, p 104). **PTCA versus coronary artery bypass graft:** We found no RCTs comparing percutaneous angioplasty versus coronary bypass grafting for people with cardiogenic shock after AMI.

Harms: The first RCT (56 people aged ≥ 75 years) found that there was a non-significant increase in 30 day mortality with early invasive cardiac revascularisation (18/24 [75%] with early invasive cardiac revascularisation v 17/32 [53%] with medical treatment alone; RR 1.41, 95% CI 0.95 to 2.11).[2,51] The first RCT also found that acute renal failure (defined as a serum creatinine level > 265 µmol/L) was significantly more common in the medical treatment alone group versus the early cardiac revascularisation group (36/150 [24%] v 20/152 [13%]; RR 1.82, 95% CI 1.1 to 3.0; NNH 9, 95% CI 5 to 48). Other harms reported by the RCT included major haemorrhage, sepsis, and peripheral vascular occlusion, although comparative data between groups for these harms were not provided. The second RCT did not report data of harms.[3]

Comment: In the first RCT, medical treatment included intra-aortic balloon counterpulsation (see glossary, p 99) and thrombolytic therapy.[2,51] In the second RCT, medical treatment was not defined.[3] The second RCT was stopped prematurely because of difficulties with recruitment. Both RCTs were conducted in centres with expertise in early invasive cardiac revascularisation and their results may not be reproducible in other settings.[2,3,51]

OPTION **THROMBOLYSIS**

One RCT found no significant reduction in mortality with thrombolysis in people with cardiogenic shock after AMI.

Benefits: We found no systematic review. We found one RCT (11 806 people within 12 hrs of AMI), which compared thrombolysis using streptokinase versus no thrombolysis (see comment, p 97).[52] Subgroup analysis of people with cardiogenic shock found no significant reduction in inpatient mortality after 21 days with thrombolysis (280 people; 102/146 [69%] with thrombolysis v 94/134 [70%] with no thrombolysis; RR 1.0, 95% CI 0.85 to 1.16).

Harms: The RCT did not report of harms in the subgroup of people with cardiogenic shock.[52] Overall, adverse reactions attributed to streptokinase were found in 12% of people (705/5860) either during or after streptokinase infusion. These adverse reactions included minor and major bleeding (3.7%), allergic reactions (2.4%), hypotension (3.0%), anaphylactic shock (0.1%), shivering/fever (1.0%), ventricular arrhythmias (1.2%), and stroke (0.2%).

Comment: The RCT was not blinded.[52] Data presented are from a retrospective subgroup analysis and randomisation was not stratified by the presence of cardiogenic shock.

| OPTION | POSITIVE INOTROPES (DOBUTAMINE, DOPAMINE, ADRENALINE [EPINEPHRINE], NOREPINEPHRINE [NORADRENALINE], AMRINONE) AND VASODILATORS (ACE INHIBITORS, NITRATES) |

We found no RCTs comparing inotropes versus placebo or comparing vasodilators versus placebo in people with cardiogenic shock after AMI.

Benefits: **Positive inotropes:** We found no systematic review or RCTs. We found three non-systematic reviews,[1,53,54] which identified no RCTs evaluating the use of positive inotropes in people with cardiogenic shock after AMI. **Vasodilators:** We found no systematic review or RCTs.

Harms: Positive inotropes may worsen cardiac ischaemia and induce ventricular arrhythmias.[1,53,54] We found no studies of harms specifically in people with cardiogenic shock after AMI (see harms of positive inotropic drugs and vasodilators under heart failure, p 72).

Comment: There is a consensus view that positive inotropes are beneficial in cardiogenic shock AMI. We found no evidence to confirm or reject this view. The risk of worsening hypotension has led to concern about the use of any vasodilator to treat acute cardiogenic shock.[54]

| OPTION | PULMONARY ARTERY CATHETERISATION |

We found no RCTs comparing pulmonary artery catheterisation versus no catheterisation in people with cardiogenic shock after AMI.

Benefits: We found no systematic review and no RCTs.

Harms: Observational studies have found an association between pulmonary artery catheterisation and increased morbidity and mortality, but it is unclear whether this arises from an adverse effect of the catheterisation or because people with a poor prognosis were selected for catheterisation.[55] Harms such as major arrhythmias, injury to the lung, thromboembolism (see thromboembolism, p 224), and sepsis occur in 0.1–0.5% of people undergoing pulmonary artery catheterisation.[55]

Comment: Pulmonary artery catheterisation helps to diagnose cardiogenic shock, guide correction of hypovolaemia, optimise filling pressures for both the left and right sides of the heart, and adjust doses of inotropic drugs.[1] There is a consensus view that pulmonary artery catheterisation is beneficial in patients with cardiogenic shock after AMI,[56,57] although we found no evidence to confirm or reject this view.

OPTION	INTRA-AORTIC BALLOON COUNTERPULSATION

We found one abstract from an RCT, which found no reduction in mortality at 6 months with intra-aortic balloon counterpulsation in people with cardiogenic shock after AMI.

Benefits: We found no systematic review. We found one abstract from an RCT (57 people), which compared intra-aortic balloon counterpulsation (see glossary, p 99) plus thrombolysis versus thrombolysis alone (see comment below).[58] The RCT found no significant reduction in mortality at 6 months' follow up (22/57 [39%] with thrombolysis plus balloon counterpulsation v 25/57 [43%] with thrombolysis alone; RR 0.9, 95% CI 0.57 to 1.37; P = 0.3).

Harms: Harms were not reported in the abstract of the RCT.[58]

Comment: The abstract from the RCT did not describe detailed methods for the trial, making interpretation of the results difficult.[58] We also found two additional small RCTs (30 people,[59] and 20 people[60]), which compared intra-aortic balloon counterpulsation versus standard treatment in people after AMI. Neither RCT specifically recruited, or identified data from, people with cardiogenic shock after AMI. Neither RCT found a reduction in mortality with intra-aortic balloon counterpulsation. There is a consensus view that intra-aortic balloon counterpulsation is beneficial in people with cardiogenic shock after AMI. We found no evidence to confirm or reject this view.

OPTION	VENTRICULAR ASSISTANCE DEVICES AND CARDIAC TRANSPLANTATION

We found no RCTs evaluating either ventricular assistance devices or cardiac transplantation in people with cardiogenic shock after AMI.

Benefits: We found no systematic review and no RCTs.

Harms: We found no evidence of harms specifically associated with the use of ventricular assistance devices (see glossary, p 99) or cardiac transplantation in people with cardiogenic shock after AMI.

Comment: Reviews of observational studies[1,54,61] and retrospective reports[62,63] have suggested that ventricular assistance devices may improve outcomes in selected people when used alone or as a bridge to cardiac transplantation. The availability of ventricular assistance devices and cardiac transplantation is limited to a few specialised centres, and results may not be applicable to other settings.

OPTION	EARLY CARDIAC SURGERY

We found no RCTs evaluating early surgical intervention for ventricular septal rupture, free wall rupture, or mitral valve regurgitation complicated by cardiogenic shock after AMI.

Benefits: We found no systematic review and no RCTs.

Harms: We found no evidence about the harms of surgery in people with cardiogenic shock caused by cardiac structural defects after AMI.

Comment: Non-systematic reviews of observational studies have suggested that death is inevitable following free wall rupture without early surgical intervention, and that surgery for both mitral valve regurgitation and ventricular septal rupture is more effective when carried out within 24–48 hours.[1,54]

GLOSSARY

Cardiac index A measure of cardiac output derived from the formula: cardiac output/unit time divided by body surface area ($L/min/m^2$).

Intra-aortic balloon counterpulsation A technique in which a balloon is placed in the aorta and inflated during diastole and deflated just before systole.

Invasive cardiac revascularisation A term used to describe either percutaneous transluminal coronary angioplasty (PTCA) or coronary artery bypass grafting (CABG).

Killip class A categorisation of the severity of heart failure based on easily obtained clinical signs. The main clinical features are Class I: no heart failure; Class II: crackles audible half way up the chest; Class III: crackles heard in all the lung fields; Class IV: cardiogenic shock.

Ventricular assistance device A mechanical device placed in parallel to a failing cardiac ventricle that pumps blood in an attempt to maintain cardiac output. Because of the risk of mechanical failure, thrombosis, and haemolysis they are normally used for short term support while preparing for a heart transplant.

REFERENCES

1. Califf RM, Bengtson JR. Cardiogenic shock. *N Engl J Med* 1994;330:1724–1730.

2. Hochman JS, Sleeper LA, Webb JG, et al, for the SHOCK investigators. Early revascularization in acute myocardial infarction complicated by cardiogenic shock. *N Engl J Med* 1999;341: 625–634.

3. Urban P, Stauffer JC, Khatchatrian N, et al. A randomized evaluation of early revascularization to treat shock complicating acute myocardial infarction. The (Swiss) Multicenter Trial of Angioplasty SHOCK - (S)MASH. *Eur Heart Journal* 1999;20:1030–1038.

4. Murray C, Lopez A. Mortality by cause for eight regions of the world: global burden of disease study. *Lancet* 1997;349:1269–1276.

5. National Heart, Lung, and Blood Institute. *Morbidity and mortality: chartbook on cardiovascular, lung, and blood diseases.* Bethesda, Maryland: US Department of Health and Human Services, Public Health Service, National Institutes of Health; May 1992.

6. Goldberg RJ, Samad NA, Yarzebski J, Gurwitz J, Bigelow C, Gore JM. Temporal trends in cardiogenic shock complicating acute myocardial infarction. *N Engl J Med* 1999;340:1162–1168.

7. Hasdai D, Califf RM, Thompson TD, et al. Predictors of cardiogenic shock after thrombolytic therapy for acute myocardial infarction. *J Am Coll Cardiol* 2000;35:136–143.

8. Hochman JS, Buller CE, Sleeper LA, et al. Cardiogenic shock complicating acute myocardial infarction – etiology, management and outcome: a report from the SHOCK trial registry. *J Am Coll Cardiol* 2000;36:1063–1070.

9. Urban P, Bernstein M, Costanza M, Simon R, Frey R, Erne P. An internet-based registry of acute myocardial infarction in Switzerland. *Kardiovasculaäre Medizin* 2000;3:430–441.

10. Berger PB, Tuttle RH, Holmes DR, et al. One year survival among patients with acute myocardial infarction complicated by cardiogenic shock, and its relation to early revascularisation: results of the GUSTO-1 trial. *Circulation* 1999;99:873–878.

11. Antiplatelet Trialists' Collaboration. Collaborative overview of randomised trials of antiplatelet therapy I: prevention of death, myocardial infarction, and stroke by prolonged antiplatelet therapy in various categories of people. *BMJ* 1994;308:81–106. Search date March 1990; primary sources Medline, and Current Contents.

12. Second International Study of Infarct Survival (ISIS-2) Collaborative Group. Randomized trial of intravenous streptokinase, oral aspirin, both or neither among 17–187 cases of suspected acute myocardial infarction. *Lancet* 1988;ii:349–360.

13. Baigent BM, Collins R. ISIS-2: four year mortality of 17 187 patients after fibrinolytic and antiplatelet therapy in suspected acute myocardial infarction study [abstract]. *Circulation* 1993(suppl I):I-291.

14. Patrignani P, Filabozzi P, Patrono C. Selective cumulative inhibition of platelet thromboxane production by low-dose aspirin in healthy subjects. *J Clin Invest* 1982;69:1366–1372.

15. Fibrinolytic Therapy Trialists' (FTT) Collaborative Group. Indications for fibrinolytic therapy in suspected acute myocardial infarction: collaborative overview of early mortality and major morbidity results of all randomized trials of more than 1000 patients. *Lancet* 1994;343:311–322.

16. French JK, Hyde TA, Patel H, et al. Survival 12 years after randomization to streptokinase: the

influence of thrombolysis in myocardial infarction flow at three to four weeks. *J Am Coll Cardiol* 1999;34:62–69.

17. Collins R, Peto R, Baigent BM, Sleight DM. Aspirin, heparin and fibrinolytic therapy in suspected acute myocardial infarction. *N Engl J Med* 1997;336:847–860.

18. Gruppo Italiano per lo studio della streptochinasi nell'infarto miocardico (GISSI). GISSI-2: a factorial randomised trial of alteplase versus streptokinase and heparin versus no heparin among 12–490 patients with acute myocardial infarction. *Lancet* 1990;336:65–71.

19. Third International Study of Infarct Survival (ISIS-3) Collaborative Group. ISIS-3: a randomised comparison of streptokinase vs tissue plasminogen activator vs anistreplase and of aspirin plus heparin vs aspirin alone among 41–299 cases of suspected acute myocardial infarction. *Lancet* 1992;339:753–770.

20. The GUSTO Investigators. An international randomized trial comparing four thrombolytic strategies for acute myocardial infarction. *N Engl J Med* 1993;329:673–682.

21. Simoons MI, Maggioni AP, Knatterud G, et al. Individual risk assessment for intracranial hemorrhage during thrombolytic therapy. *Lancet* 1993;342:523–528.

22. Gore JM, Granger CB, Simoons MI, et al. Stroke after thrombolysis: mortality and functional outcomes in the GUSTO-1 trial. *Circulation* 1995; 92:2811–2818.

23. Berkowitz SD, Granger CB, Pieper KS, et al. Incidence and predictors of bleeding after contemporary thrombolytic therapy for myocardial infarction. *Circulation* 1997;95:2508–2516.

24. Freemantle N, Cleland J, Young P, Mason J, Harrison J. Beta blockade after myocardial infarction: systematic review and meta regression analysis. *BMJ* 1999;318:1730–1737. Search date 1997; primary sources Medline, Embase, Biosis, Healthstar, Sigle, IHTA, Derwent drug file, dissertation abstracts, Pascal, international pharmaceutical abstracts, science citation index, and handsearch of reference lists.

25. Yusuf S, Peto R, Lewis S, et al. Beta-blockade during and after myocardial infarction: an overview of the randomized trials. *Prog Cardiovasc Dis* 1985;27:355–371. Search date not stated; primary sources computer-aided search of the literature, manual search of reference lists, and enquiries to colleagues about relevant papers.

26. Sleight P for the ISIS Study Group. Beta blockade early in acute myocardial infarction. *Am J Cardiol* 1987;60:6A–12A.

27. First International Study of Infarct Survival (ISIS-1). Randomised trial of intravenous atenolol among 16 027 cases of suspected acute myocardial infarction. *Lancet* 1986;ii:57–66.

28. Roberts R, Rogers WJ, Mueller HS, et al. Immediate versus deferred beta-blockade following thrombolytic therapy in patients with acute myocardial infarction: results of the thrombolysis in myocardial infarction (TIMI) II-B study. *Circulation* 1991;83:422–437.

29. ACE Inhibitor Myocardial Infarction Collaborative Group. Indications for ACE inhibitors in the early treatment of acute myocardial infarction: systematic overview of individual data from 100 000 patients in randomised trials. *Circulation* 1998;97:2202–2212. Search date not stated; primary source collaboration group of principal investigators of all randomised trials who collated individual patient data.

30. Domanski MJ, Exner DV, Borkowf CB, Geller NL, Rosenberg Y, Pfeffer MA. Effect of angiotensin converting enzyme inhibition on sudden cardiac death in patients following acute myocardial infarction. A meta-analysis of randomized clinical trials. *J Am Coll Cardiol* 1999;33:598–604. Search date August 1997; primary sources Medline and hand searches of reference lists.

31. Pfeffer MA, Braunwald E, Moye LA, et al. Effect of captopril on mortality and morbidity in patients with left ventricular dysfunction after myocardial infarction. *N Engl J Med* 1992;327:669–677.

32. The Acute Infarction Ramipril Efficacy (AIRE) Study Investigators. Effect of ramipril on mortality and morbidity of survivors of acute myocardial infarction with clinical evidence of heart failure. *Lancet* 1993;342:821–828.

33. The Trandolapril Cardiac Evaluation (TRACE) Study Group. A clinical trial of the angiotensin-converting-enzyme inhibitor trandolapril in patients with left ventricular dysfunction after myocardial infarction. *N Engl J Med* 1995;333:1670–1676.

34. Latini R, Tognoni G, Maggioni AP, et al. Clinical effects of early angiotensin-converting enzyme inhibitor treatment for acute myocardial infarction are similar in the presence and absence of aspirin. Systematic overview of individual data from 96 712 randomized patients. *J Am Coll Cardiol* 2000;35:1801–1807. Search date not stated; primary sources individual patient data on all trials involving more than 1000 patients.

35. Yusuf S, Collins R, MacMahon S, Peto R. Effect of intravenous nitrates on mortality in acute myocardial infarction: an overview of the randomised trials. *Lancet* 1988;1:1088–1092. Search date not stated; primary sources literature, colleagues, investigators, and pharmaceutical companies.

36. Fourth International Study of Infarct Survival (ISIS-4) Collaborative Group. ISIS-4: a randomised factorial trial assessing early oral captopril, oral mononitrate, and intravenous magnesium sulphate in 58 050 patients with suspected acute myocardial infarction. *Lancet* 1995;345: 669–685.

37. Gruppo Italiano per lo studio della streptochinasi nell'infarto miocardico (GISSI). GISSI-3: effects of lisinopril and transdermal glyceryl trinitrate singly and together on 6-week mortality and ventricular function after acute myocardial infarction. *Lancet* 1994;343:1115–1122.

38. Opie LH, Yusuf S, Kubler W. Current status of safety and efficacy of calcium channel blockers in cardiovascular diseases: a critical analysis based on 100 studies. *Prog Cardiovasc Dis* 2000;43: 171–196.

39. Wilcox RG, Hampton JR, Banks DC, et al. Early nifedipine in acute myocardial infarction: the TRENT study. *BMJ* 1986;293:1204–1208.

40. Goldbourt U, Behar S, Reicher-Reiss H, et al. Early administration of nifedipine in suspected acute myocardial infarction: the secondary prevention reinfarction Israel nifedipine trial 2 study. *Arch Intern Med* 1993;153:345–353.

41. Pepine CJ, Faich G, Makuch R. Verapamil use in patients with cardiovascular disease: an overview of randomized trials. *Clin Cardiol* 1998;21: 633–641. Search date 1997; primary sources Medline, Science Citation Index, Current Contents, and hand searches of reference lists.

42. Yusuf S, Furberg CD. Effects of calcium channel blockers on survival after myocardial infarction. *Cardiovasc Drugs Ther* 1987;1:343–344. Search dates and primary sources not stated.

43. Teo KK, Yusuf S, Furberg CD. Effects of prophylactic antiarrhythmic drug therapy in acute myocardial infarction: an overview of results from randomized controlled trials. *JAMA* 1993;270: 1589–1595. Search date not stated; primary

sources Medline and correspondence with investigators and pharmaceutical companies.

44. The Multicenter Diltiazem Post Infarction Trial Research Group. The effect of diltiazem on mortality and reinfarction after myocardial infarction. *N Engl J Med* 1988;319:385–392.

45. Weaver WD, Simes RJ, Betriu A, et al. Comparison of primary coronary angioplasty and intravenous thrombolytic therapy for acute myocardial infarction: a quantitative review. *JAMA* 1997;278: 2093–2098. Search date March 1996; primary sources Medline and scientific session abstracts of stated journals.

46. Cucherat M, Bonnefoy E, Tremeau G. Primary angioplasty versus intravenous thrombolysis for acute myocardial infarction. In: The Cochrane Library, Issue 1, 2001. Oxford: Update Software. Search date January 1998; primary sources The Cochrane Library, Medline, references from reviews, and experts.

47. The GUSTO IIb Angioplasty Substudy Investigators. A clinical trial comparing primary coronary angioplasty with tissue plasminogen activator for acute myocardial infarction. *N Engl J Med* 1997; 336:1621–1628.

48. Zijlstra F, Hoorntje JC, de Boer MJ, et al. Long-term benefit of primary angioplasty as compared with thrombolytic therapy for acute myocardial infarction. *N Engl J Med* 1999 341:1413–1419.

49. Yusuf S, Pogue J. Primary angioplasty compared to thrombolytic therapy for acute myocardial infarction [editorial]. *JAMA* 1997;278: 2110–2111.

50. Van de Werf F, Topol EJ, Lee KL, et al. Variations in patient management and outcomes for acute myocardial infarction in the United States and other countries: results from the GUSTO trial. *JAMA* 1995;273:1586–1591.

51. Hochman JS, Sleeper LA, White HD et al. One year survival following early revascularization for cardiogenic shock. *JAMA* 2001;285:190–192.

52. GISSI-1. Effectiveness of intravenous thrombolytic treatment in acute myocardial infarction. *Lancet* 1986;1:397–401.

53. Herbert P, Tinker J. Inotropic drugs in acute circulatory failure. *Intensive Care Med* 1980;6: 101–111.

54. Hollenberg SM, Kavinsky CJ, Parrillo JE. Cardiogenic shock. *Ann Int Med* 1999;131: 47–59. Search date 1998; primary sources Medline and hand searches of bibliographies of relevant papers.

55. Bernard GR, Sopko G, Cerra F, et al. Pulmonary artery catheterization and clinical outcomes. *JAMA* 2000;283:2568–2562.

56. Hollenberg SM, Hoyt J. Pulmonary artery catheters in cardiovascular disease. *New Horiz* 1977;5: 207–213. Search date 1996; primary sources not stated.

57. Participants. Pulmonary artery catheter consensus Conference: consensus statement. *Crit Care Med* 1997;25:910–925.

58. Ohman EM, Nanas J, Stomel R, et al. Thrombolysis and counterpulsation to improve cardiogenic shock survival (Tactics): results of a prospective randomized trial [abstract]. *Circulation* 2000;102(suppl II):II-600.

59. O'Rourke, MF, Norris RM, Campbell TJ, Chang VP, Sammel NL. Randomized controlled trial of intraaortic balloon counterpulsation in early myocardial infarction with acute heart failure. *Am J Cardiol* 1981;47:815–820.

60. Flaherty JT, Becker LC, Weiss JL, et al. Results of a randomized prospective trial of intraaortic balloon counterpulsation and intravenous nitroglycerin in patients with acute myocardial infarction. *J Am Coll Cardiol* 1985;6:434–446.

61. Frazier OH. Future directions of cardiac assistance. *Semin Thorac Cardiovasc Surg* 2000;12: 251–258.

62. Pagani FD, Lynch W, Swaniker F, et al. Extracorporal life support to left ventricular assist device bridge to cardiac transplantation. *Circulation* 1999;100(suppl 19):II206–210.

63. Mavroidis D, Sun BC, Pae WE. Bridge to transplantation: the Penn State experience. *Ann Thorac Surg* 1999;68:684–687.

Shamir Mehta
Assistant Professor of Medicine
Faculty of Health Sciences
McMaster University
Hamilton
Ontario
Canada

Philip Urban
Director, Interventional Cardiology
Hôpital de la Tour
Meyrin-Geneva
Switzerland

Edoardo De Benedetti
Cardiologist
C.H.U.V.
Lausanne
Switzerland

Competing interests: SM has received honoraria from various sources for educational speaking engagements. PU has received funds for research and public speaking from a variety of pharmaceutical and device companies, both related and unrelated to products discussed here.

Cardiovascular disorders

TABLE 1 Direct randomised comparisons of the standard streptokinase regimen with various tPA based fibrinolytic regimens in patients with suspected AMI in the GISSI-2, ISIS-3, and GUSTO-1 trials (see text, p 89).[18-20]

Trial and treatment	Number of participants randomised	Any stroke Absolute number (%)	Any death Absolute number (%)	Death not related to stroke* Absolute number (%)	Stroke or death Absolute number (%)
GISSI-2†					
Streptokinase	10 396	98 (0.9)	958 (9.2)	916 (8.8)	1014 (9.8)
t-PA	10 372	136 (1.3)	993 (9.6)	931 (9.0)	1067 (10.3)
Effect/1000 people treated with t-PA instead of streptokinase		3.7 ± 1.5 more	3.6 ± 4.0 more	1.7 ± 4.0 more	5.3 ± 4.2 more
ISIS-3‡					
Streptokinase	13 780	141 (1.0)	1455 (10.6)	1389 (10.1)	1530 (11.1)
t-PA	13 746	188 (1.4)	1418 (10.3)	1325 (9.6)	1513 (11.0)
Effect/1000 people treated with t-PA instead of streptokinase		3.5 ± 1.3 more	2.4 ± 3.7 fewer	4.4 ± 3.6 fewer	1.0 ± 3.8 fewer
GUSTO-1§					
Streptokinase (sc heparin)	9841	117 (1.2)	712 (7.3)	666 (6.8)	783 (8.0)
Streptokinase (iv heparin)	10 410	144 (1.4)	763 (7.4)	709 (6.8)	853 (8.2)
t-PA alone	10 396	161 (1.6)	653 (6.3)	585 (5.6)	746 (7.2)
t-PA plus streptokinase	10 374	170 (1.6)	723 (7.0)	647 (6.2)	817 (7.9)
Effect/1000 people treated with t-PA-based regimens instead of streptinokinase		3.0 ± 1.2 more	6.6 ± 2.5 fewer	8.6 ± 2.4 fewer	5.5 ± 2.6 fewer

TABLE 1 continued

$\chi^2/2$ heterogeneity of effects between 3 trials	0.7	5.6	7.0	5.4
P value	0.3	0.06	0.03	0.07
Weighted average of all 3 trials¶ Effect/1000 patient treated with t-PA-based regimens instead of streptokinase	3.3 ± 0.8 more	2.9 ± 1.9 fewer	4.9 ± 1.8 fewer	1.6 ± 1.9 fewer
P value	< 0.001	> 0.1	0.01	0.4

Values are numbers (%). This table should not be used to make direct non-randomised comparisons between the absolute event rates in different trials, because the patient populations may have differed substantially in age and other characteristics. Deaths recorded throughout the first 35 days are included for GISSI-2 and ISIS-3 and throughout the first 30 days for GUSTO-1. Numbers randomised and numbers with follow up are from the ISIS-3 report[19] and GUSTO-1[20] (supplemented with revised GUSTO-1 data from the National Auxiliary Publications Service), and numbers with events and the percentages (based on participants with follow up) are from the ISIS-3 report[20] and Van de Werf, etal.[50] Plus-minus values are ± standard deviation. In all three trials, streptokinase was given in intravenous infusions of 1.5 MU over a period of 1 hour. iv, intravenous; t-PA, tissue plasminogen activator; sc, subcutaneous.

*Death not related to stroke was defined as death without recorded stroke.

†In the GISSI-2 trial, the t-PA regimen involved an initial bolus of 10 mg, followed by 50 mg in the first hour and 20 mg in each of the second and third hours.

‡In the ISIS-3 trial, the t-PA regimen involved 40 000 clot-lysis units/kg of body weight as an initial bolus, followed by 360 000 units/kg in the first hour and 67 000 units/kg in each of the next 3 hours.

§In the GUSTO-1 trial, the t-PA alone regimen involved an initial bolus of 15 mg, followed by 0.75 mg/kg (up to 50 mg) in the first 30 minutes and 0.5 mg/kg (up to 35 mg) in the next hour; in the GUSTO-1 trial the other t-PA based regimen involved 0.1 mg of t-PA/kg (up to 9 mg) as an initial bolus and 0.9 mg/kg (up to 81 mg) in the remainder of the first hour, plus 1 MU of streptokinase in the first hour.

¶The weights are proportional to the sample sizes of the trials, so this average gives most weight to the GUSTO-1 trial and least to the GISSI-2 trials.[17] Reproduced from Collins R, Peto R, Baigent BM, Sleight DM. Aspirin, heparin and fibrinolytic therapy in suspected AMI. *N Engl J Med* 1997;336:847–860, with permission of the publisher.

Cardiovascular disorders

TABLE 2 Comparison of early invasive cardiac revascularisation versus initial medical treatment on mortality at 30 days, 6 months, and 12 months (see text, p 96).[2,3,51]

Time after AMI	Mortality in early invasive cardiac revascularisation group Number dead/total number (%)	Mortality in medical therapy alone group Number dead/total number (%)	ARR (95% CI)	RR (95% CI)	NNT (95% CI)
SHOCK study[2,51]					
30 days	71/152 (47)	84/150 (56)	9.3% (−2 to +20.2)	0.83 (0.67 to 1.04)	NA
6 months	76/152 (50)	94/150 (63)	12.7% (1.5 to 23.4)	0.80 (0.65 to 0.98)	8 (5 to 68)
12 months	81/52 (53)	99/150 (66)	12.7% (1.6 to 23.3)	0.80 (0.67 to 0.97)	8 (5 to 61)
SMASH study[3]					
30 days	22/32 (69)	18/23 (78)	9.5% (−14.6 to +30.6)	0.88 (0.64 to 1.2)	NA
12 months	23/32 (74)	19/23 (83)	10.7% (−12.7 to +30.9)	0.87 (0.65 to 1.16)	NA

AMI, acute myocardial infarction; NA, not applicable.

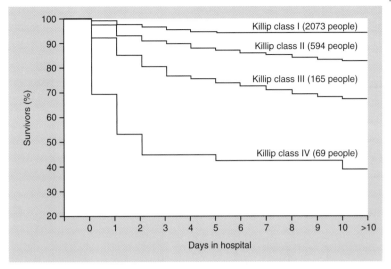

FIGURE 1 The AMIS registry Kaplan–Meier survival curves as a function of Killip class at hospital admission for 3138 people admitted in 50 Swiss hospitals between 1977 and 1998. Published with permission (see text, p 87).[9]

Cardiovascular disorders

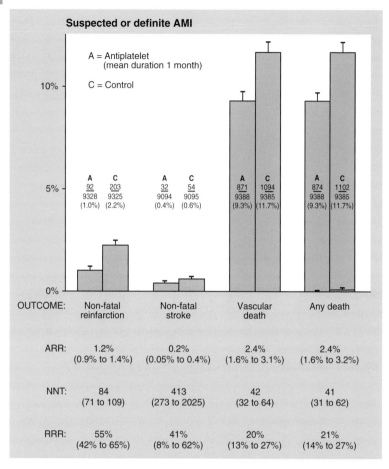

Suspected or definite AMI

A = Antiplatelet (mean duration 1 month)

C = Control

OUTCOME:	Non-fatal reinfarction	Non-fatal stroke	Vascular death	Any death
A	92	32	871	874
	9328	9094	9388	9388
	(1.0%)	(0.4%)	(9.3%)	(9.3%)
C	203	54	1094	1102
	9325	9095	9385	9385
	(2.2%)	(0.6%)	(11.7%)	(11.7%)
ARR:	1.2% (0.9% to 1.4%)	0.2% (0.05% to 0.4%)	2.4% (1.6% to 3.1%)	2.4% (1.6% to 3.2%)
NNT:	84 (71 to 109)	413 (273 to 2025)	42 (32 to 64)	41 (31 to 62)
RRR:	55% (42% to 65%)	41% (8% to 62%)	20% (13% to 27%)	21% (14% to 27%)

FIGURE 2 Absolute effects of antiplatelet treatment on various outcomes in people with a prior suspected or definite AMI.[11] The columns show the absolute risks over 1 month for each category; the error bars are the upper 95% confidence interval. In "any death" column, non-vascular deaths are represented by lower horizontal lines. The table displays for each outcome the absolute risk reduction (ARR), the number of people needing treatment for 1 month to avoid one additional event (NNT), and the relative risk reduction (RRR), with their 95% CIs (see text, p 88). Published with permission.[11]

Cardiovascular disorders

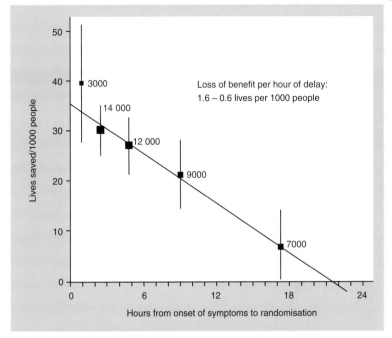

FIGURE 3   Absolute number of lives saved at 1 month/1000 people receiving thrombolytic treatment plotted against the time from the onset of symptoms to randomisation among 45 000 people with ST segment elevation or bundle branch block.[15] Numbers along the curve are the number of people treated at different times (see text, p 89). Published with permission.[17]

Obesity

Search date January 2001

David Arterburn and Polly Hitchcock Noel

INTERVENTIONS

Key Messages

Centrally acting agents

- We found limited evidence from seven RCTs that sibutramine is more effective than placebo in promoting modest weight loss in healthy obese adults and obese adults with controlled hypertension (body mass index [BMI] 25–40 kg/m^2). Weight regain occurs after stopping treatment. We found insufficient evidence about short term safety and no evidence about long term safety.

- Small RCTs found that phentermine and mazindol versus placebo cause modest weight loss in adults more than 15% overweight. We found insufficient evidence on weight regain and long term safety.

- Small RCTs found limited and conflicting evidence on the efficacy of diethylproprion and fluoxetine for weight loss when compared with placebo.

- Dexfenfluramine and fenfluramine have been associated with valvular heart disease and pulmonary hypertension and are no longer marketed. Phenylpropanolamine has recently been linked with increased risk of haemorrhagic stroke.

Orlistat (lipase inhibitor)

- One systematic review and three subsequent RCTs have found that orlistat plus a low calorie diet has a modest effect on body weight compared with placebo plus diet in people with a BMI between 28–47 kg/m^2. We found no evidence on weight regain after stopping treatment, and no evidence on long term safety.

DEFINITION	Obesity is a chronic condition characterised by an excess of body fat. It is most often defined by the BMI (see glossary, p 114), a mathematical formula that is highly correlated with body fat. BMI is weight in kilograms divided by height in metres squared (kg/m^2). In the USA and the UK, people with BMIs between 25–30 kg/m^2 are categorised as overweight, and those with BMIs above 30 kg/m^2 are categorised as obese.[1]
INCIDENCE/ PREVALENCE	Obesity has increased steadily in many countries since 1900. In England, in 1994, it was estimated that 13% of men and 16% of women were obese.[1,2] In the past decade alone, the prevalence of obesity in the USA has increased from 12.0% in 1991 to 17.9% in 1998.[3]
AETIOLOGY/ RISK FACTORS	The aetiology of obesity includes both genetic and environmental factors. Obesity may also be induced by drugs (e.g. high dose glucocorticoids), or be secondary to a variety of neuroendocrine disorders such as Cushing's syndrome and polycystic ovary syndrome.[4]
PROGNOSIS	Obesity is a risk factor for several chronic diseases, including hypertension, dyslipidaemia, diabetes, cardiovascular disease, sleep apnoea, osteoarthritis, and some cancers.[1] The relation between increasing body weight and the mortality rate is curvilinear, with mortality rate increasing in people with low body weight. Whether this is caused by increased mortality risk at low body weights or by unintentional weight loss is not clear.[5] Results from five prospective cohort studies and 1991 national statistics suggest that the number of annual deaths attributable to obesity among US adults is approximately 280 000.[6]
AIMS	To achieve realistic gradual weight loss and prevent the morbidity and mortality associated with obesity, without undue adverse effects.
OUTCOMES	We found no studies that used the primary outcomes of functional morbidity or mortality. Proxy measures include mean weight loss (kg), number of people losing 5% or more of baseline body weight, and number of people maintaining weight loss.
METHODS	*Clinical Evidence* search and appraisal January 2001.

QUESTION What are the effects of drug treatments in adults?

OPTION CENTRALLY ACTING AGENTS

We found limited evidence from six RCTs that sibutramine is more effective than placebo at promoting modest weight loss in adults with BMIs between 25–40 kg/m^2. The weight loss stabilised after 6 months of treatment and was not sustained after stopping treatment. One RCT found that sibutramine caused modest weight loss in obese adults with controlled hypertension, but we found insufficient evidence about short term safety and no evidence of long term safety. Limited evidence suggests that phentermine and mazindol, compared with placebo, result in modest weight loss over short periods in people more than 15% overweight. Weight regain was found after stopping treatment and after longer treatment periods. We found no strong evidence of serious

Obesity

adverse events associated with either phentermine or mazindol. We found insufficient evidence about either diethylproprion or fluoxetine for weight loss. Dexfenfluramine, fenfluramine, and the combination of fenfluramine plus phentermine have been associated with valvular heart disease and pulmonary hypertension. Phenylpropanolamine has been associated with increased risk of haemorrhagic stroke.

Benefits: We found no systematic review or RCTs examining effects of centrally acting drugs on functional morbidity and mortality. **Sibutramine:** We found one systematic review (search date 1998, 6 RCTs, adults aged 18–65 years with BMIs 25–40 kg/m^2)[7] and one subsequent RCT[8] comparing the effect of sibutramine versus placebo on weight loss. The systematic review did not report a quantitative summary. The studies usually excluded people with other illnesses, described participants as healthy, or did not specify participants' health status. In three of the six RCTs in the systematic review, both sibutramine and placebo groups received other interventions such as diet or calorie restriction, behaviour modification, or exercise.[9-11] In a fourth RCT, participants received a diet of 220–800 kcal/day for 4 weeks before randomisation.[12] Four RCTs were 8–24 weeks and two were 12 months long. The largest RCT (1024 people) found that sibutramine (5–30 mg/day) versus placebo reduced mean weight loss at 24 weeks (5.3 kg with sibutramine 15 mg/day v 0.9 kg with placebo, 95% CI not reported, P < 0.001) and increased the percentage of people losing 5% or more of body weight at 24 weeks (53% with sibutramine 15 mg/day v 13% with placebo, 95% CI not reported; NNT 3, P < 0.001).[9] Mean weight losses for the two 12 month trials were 4.4 and 5.2 kg for people on 15 and 10 mg sibutramine versus maximal weight losses of 1.6 kg with placebo.[12,13] Weight regain of up to 25% of previously lost weight was observed within 1–6 weeks of stopping treatment in three of the RCTs.[9-11] Weight regain of up to 80% was observed within 3 months after stopping medication in one RCT.[12] The subsequent RCT (224 obese people with a diagnosis of controlled hypertension for at least 12 months, BMIs 27–40 kg/m^2) found sibutramine 20 mg/day versus placebo increased mean weight loss after treatment for 12 months (4.4 kg with sibutramine v 0.5 kg placebo, 95% CI not reported, P < 0.05).[8] In all the 12 month trials, weight loss stabilised after 6 months of sibutramine.[8,12,13] **Phentermine:** We found one RCT (108 people who were more than 20% overweight), which compared phentermine (30 mg/day) versus placebo.[14] All participants were placed on a diet of 1000 kcal/day. It found that, after 9 months, phentermine reduced weight more than placebo (–12.2 kg with phentermine v –4.8 kg with placebo; mean difference –7.4 kg, 95% CI –11.2 to –4.6 kg). **Mazindol:** We found one RCT (65 people who were more than 15% overweight), which found that mazindol (3 mg/day) reduced weight more than placebo after 3 months' treatment (–6.4 kg with mazindol v –2.6 kg with placebo; mean difference –3.8 kg, 95% CI not reported, P < 0.001). Weight loss was not sustained when treatment was discontinued.[15] **Diethylproprion:** We found two small RCTs with conflicting results. The first (20 people who were 15–20% overweight) found that diethylproprion 75 mg/day reduced weight more than placebo at 6 months

(–11.6 kg with diethylproprion v –2.5 kg with placebo; mean difference –9.1 kg, 95% CI not reported). Both groups were placed on a "strict diet".[16] The second trial (32 people with mean weight 13 kg above ideal body weight) found no significant difference in weight loss between diethylproprion (75 mg/day) and placebo after treatment for 12 months (–8.9 kg with diethylproprion v –10.5 kg with placebo; mean difference +1.6 kg, 95% CI not reported). Both groups were placed on a "low carbohydrate diet".[17] **Fluoxetine:** We found three systematic reviews (search dates 1995, 1996, 1998), which identified two RCTs of at least 1 year's duration evaluating fluoxetine, a selective serotonin reuptake inhibitor.[2,18,19] One RCT (458 people, mean BMI 35 kg/m^2) found no significant difference in weight loss between fluoxetine 60 mg/day and placebo after treatment for 1 year (–1.4 kg with fluoxetine v –1.2 kg with placebo; mean difference –0.2 kg, 95% CI not reported).[20] The second small RCT (19 people with diabetes and BMI > 30 kg/m^2) found that fluoxetine (60 mg/day) reduced weight more than placebo after treatment for 12 months (–4.3 kg with fluoxetine v +1.5 kg with placebo; mean difference –5.8 kg, 95% CI not reported).[21] **Fenfluramine:** We found two RCTs (45 and 134 people who were more than 15% overweight), which found no significant difference between fenfluramine alone, fenfluramine with behavioural therapy, and behavioural therapy or diet alone (results not pooled).[22,23] **Dexfenfluramine:** We found one systematic review (search date 1995, 5 RCTs), which found that dexfenfluramine (30–120 mg/day) reduced weight more than placebo after 1 year of treatment. The review pooled data from four trials in a total of 634 adults who were at least 20% overweight. The mean difference in weight at 1 year for dexfenfluramine versus placebo was –2.6 kg (95% CI –3.8 to –1.3 kg). All participants were also prescribed a calorie restricted diet.[2] **Fenfluramine plus phentermine:** We found one RCT (121 people, 30–80% overweight), which found that a combination of phentermine (15 mg/day) plus fenfluramine (60 mg/day) reduced weight more than placebo after treatment for 6 months (–14.3 kg with phentermine/fenfluramine v –4.6 kg with placebo; mean difference –9.7 kg, 95% CI –12.0 to –7.4 kg). The trial found that weight loss ceased at 18 weeks of treatment; weight regain was noted after 60 weeks of treatment.[24] **Phenylpropanolamine:** We found one non-systematic meta-analysis (7 trials, 643 obese people, BMI not stated), which found that phenylpropanolamine (dose not specified) compared with placebo reduced weight after treatment for 4 weeks (0.21 kg/week).[25] At the end of these trials (duration not specified), there was an additional weight loss of 0.14 kg/week compared with placebo.[25]

Harms: **Sibutramine:** Common adverse effects were headache, dry mouth, anorexia, constipation, insomnia, rhinitis, and pharyngitis occurring in 10–30% of people taking sibutramine versus 8–19% of people on placebo (significance of difference not reported).[7] Mean increases in systolic and diastolic blood pressure (1–3 mmHg) and heart rate (4–5 beats/minute) have been reported in people taking sibutramine at doses of 5–20 mg/day.[7] In people with controlled hypertension, the proportion who experienced a clinically significant increase in baseline systolic or diastolic blood pressure (> 10 mmHg at 3 consecutive visits) was comparable with placebo (17.6% with sibutramine v 14.5% with placebo, P value and 95% CI not reported; NNH 32). However, hypertension was the most common adverse event causing withdrawal from the study (5.3% with sibutramine v 1.4% with placebo). No serious adverse events were reported.[8] We found no evidence on long term safety. **Phentermine:** We found no evidence of serious adverse reactions. Phentermine given alone has not been associated with valvular heart disease.[26] **Mazindol and diethylproprion:** We found a single case report of pulmonary hypertension diagnosed 12 months after stopping mazindol that had been taken for 10 weeks.[27] Case reports have described pulmonary hypertension and psychosis in users of diethylproprion.[28,29] The frequency of serious adverse events with these agents is not clear. **Fluoxetine:** One RCT comparing fluoxetine versus placebo for obesity reported more frequent gastrointestinal symptoms, sleep disturbance, sweating, tremor, amnesia, and thirst in the active treatment groups (frequency of events not provided).[20] One systematic review of antidepressant treatment found that selective serotonin reuptake inhibitors were associated with a 10–15% incidence of anxiety, diarrhoea, dry mouth, headache, and nausea.[30] **Dexfenfluramine, fenfluramine, fenfluramine plus phentermine:** These agents have been associated with valvular heart disease and primary pulmonary hypertension,[31,32] and are no longer marketed.[33] One 25 centre retrospective cohort study in 1473 people found prevalence rates and relative risk of aortic regurgitation of 8.9% with dexfenfluramine (RR 2.18, 95% CI 1.32 to 3.59; NNH 20) and 13.7% with phentermine plus fenfluramine (RR 3.34, 95% CI 2.09 to 5.35; NNH 10), compared with 4.1% with no treatment.[34] One prospective study in 1072 participants found no greater risk of valvular heart disease in people taking dexfenfluramine less than 3 months than in those taking placebo (sustained release dexfenfluramine RR 1.6, 95% CI 0.8 to 3.4, regular dexfenfluramine RR 1.4, 95% CI 0.7 to 3.0, when compared with placebo).[35] One case control study in 95 people with primary pulmonary hypertension and 355 matched controls found a history of fenfluramine use was associated with increased risk of primary pulmonary hypertension (OR 6.3, 95% CI 3.0 to 13.2). The odds ratio was higher among people who had taken fenfluramine in the past year (OR 10.1, 95% CI 3.4 to 29.9), and among people treated for more than 3 months (OR 23.1, 95% CI 6.9 to 77.7).[36] **Phenylpropanolamine:** A recent case control study (men and women aged 18–49 years) found that phenylpropanolamine used as an appetite suppressant increased the risk of haemorrhagic stroke within the first 3 days of use (adjusted OR 15.9, lower confidence limit 2.04, P = 0.013). For the association between phenylpropanolamine in appetite suppressants and risk for haemorrhagic stroke among women, the adjusted odds ratio was 16.6 (lower confidence limit 2.2, P = 0.011).[37] Phenylpropanolamine is no longer marketed in the USA.[38]

Comment: **Phenylpropanolamine, phentermine, mazindol, and diethylpropion:** The few trials that we identified were small, with short duration of follow up, and high withdrawal rates. Nearly 5 million US adults used prescription weight loss pills in 1996–1998. A quarter of users were not overweight, suggesting that weight loss pills may be inappropriately used, especially among women, white people, and Hispanic people.[39]

OPTION	ORLISTAT

One systematic review and three subsequent RCTs have found that orlistat combined with a low calorie diet modestly increases weight loss in adults with obesity, compared with placebo plus diet. We found no evidence on weight gain following discontinuation, or on long term adverse effects.

Benefits: We found no systematic reviews or RCTs examining effects of orlistat on functional morbidity and mortality. We found one systematic review (search date 1999, 7 RCTs, 4188 adults with BMIs between 28–47 kg/m^2)[40] and three subsequent RCTs comparing orlistat versus placebo.[41-43] Trials lasted 1–2 years. Meta-analysis of five of the trials found that orlistat combined with a low calorie diet (below 1500 kcal/day) reduced weight more than placebo plus diet after treatment for 1 year (mean weight loss 6.1 kg with orlistat 120 mg three times daily v 2.6 kg with placebo; P < 0.001, 95% CI not reported).[44] A greater proportion of the participants lost 10% or more of their initial weight in the orlistat groups than in the placebo groups at 12 months (20.2% v 8.3%, P < 0.001). In a 1 year trial (322 people with type 2 diabetes included in the review but not the meta-analysis), 30.2% of the orlistat plus diet group, and 13.2% of the placebo plus diet group lost 5% or more of their initial body weight.[45] We found three subsequent multicentre trials with over 30 people per trial (placebo controlled, double blind, 796,[41] 783,[42] and 376[43] people) whose results were consistent with the earlier systematic review. In the two larger trials, generally healthy obese adults (BMI 28–44 kg/m^2) were randomised to placebo or orlistat (60 or 120 mg) three times a day for 2 years after a 4 week placebo and reduced energy diet run-in, which 54 of the 796 and 161 of the 783 participants did not complete. Participants in both trials followed a reduced energy diet for the first year and a weight maintenance diet for the second year. People taking orlistat were significantly more likely to lose 10% or more of initial body weight compared with those taking placebo at the end of the first year (28.6–38.2% with orlistat 60 mg v 11.3–18.6% with placebo), and to maintain this weight loss after 2 years (28.2–33.0% with orlistat 60 mg v 6.6–18.6% with placebo). One of the trials reported significantly improved "quality of life" on orlistat compared with placebo, but this consisted of reduced obesity specific distress and reduced treatment dissatisfaction.[42] The third RCT (376 obese adults, BMI 28–38 kg/m^2 with type 2 diabetes, hypercholesterolaemia, or hypertension) compared orlistat (120 mg) versus placebo three times daily in conjunction with dietary intervention for 1 year.[43] All participants were given placebo for 2 weeks before randomisation. Orlistat versus placebo significantly increased the proportion of people who lost 5% or more of their initial body weight (54% with orlistat v 41% with placebo; P < 0.001), but did not significantly increase weight reduction of 10% or more (19.2% with orlistat v 14.6% with placebo).

Harms: Common adverse effects included oily spotting from the rectum, flatulence, and faecal urgency in 22–27% of people taking orlistat versus 1–7% of people taking placebo.[40] Four RCTs reported monitoring plasma levels of fat soluble vitamins and found a higher percentage of people treated with orlistat required vitamin supplements compared with placebo.[45-48] In the largest RCT (892 people), vitamin supplements were given to 14.1% with orlistat versus 6.5% with placebo.[47] A single case study suggests that orlistat may also reduce the intestinal absorption of contraceptive pills.[49] In the RCT of people with obesity associated coronary heart disease risk factors, more unidentified serious adverse events occurred with orlistat than with placebo (10% with orlistat v 2.6%).[43]

Comment: People in six of the seven trials in the systematic review were selected for participation after losing weight on a preliminary low calorie diet with placebo for 4–5 weeks before randomisation.[40]

GLOSSARY

Body mass index (BMI) Expressed as weight in kilograms divided by height in metres squared (kg/m^2). In the USA and UK, individuals with BMIs between 25–30 kg/m^2 are considered overweight; those with BMIs above 30 kg/m^2 are considered obese.

REFERENCES

1. National Institutes of Health. *Clinical guidelines on the identification, evaluation, and treatment of overweight and obesity in adults: the Evidence Report.* Bethesda, Maryland: US Department of Health and Human Services, 1998.

2. University of York, NHS Centre for Reviews and Dissemination. *A systematic review of the interventions for the prevention and treatment of obesity, and the maintenance of weight loss.* York, England: NHS Centre for Reviews and Dissemination, 1997. Search date 1995; primary sources Medline, Embase, Bids, Dare, Psychlit, bibliographies of review articles, and contributions from peer reviewers.

3. Mokdad AH, Serdula MK, Dietz WH, Bowman BA, Marks JS, Koplan JP. The spread of the obesity epidemic in the United States 1991–1998. *JAMA* 1999;282:1519–1522.

4. Bray GA. Obesity: etiology. *UpToDate* [serial on CD-ROM] 2000;8(1). UpToDate, Inc, Wellesley, Massachusetts, USA.

5. Bray GA. Obesity: Overview of therapy for obesity. *UpToDate* [serial on CD-ROM] 2000;8(1). UpToDate, Inc, Wellesley, Massachusetts, USA.

6. Allison DB, Fontaine KR, Manson JE, Stevens J, Vanitallie TB. Annual deaths attributable to obesity in the United States. *JAMA* 1999;282: 1530–1538.

7. Luque CA, Rey JA. Sibutramine: a serotonin-norepinephrine reuptake-inhibitor for the treatment of obesity. *Ann Pharmacother* 1999;33: 968–978. Search date 1998; primary sources Medline, Embase, manual search, and reference lists of relevant articles.

8. McMahon FG, Fujioka K, Singh BN, et al. Efficacy and safety of sibutramine in obese white and African American patients with hypertension: a 1-year, double-blind, placebo-controlled multicenter trial. *Arch Int Med* 2000;160: 2185–2191.

9. Bray GA, Blackburn GL, Ferguson JM, et al. Sibutramine produces dose-related weight loss. *Obes Res* 1999;7:189–198.

10. Hanotin C, Thomas F, Jones SP, Leutenegger E, Drouin P. Efficacy and tolerability of sibutramine in obese patients: a dose-ranging study. *Int J Obes Relat Metab Disord* 1998;22:32–38.

11. Weintraub M, Rubio A, Golik A, Byrne L, Scheinbaum ML. Sibutramine in weight control: a dose-ranging, efficacy study. *Clin Pharmacol Ther* 1991;50:330–337.

12. Apfelbaum M, Vague P, Ziegler O, Hanotin C, Thomas F, Leutnegger E. Long-term maintenance of weight loss after a very-low calorie diet: a randomized blinded trial of the efficacy and tolerability of sibutramine. *Am J Med* 1999;106:179–184.

13. Jones SP, Smith IG, Kelly F, Gray JA. Long-term weight loss with sibutramine [abstract]. *Int J Obes Relat Metab Disord* 1995;19(suppl 2):41.

14. Munro JF, MacCuish AC, Wilson EM, et al. Comparison of continuous and intermittent anorectic therapy in obesity. *BMJ* 1968;1:352–354.

15. Vernace BJ. Controlled comparative investigation of mazindol, D-amphetamine, and placebo. *Obesity Bariatric Med* 1974;3:124–129.

16. McKay RHG. Long-term use of diethlypropion in obesity. *Curr Med Res Opin* 1973;1:489–493.

17. Silverstone JT, Solomon T. The long-term management of obesity in general practice. *Br J Clin Pract* 1965;19:395–398.

18. Douketis JD, Feightner JW, Attia J, et al. Periodic health examination, 1999 update: 1. Detection, prevention and treatment of obesity. Canadian Task Force on Preventive Health Care. *Can Med Assoc J* 1999;160:513–525. Search date 1998; primary sources Medline, bibliographies of review articles, and Current Contents listings.

19. National Task Force on the Prevention and Treatment of Obesity. Long-term pharmacotherapy in the management of obesity. *JAMA* 1996;276: 1907–1915. Search date 1996; primary sources Medline and manual search of bibliographies.

20. Goldstein DJ, Rampey AH Jr, Enas GG, et al. Fluoxetine: a randomized clinical trial in the treatment of obesity. *Int J Obes* 1994;18: 129–135.

21. O'Kane M, Wiles PG, Wales JK. Fluoxetine in the treatment of obese type II diabetic patients. *Diabet Med* 1994;11:105–110.

22. Ost LG, Gotestam KG. Behavioral and pharmacological treatments for obesity: an experimental comparison. *Addict Behav* 1976;1: 331–338.

23. Stunkard AJ, Craighead LW, O'Brien R. Controlled trial of behavior therapy, pharmacotherapy, and their combination in the treatment of obesity. *Lancet* 1980;2:1045–1047.

24. Weintraub M. Long term weight control study: the National Heart, Lung, and Blood Institute funded multimodal intervention study. *Clin Pharmacol Ther* 1992;51:581–646.

25. Greenway FL. Clinical studies with phenylpropanolamine: a metaanalysis. *Am J Clin Nutr* 1992;55(suppl 1):203–205.

26. Gaasch WH, Aurigemma GP. Valvular heart disease induced by anorectic drugs. *UpToDate* [serial on CD-ROM][2000;8(3). UpToDate, Inc, Wellesley, Massachusetts, USA.

27. Hagiwara M, Tsuchida A, Hyakkoku M, et al. Delayed onset of pulmonary hypertension associated with an appetite suppressant, mazindol: a case report. *Jpn Circ* 2000;64: 218–221.

28. Thomas SH, Butt AY, Corris PA, et al. Appetite suppressants and primary pulmonary hypertension in the United Kingdom. *Br Heart J* 1995;74: 660–663.

29. Little JD, Romans SE. Psychosis following readministration of diethylproprion: a possible role for kindling? *Int Clin Psychopharmacol* 1993;8: 67–70.

30. Mulrow CD, Williams JW Jr, Trivedi M, et al. Treatment of depression – newer pharmacotherapies. *Psychopharmacol Bull* 1998; 34:409–795. Search date 1998; primary sources the Cochrane and collaboration depression, anxiety and neurosis (CCDAN) Review Group's registry, and bibliographies of trial and review articles.

31. Poston WS, Foreyt JP. Scientific and legal issues in fenfluramine/dexfenfluramine litigation. *J Texas Med* 2000;96:48–56.

32. Connolly HM, Crary JL, McGoon MD, et al. Valvular heart disease associated with fenfluramine-phentermine. *N Engl J Med* 1997;337:581–588.

33. Scheen AJ, Lefebvre PJ. Pharmacological treatment of obesity: present status. *Intl J Obes Relat Metab Disord* 1999;23(suppl 1):47–53.

34. Gardin JM, Schumacher J, Constantine G, et al. Valvular abnormalities and cardiovascular status following exposure to dexfenfluramine and phentermine/fenfluramine. *JAMA* 2000;283: 703–709.

35. Weissman NJ, Tighe JF, Gottdiener JS, Gwynne JT. An assessment of heart-valve abnormalities in obese patients taking dexfenfluramine, sustained-release dexfenfluramine, or placebo. Sustained release dexfenfluramine study group. *N Engl J Med* 1998;339:725–732.

36. Abenhaim L, Moride Y, Brenot F, et al. Appetite-suppressant drugs and the risk of primary pulmonary hypertension. International primary pulmonary hypertension study group. *N Engl J Med* 1996;335:609–616.

37. Horwitz RI, Brass LM, Kernan WN, Viscoli CM. Phenylpropanolamine and risk of hemorrhagic stroke: final report of the hemorrhagic stroke project. http://www.fda.gov/ohrms/dockets/ac/00/backgrd/3647b1_tab19.doc (accessed 2 Mar 2001).

38. U.S. Food and Drug Administration. Center for Drug Evaluation and Research. Phenylpropanolamine (PPA) information page. http://www.fda.gov/cder/drug/infopage/ppa/ (accessed 2 Mar 2001).

39. Khan LK, Serdula MK, Bowman BA, Williamson DF. Use of Prescription Weight Loss Pills among U.S. Adults in 1996–1998. *Ann Int Med* 2001; 134:282–286.

40. Anonymous. Orlistat: no hurry. *Can Fam Physician* 1999;45:2331–2351. Search date 1999; primary sources Medline, Embase, Reactions, Cochrane; hand searches of international journals, the Prescribe Library, and clinical pharmacology reference texts and personal contact with Produits Roche, the European Medicines Evaluation Agency, and Food and Drug Administration committees.

41. Hauptman J, Lucas C, Boldrin MN, Collins H, Segal KR. Orlistat in the long-term treatment of obesity in primary care settings. *Arch Fam Med* 2000;9:160–167.

42. Rossner S, Sjöstrom L, Noack R, Meinders AE, Noseda G. Weight loss, weight maintenance, and improved cardiovascular risk factors after 2 years treatment with orlistat for obesity. *Obes Res* 2000; 8:49–61.

43. Lindgarde F. The effect of orlistat on body weight and coronary heart disease risk profile in obese patients: the Swedish Multimorbidity Study. *J Int Med* 2000;248:245–254.

44. European Agency for the Evaluation of Medicinal Products. *Committee for proprietary medicinal products. European public assessment report (EPAR) – Xenical.* London: European Agency for the Evaluation of Medicinal Products, 1998.

45. Hollander PA, Elbein SC, Hirsch IR, et al. Role of orlistat in the treatment of obese patients with type 2 diabetes: a 1-year randomized double-blind study. *Diabetes Care* 1998;21:1288–1294.

46. Sjostrom L, Rissanen A, Anderson T, et al. Randomised placebo-controlled trial of orlistat for weight loss and prevention of weight regain in obese patients. *Lancet* 1998;352:167–173.

47. Davidson MH, Hauptman J, DiGirolamo M, et al. Weight control and risk factor reduction in obese subjects treated for 2 years with orlistat: a randomized controlled trial. *JAMA* 1999;281: 235–242.

48. Finer N, James WPT, Kopelman PG, Lean MEJ, Williams G. One-year treatment of obesity: a randomized, double-blind, placebo-controlled, multicentre study of orlistat, a gastrointestinal lipase inhibitor. *Int J Obes* 2000;24:306–313.

49. Peleg R. Caution when using oral contraceptive pills with Orlistat [letter]. *Isr Med Assoc J* 2000;2: 712.

David Arterburn
Chief Resident/Instructor
University of Texas
Health Science Center at San Antonio
San Antonio
USA

Polly Hitchcock Noel
Associate Director
VERDICT
a VA HSR&D Center of Excellence
South Texas Veterans Health Care System
US Department of Veterans Affairs
San Antonio, Texas
USA

Competing interests: None declared. The views expressed in this article are those of the authors and do not necessarily represent the views of the US Department of Veterans Affairs.

Peripheral arterial disease

Search date May 2001

Sonia Anand and Mark Creager

INTERVENTIONS

Key Messages

- One systematic review has found strong evidence that antiplatelet agents versus control treatments reduce the rate of major cardiovascular events and local arterial occlusion in people with peripheral arterial disease. The balance of benefits and harms is in favour of treatment for most people with symptomatic peripheral arterial disease, because as a group they are at much greater risk of cardiovascular events.

- Systematic reviews have found that regular exercise three times a week for 30 minute sessions significantly improves the limitation of walking by claudication.

- Observation studies have found that people with arterial disease who stop smoking rapidly reduce their risk of cardiovascular death, myocardial infarction (MI), and stroke (see smoking cessation under secondary prevention of ischaemic cardiac events, p 179). One systematic review has found observational evidence that continued cigarette smoking by people with intermittent claudication is associated with progression of symptoms, poor prognosis after bypass surgery, amputation, and need for reconstructive surgery. Another systematic review found no good evidence from controlled studies about the effects of advice to stop smoking.

- Four RCTs of cilostazol versus placebo in people with intermittent claudication have found improved initial claudication distance and absolute claudication distance measured on a treadmill, and a reduced proportion of people with symptoms that did not improve compared with people treated with placebo.

- Systematic reviews of small RCTs of variable quality have found that pentoxifylline versus placebo increases the walking distance by a small amount in people with intermittent claudication. One recently published RCT with a high withdrawal rate found no convincing benefit with pentoxifylline versus placebo in people with intermittent claudication. The available evidence is not good enough to define clearly the effects of pentoxifylline.

- One systematic review of two small RCTs found limited evidence that angioplasty versus no angioplasty transiently improved total walking distance.
- We found limited evidence from small RCTs about the effects of bypass surgery versus other treatments for people with debilitating symptomatic peripheral arterial disease.

DEFINITION   Peripheral arterial disease arises when there is significant narrowing of arteries distal to the arch of the aorta. Narrowing can arise from atheroma, arteritis, local thrombus formation, or embolisation from the heart or more central arteries. This topic includes treatment options for people with symptoms of reduced blood flow to the leg that are likely to arise from atheroma. These symptoms range from calf pain on exercise (intermittent claudication), to rest pain, skin ulceration, or ischaemic necrosis (gangrene) in people with critical ischaemia.

INCIDENCE/   Peripheral arterial disease is more common in people aged over 50
PREVALENCE   years than young people, and is more common in men than women. The prevalence of peripheral arterial disease of the legs (assessed by non-invasive tests) is about 3% in people under the age of 60 years, but rises to over 20% in people over 75 years.[1] The overall annual incidence of intermittent claudication is 1.5–2.6/1000 men a year and 1.2–3.6/1000 women a year.[2]

AETIOLOGY/   Factors associated with the development of peripheral arterial
RISK FACTORS disease include age, gender, cigarette smoking, diabetes mellitus, hypertension, hyperlipidaemia, obesity, and physical inactivity. The strongest association is with smoking (RR 2.0–4.0) and diabetes (RR 2.0–3.0).[3] Acute limb ischaemia may result from thrombosis arising within a peripheral artery or embolic occlusion.

PROGNOSIS   The symptom of intermittent claudication can resolve spontaneously, remain stable over many years, or progress rapidly to critical limb ischaemia. The incidence of critical limb ischaemia in Denmark and Italy in 1990 was 0.25–0.45/1000 people a year.[4,5] About 15% of people with intermittent claudication eventually develop critical leg ischaemia, which endangers the viability of the limb. Coronary heart disease is the major cause of death in people with peripheral arterial disease of the legs. Over 5 years, about 20% of people with intermittent claudication have a non-fatal cardiovascular event, MI, or stroke.[6] The mortality rate of people with peripheral arterial disease is two to three times higher than that of age and sex matched controls. Overall mortality after the diagnosis of peripheral arterial disease is about 30% after 5 years and 70% after 15 years.[6]

AIMS   To reduce symptoms (intermittent claudication), local complications (arterial leg ulcers, critical leg ischaemia), and general complications (MI and stroke).

OUTCOMES   **Local outcomes:** Proportion of people with adverse outcomes (decline in claudication distance, amputation, adverse effects of treatment), the mean improvement in claudication distance measured on a treadmill or by some other specified means. We did not include studies that reported other measures such as patency assessed by angiography or ultrasound. **General outcomes:** Rates of MI, stroke, and other major cardiovascular events.

METHODS   *Clinical Evidence* search and appraisal May 2001.

QUESTION   **What are the effects of treatments for people with chronic peripheral arterial disease?**

OPTION   **ANTIPLATELET AGENTS**

One systematic review has found strong evidence that antiplatelet agents versus control treatments reduce the rate of major cardiovascular events and local arterial occlusion in people with peripheral arterial disease. The balance of benefits and harms is in favour of treatment for most people with peripheral arterial disease because they are at greater risk of cardiovascular events.

Benefits: **Peripheral arterial disease complications:** We found two systematic reviews.[7,8] The first systematic review (search date 1990; 11 RCTs; 1990 people with intermittent claudication [see glossary, p 125], bypass surgery of the leg, or peripheral artery angioplasty)[7] found that antiplatelet compared with no additional treatment reduced the risk of arterial occlusion over 19 months (RRR 0.30; P < 0.00001).[9] The second systematic review (search date 1998, 54 RCTs)[8] found that, in people with intermittent claudication, aspirin versus placebo reduced the number of arterial occlusions and ticlopidine reduced the risk of revascularisation procedures. **Cardiovascular events:** We found one systematic review[7] (search date 1990; 39 RCTs; 9000 people with intermittent claudication, arterial reconstruction of the lower limb, or peripheral angioplasty) and one subsequent RCT.[10] The systematic review found that, over an average of about 2 years, antiplatelet versus control treatment reduced the combined outcome of vascular death, MI, or stroke (AR 273/4361 [6.3%] with antiplatelet therapy *v* 329/4362 [7.5%] with control; RR 0.83, 95% CI 0.71 to 0.97; ARR 1.2%, 95% CI 0.2% to 2.3%; NNT 79, 95% CI 44 to 455).[9] The subsequent RCT found in a subgroup analysis that over a mean of 1.8 years, clopidogrel versus aspirin reduced vascular death, MI, and stroke in people with peripheral arterial disease (215/3223 [6.7%] with clopidogrel *v* 277/3229 [8.6%] with aspirin; RR 0.78, 95% CI 0.66 to 0.92; ARR 1.9%, 95% CI 0.6% to 3.2%; NNT 53, 95% CI 32 to 164 over 1.8 years).[10]

Harms: In the systematic review (search date 1990; 35 RCTs; 8098 people with peripheral arterial disease), antiplatelet treatment versus control treatment increased the risk of non-fatal major bleeds (14/2545 [0.55%] *v* 9/2243 [0.40%]; RR 1.37, 95% CI 0.60 to 3.16).[7] The number of events was too low to exclude a clinically important increase in major bleeding. Across a wide range of people, antiplatelet agents have been found to increase significantly the risk of major haemorrhage (see harms of antiplatelet agents under primary prevention, p 147).

Comment: In the subsequent RCT,[10] figures were presented for number of events per person year. *Clinical Evidence* has recalculated the figures assuming that no individual had more than one event; this assumption has minimal impact on the results because the RR reported by the RCT authors (0.76, 95% CI 0.64 to 0.91) is very close to that given above. We found no evidence about the effects of combined clopidogrel and aspirin versus a single antiplatelet agent in people with peripheral arterial disease. Peripheral arterial disease increases the risk of cardiovascular events, so for most people the risk of bleeding is outweighed by the benefits of regular antiplatelet use.

| OPTION | EXERCISE |

Systematic reviews have found that regular exercise three times a week for 30 minute sessions significantly improves the limitation of walking by claudication.

Benefits: **Walking exercise versus no exercise:** We found two systematic reviews of exercise versus no exercise in people with chronic stable intermittent claudication (see glossary, p 125) (search dates 1996[11] and not stated[12]). The first systematic review found that exercise programmes (at least 30 min walking as far as claudication permits, at least 3 times weekly, for 3–6 months) versus no exercise increased both the initial claudication distance (see glossary, p 125) (4 RCTs; 94 people; difference of means 139 m, 95% CI 31 m to 247 m) and the absolute claudication distance (see glossary, p 125) (5 RCTs; 115 people; difference of means 179 m, 95% CI 60 m to 298 m).[11] Outcomes were evaluated after 3–12 months. The RCTs measured the effects of exercise in people also being treated with surgery, aspirin, or dipyridamole. Control treatments were placebo tablets (2 RCTs) or "instructed to continue with normal lifestyle". The second systematic review (10 RCTs, including all those in the first review) found that exercise versus no exercise increased maximal exercise time (3 RCTs; 53 people; WMD 6.5 min, 95% CI 4.4 to 8.7 min).[12] **Different types of exercise:** All the RCTs in the systematic reviews involved walking exercise. We found one RCT (67 people with moderate to severe intermittent claudication), which compared arm versus leg exercise of similar intensity.[13] A third group of 15 people was given no exercise, but this group was not created by random allocation. After 6 weeks, both training groups had similar improvements in initial claudication distance (122% with arm exercise *v* 93% with leg exercise) and absolute claudication distance (47% with arm exercise *v* 50% with leg exercise), and there were no significant changes in the control group.

Harms: Neither review gave details of any observed harms of the exercise programmes.[11,12]

Cardiovascular disorders

Peripheral arterial disease

Comment: The RCTs in the systematic reviews had low drop out rates. Blinding of participants was not possible. Blinding of assessors is not clear from the reviews. We found one further systematic review of 21 observational studies or RCTs of exercise in 564 people with peripheral arterial disease.[14] This review calculated effects based on the differences in claudication difference after and before exercise treatment, but it made no allowance for any spontaneous improvement that might have occurred in the participants. It reported large increases with exercise in the initial claudication distance (126–351 m) and in the absolute claudication distance (325–723 m), but these estimates were based on observational data. Most (5/6) exercise programmes in the second systematic review[11] occurred under supervision. An Australian RCT is examining the effect of exercise treatment in 1400 men.[12] The benefit from arm exercise remains unconfirmed, but suggests that improved walking may be caused by generally improved cardiovascular function rather than local changes of the peripheral circulation.

OPTION **SMOKING CESSATION**

An old systematic review found observational evidence that continued cigarette smoking by people with intermittent claudication is associated with an increased rate of cardiovascular outcomes such as MI, stroke, and death. Another systematic review has found no good evidence from controlled studies about advice to stop smoking in people intermittent claudication.

Benefits: We found one systematic review of advice to quit cigarette smoking versus no advice (search date 1996; no specific RCTs; 4 observational studies; 866 people).[11]

Harms: The systematic review presented no evidence about the harms of strong advice to quit smoking versus no advice.

Comment: The intervention in all the studies was strong advice to stop smoking. One large observational study in the systematic review found no significant increase in absolute claudication distance (see glossary, p 125) after cessation of smoking.[11] Two other studies found conflicting results about the risk of deteriorating from moderate to severe claudication in people who successfully quit smoking compared with current smokers. The fourth study provided no numerical results. Overall, the review found no good evidence to confirm or refute the consensus view that advice to stop smoking improves symptoms in people with intermittent claudication (see glossary, p 125). An older systematic review (search date 1989) concluded that most of the evidence on the effects of smoking cessation derives from observational studies that have found among cigarette smokers increased risk of onset of intermittent claudication, progression of symptoms, poor progress after bypass surgery, amputation, and the need for reconstructive surgery.[15]

OPTION	CILOSTAZOL

Four RCTs of cilostazol versus placebo in people with intermittent claudication have found improved initial claudication distance and absolute claudication distance measured on a treadmill, and a reduced proportion of people whose symptoms did not improve. The moderate withdrawal rate in the cilostazol arm of the RCTs reduces confidence in these conclusions.

Benefits: We found no systematic review. **Versus placebo:** We found four RCTs comparing cilostazol versus placebo (see table 1, p 127).[16-19] The RCTs found that cilostazol versus placebo reduced the risk of being rated as unchanged, worsened, or unsure at the end of each trial (4 RCTs; 1091 people; no heterogeneity; combined RR using fixed effects model 0.71, 95% CI 0.63 to 0.81), and significantly improved the initial claudication distance (see glossary, p 125) (by 38–80 m) and the absolute claudication distance (see glossary, p 125) (by 28–84 m). Cilostazol also caused small increases in ankle–brachial index (see glossary, p 125) values and raised serum high density lipoprotein cholesterol concentrations.[17] None of the trials evaluated cilostazol beyond 24 weeks. Although the overall results of cilostazol versus placebo indicate a significant effect of cilostazol on increasing walking distance, the trials have some weakness of their methods, which impedes interpretation (see comment below).

Harms: More people withdrew from the most recent RCT[16] because of adverse effects or concerns about safety with cilostazol than with placebo (39/227 [17%] with cilostazol v 24/239 [10%] with placebo; RR 1.71, 95% CI 1.06 to 2.75; ARI 7.1%, 95% CI 0.9% to 13.3%; NNH 14, 95% CI 8 to 111). Side effects of cilostazol included headache (28% v 12% with placebo; NNH 7), diarrhoea (19% v 8%; NNH 9), abnormal stools (15% v 5%; NNH 10), palpitations (17% v 2%; NNH 6), and dizziness. Cilostazol is a phosphodiesterase inhibitor; RCTs have found that other phosphodiesterase inhibitors (milrinone, vesnarinone) are associated with increased mortality in people with heart failure. The trial was too small to assess reliably the effect of cilostazol on cardiovascular morbidity. Results aggregated from other studies have not found an excess of cardiovascular events with cilostazol (see comment below).[20]

Comment: The RCTs all had moderate withdrawal rates after randomisation (up to 28.9%).[17] For example, in the most recent RCT,[16] some people had protocol violations caused by no treadmill test (22/227 [9.7%] with cilostazol v 13/239 [5.4%]), and others withdrew before completing the trial (39/227 [17%] with cilostazol v 25/239 [10%] with placebo). In all RCTs, withdrawals were more common with cilostazol (61/227 [27%] v 38/239 [16%] with placebo; RR 1.69, 95% CI 1.18 to 2.43; ARI 11%, 95% CI 4% to 18%). To allow for these problems, the authors performed an intention to treat analysis using "last available observation carried forward". However, the analysis did not include the 35 people with no observations to carry forward, and the effects of the difference in withdrawals between the groups was not explored adequately (e.g. if people with worsening claudication were more likely to withdraw, then the observed differences may be artefactual). Although cilostazol appears promising, the exact balance of its benefits and harms remains unclear. Given the concerns about milrinone, cilostazol is not recommended for use in people with congestive heart failure.

| OPTION | PENTOXIFYLLINE |

Systematic reviews of many small RCTs of variable quality have found that pentoxifylline versus placebo increases the walking distance in people with intermittent claudication. One recently published RCT with a high withdrawal rate found no convincing benefit with pentoxifylline versus placebo in people with intermittent claudication. The available evidence is not good enough to define clearly the effects of pentoxifylline.

Benefits: We found two systematic reviews[11,21] and one subsequent RCT.[16] The first review (search date 1994, 29 RCTs of people with Fontaine's classification stage II or III intermittent claudication [see glossary, p 125] for at least 3 months)[21] included RCTs only if they were placebo controlled and double blinded, and used pentoxifylline 600–1800 mg daily for 2–26 weeks. A meta-analysis found that pentoxifylline versus placebo significantly increased both the initial claudication distance (see glossary, p 125) and the absolute claudication distance (see glossary, p 125 and see table 2, p 127). The second systematic review[11] found similar results (see table 1, p 127). The subsequent RCT found that pentoxifylline versus placebo had no significant effect after 24 weeks in the number of people who had no change or deterioration in the claudication distance (72/212 [34%] with pentoxifylline v 68/226 [30%] with placebo; RR 1.13, 95% CI 0.86 to 1.48), the initial claudication distance (202 m with pentoxifylline v 180 m with placebo; mean difference 22 m; P for change from baseline = 0.07), or the absolute claudication distance (308 m with pentoxifylline v 300 m with placebo; mean difference 8 m; P for change from baseline = 0.82).[16] **Versus cilostazol:** The same RCT found that pentoxifylline versus cilostazol after 24 weeks significantly worsened the number of people who had no change or deterioration in the claudication distance (72/212 [34%] with pentoxifylline v 47/205 [23%] with cilostazol; RR 1.48, 95% CI 1.08 to 2.03; ARR 11%, 95% CI 2.4% to 20%; NNT 9, 95% CI 5 to 42), the initial claudication distance (202 m with pentoxifylline v 218 m with cilostazol; mean difference –16 m; P = 0.0001), and the absolute claudication distance (308 m with pentoxifylline v 350 m with cilostazol; mean difference –42 m; P = 0.0005). However, this RCT had a high withdrawal rate after randomisation (26% [60/232] with pentoxifylline v 26% [61/237] with cilostazol), which may have biased the results.

Harms: More people withdrew from the RCT because of adverse effects or concerns about safety with pentoxifylline than with placebo (44/232 [19%] with pentoxifylline v 24/239 [10%] with placebo; RR 1.89, 95% CI 1.19 to 3.00; ARI 8.9%, 95% CI 2.6% to 15.3%; NNH 12, 95% CI 7 to 39).[16] Side effects of pentoxifylline included sore throat (14% v 7%; NNH 15), dyspepsia, nausea, diarrhoea (8% v 5% with placebo; P = 0.31), and vomiting.[16] No life threatening side effects of pentoxifylline have been reported, although RCTs have been too small to date to assess this reliably.

Comment: The systematic reviews contained many RCTs in common. Results of the subsequent RCT[16] have been published in numerous articles without stating clearly whether any contain additional results.[17-19] The RCT had a high withdrawal rate after randomisation. Some people had protocol violations caused by no treadmill test. In all RCTs, withdrawals were more common with pentoxifylline (60/232 [26%] v 38/239 [16%] with placebo; RR 1.63, 95% CI 1.13 to 2.34; ARI 10%, 95% CI 3% to 17%). To allow for these problems, the published analysis performed an intention to treat analysis using "last available observation carried forward". However, the analysis did not include the 33 people with no observations to carry forward, and the effects of the difference in withdrawals between the groups was not explored adequately (e.g. if people with worsening claudication were more likely to withdraw, then the observed differences may be artefactual). The available evidence is not good enough to define clearly the effects of pentoxifylline.

OPTION	PERCUTANEOUS TRANSLUMINAL ANGIOPLASTY (PTA)

One systematic review of two small RCTs found limited evidence that angioplasty versus no angioplasty improved total walking distance in the short term, but had no long term benefits.

Benefits: **Angioplasty versus no angioplasty:** We found one systematic review[22] (search date not stated; 2 RCTs;[23,24] 78 men and 20 women with mild to moderate intermittent claudication [see glossary, p 125]) of percutaneous transluminal angioplasty (PTA) of the aortoiliac or femoral-popliteal arteries versus no angioplasty. The first RCT found that angioplasty versus no angioplasty significantly increased the median claudicating distance after 6 months (667 m v 172 m; P < 0.05), but after 2 years the difference was no longer significant and there were no significant differences in quality of life measures.[23] The second RCT[24] found that angioplasty versus an exercise programme significantly increased the absolute claudication distance (see glossary, p 125) at 6 months (130 m v 50 m; WMD 80 m), but after 6 years the difference was not significant (180 m v 130 m; WMD 50 m; P > 0.05).[25] **Angioplasty versus stents:** We found no systematic review, but we found two RCTs.[26,27] The first RCT (279 people) compared angioplasty plus routine stent placement versus angioplasty plus selective stent placement in people with intermittent claudication and iliac artery stenosis.[26] The trial found no significant difference in short or long term patency rates. The second RCT (51 people with symptomatic femoral-popliteal disease) compared angioplasty plus selective stent placement versus angioplasty alone.[27] There were no significant differences in primary patency assessed by colour flow duplex ultrasound (62% with angioplasty plus stent v 74% with angioplasty alone; P = 0.22) or in the occlusion rate (5/24 [21%] with angioplasty plus stent v 7% [2/27] with angioplasty alone; P = 0.16).

Harms: Prospective cohort studies have found that PTA complications include puncture site major bleeding (3.4%), pseudoaneurysms (0.5%), limb loss (0.2%), renal failure secondary to intravenous contrast (0.2%), cardiac complications such as MI (0.2%), and death (0.2%).[28,29]

Comment: The limited evidence suggests transient benefit from angioplasty versus no angioplasty. The longer term effects of angioplasty or stent placement on symptoms, bypass surgery, and amputation remain unclear.

OPTION	BYPASS SURGERY

We found only limited evidence from small RCTs using proxy outcomes for the consensus view that bypass surgery is the most effective treatment for people with debilitating symptomatic peripheral arterial disease.

Benefits: **Surgery versus medical treatment:** We found no systematic review and no RCTs on people with atheromatous perihperal vascular disease. **Surgery versus PTA:** We found no systematic review, but we found two RCTs (365 people with chronic progressive peripheral arterial disease) of surgery versus PTA.[30,31] The first RCT (255 people with symptomatic peripheral arterial disease and ≥ 80% stenosis of the iliac, femoral, or popliteal vessels) found that bypass surgery versus PTA had no significant effect on patency rates after 4 years (64% v 68%; P = 0.14) or on overall survival.[30] The second RCT (102 people with rest pain, ischaemia ulcers, or severe intermittent claudication [see glossary, p 125]) found that surgery versus PTA had no significant effect on patency rates after 1 year (62% with surgery v 60% with PTA).[31] **Surgery versus PTA plus stent placement:** We found no RCTs of surgery versus PTA plus stent placement that reported long term harms.

Harms: Surgery versus PTA increased early procedural complications. Among people having aortoiliac surgery, perioperative mortality (within 30 days of the procedure) was 3.3%, and complications having a major health impact occurred in 8.3%.[32] Among people having infrainguinal bypass surgery, perioperative mortality was about 2% and serious complications occurred in 8%.[33] Among people having PTA with or without stent placement, perioperative mortality was about 1% and serious complications occurred in about 5%.[34]

Comment: The RCTs are small, have different follow up periods, and assessed different outcomes. Indirect comparisons from observational studies of proxy outcomes (primary patency rates) suggest that for aortoiliac stenosis or occlusion, greater patency rates 5 years after intervention are achieved with surgery (6250 [89%] people) compared with PTA (1300 [34–85%] people) or compared with combined PTA and stent placement (816 [54–74%] people).[32-34] Too few people with infrainguinal lesions were included in the RCTs to provide good evidence about surgical management. Indirect comparisons of proxy outcomes in people with infrainguinal lesions suggest worse results after PTA (after 5 years patency 38%, range 34–42%) compared with surgery (patency 80%).[35] Although there is consensus that bypass surgery is the most effective treatment for people with debilitating symptomatic peripheral arterial disease, we found inadequate evidence from RCTs reporting long term clinical outcomes to confirm this view.

GLOSSARY

Absolute claudication distance Also known as the total walking distance; the maximum distance a person can walk before stopping.

Ankle–brachial index The ratio of the systolic blood pressure in the leg over the systolic blood pressure in the arm.

Fontaine's classification I: asymptomatic; II: intermittent claudication; II-a: pain free, claudication walking > 200 metres; II-b: pain free, claudication walking < 200 metres; III: rest/nocturnal pain; IV: necrosis/gangrene.

Initial claudication distance The distance a person can walk before the onset of claudication symptoms.

Intermittent claudication Pain, stiffness, or weakness in the leg that develops on walking, intensifies with continued walking until further walking is impossible, and is relieved by rest.

REFERENCES

1. Fowkes FGR, Housely E, Cawood EH, et al. Edinburgh Artery Study: prevalence of asymptomatic and symptomatic peripheral arterial disease in the general population. *Int J Epidemiol* 1991;20:384–392.
2. Kannel WB, McGee DL. Update on some epidemiological features of intermittent claudication. *J Am Geriatr Soc* 1985;33:13–18.
3. Maurabito JM, D'Agostino RB, Sibersschatz, et al. Intermittent claudication: a risk profile from the Framingham Heart Study. *Circulation* 1997;96:44–49.
4. Catalano M. Epidemiology of critical limb ischemia: north Italian data. *Eur J Med* 1993;2:11–14.
5. Ebskov L, Schroeder T, Holstein P. Epidemiology of leg amputation: the influence of vascular surgery. *Br J Surg* 1994;81:1600–1603.
6. Leng GC, Lee AJ, Fowkes FG, et al. Incidence, natural history and cardiovascular events in symptomatic and asymptomatic peripheral arterial disease in the general population. *Int J Epidemiol* 1996;25:1172–181.
7. Antiplatelet Trialists' Collaborative overview of randomized trials of antiplatelet therapy. I: prevention of death, myocardial infarction, and stroke by prolonged antiplatelet therapy in various categories of patients. *BMJ* 1994;308:81–106. Search date 1990; primary sources Medline, Current Contents, hand searches of reference lists of trials and review articles, journal abstracts and meeting proceedings, trial register of the International Committee on Thrombosis and Haemostasis, and personal contacts with colleagues and antiplatelet manufacturers.
8. Girolami B, Bernardi E, Prins MH, et al. Antithrombotic drugs in the primary medical management of intermittent claudication: a meta-analysis. *Thromb Haemost* 1999;81:715–722. Search date 1998; primary sources Medline and hand searches.
9. Antiplatelet Trialists' Collaboration overview of randomized trials of antiplatelet therapy. I: prevention of death, myocardial infarction, and stroke by prolonged antiplatelet therapy in various categories of patients. Antithrombotic Trialists Conference, Oxford, UK, September 1997.
10. CAPRIE Steering Committee. A randomized, blinded, trial of clopidogrel versus aspirin in patients at risk of ischemic events (CAPRIE). *Lancet* 1996;348:1329–1339.
11. Girolami B, Bernardi E, Prins M, et al. Treatment of intermittent claudication with physical training, smoking cessation, pentoxifylline, or nafronyl: a meta-analysis. *Arch Intern Med* 1999;159:337–345. Search date 1996; primary sources Medline and hand searches of reference lists.
12. Leng GC, Fowler B, Ernst E. Exercise for intermittent claudication In: The Cochrane Library, Issue 3, 2000. Oxford: Update Software. Search date not stated; primary sources Cochrane Peripheral Vascular Diseases Group trials register, Embase, reference lists of relevant articles, and personal contact with principal investigators of trials.
13. Walker RD, Nawaz S, Wilkinson CH, Saxton JM, Pockley AG, Wood RF. Influence of upper- and lower-limb exercise training on cardiovascular function and walking distances in patients with intermittent claudication. *J Vasc Surg* 2000;31:662–669.
14. Gardner A, Poehlman E. Exercise rehabilitation programs for the treatment of claudication pain. *JAMA* 1995;274:975–980. Search date 1993; primary sources Medline and hand searches of bibliographies of reviews, textbooks, and studies located through the computer search.
15. Radack K, Wyderski RJ. Conservative management in intermittent claudication. *Ann Intern Med* 1990;113:135–146. Search date 1989; primary sources Index Medicus, Medline, textbooks, and experts.
16. Dawson DL, Cutler BS, Hiatt WR, et al. A comparison of cilostazol and pentoxifylline for treating intermittent claudication. *Am J Med* 2000;109:523–530.
17. Money SR, Herd A, Isaacsohn JL, et al. Effect of cilostazol on walking distances in patients with intermittent claudication cause by peripheral vascular disease. *J Vasc Surg* 1998;27:267–275.
18. Beebe HG, Dawson D, Cutler B, et al A new pharmacological treatment for intermittent claudication. *Arch Intern Med* 1999;159:2041–2050.
19. Dawson D, Cutler B, Meeisner M, Strandness E. Cilostazol has beneficial effects in treatment of intermittent claudication. *Circulation* 1998;98:678–686.
20. Hiatt WR. Medical treatment of peripheral arterial disease and claudication. *N Engl J Med* 2001;344:1608–1621.

21. Hood S, Moher D, Barber G. Management of intermittent claudication with pentoxifylline: a meta-analysis of randomized controlled trials. *Can Med Assoc J* 1996;155:1053–1059. Search date 1994; primary sources Medline and hand searches of references lists.

22. Fowkes FG, Gillespie IN. Angioplasty (versus non surgical management) for intermittent claudication. In: The Cochrane Library, Issue 3, 2000. Oxford: Update Software. Search date not stated; primary sources Cochrane Peripheral Vascular Diseases Group Trials Register, Embase, reference lists of relevant articles and conference proceedings, and personal contact with principal investigators of trials.

23. Whyman MR, Fowkes FGR, Kerracher EMG, et al. Randomized controlled trial of percutaneous transluminal angioplasty for intermittent claudication. *Eur J Vasc Endovasc Surg* 1996;12: 167–172.

24. Creasy TS, McMillan PJ, Fletcher EWL, Collin J, Morris PJ. Is percutaneous transluminal angioplasty better than exercise for claudication? Preliminary results of a prospective randomized trial. *Eur J Vasc Surg* 1990;4:135–140.

25. Perkins JMT, Collin J, Creasy TS, Fletcher EWL, Morris PJ. Exercise training versus angioplasty for stable claudication. Long and medium term results of a prospective, randomized trial. *Eur J Vasc Endovasc Surg* 1996;11:409–413.

26. Teteroo E, van der Graef Y, Bosch J, et al. Randomized comparison of primary stent placement versus primary angioplasty followed by selective stent placement in patients with iliac artery occlusive disease. *Lancet* 1998;351: 1153–1159.

27. Vroegindeweij D, Vos L, Tielbeek A, et al. Balloon angioplasty combined with primary stenting versus balloon angioplasty alone in femoropopliteal obstructions: a comparative randomized study. *Cardiovasc Intervent Radiol* 1997;20:420–425.

28. Becker GJ, Katzen BT, Dake MD. Noncoronary angioplasty. *Radiology* 1989;170:921–940.

29. Matsi PJ, Manninen HI. Complications of lower-limb percutaneous transluminal angioplasty: a prospective analysis of 410 procedures on 295 consecutive patients. *Cardiovasc Intervent Radiol* 1998;21:361–366.

30. Wilson SE, Wolf G, Cross AP. Percutaneous transluminal angioplasty versus operation for peripheral arteriosclerosis. *J Vasc Surg* 1989;9: 1–9.

31. Holm J, Arfvidsson B, Jivegard L, et al. Chronic lower limb ischemia. *Eur J Vasc Surg* 1991;5: 517–522.

32. De Vries SO, Hunink MG. Results of aortic bifurcation grafts for aortoiliac occlusive disease: a meta-analysis. *J Vasc Surg* 1997;26:558–569. Search date 1996; primary sources Medline and hand searches of review articles, original studies, and a vascular surgery textbook.

33. Johnston KW, Rae M, Hogg-Johnston SA, et al. Five-year results of a prospective study of percutaneous transluminal angioplasty. *Ann Surg* 1987;206:403–413.

34. Bosch J, Hunink M. Meta-analysis of the results of percutaneous transluminal angioplasty and stent placement for aortoiliac occlusive disease. *Radiology* 1997;204:87–96. Search date not stated; primary sources Medline and hand searches of reference lists.

35. Johnson KW. Femoral and popliteal arteries: reanalysis of results of balloon angioplasty. *Radiology* 1992;183:767–771.

Sonia Anand
Assistant Professor of Medicine
McMaster University
Hamilton
Canada

Mark Creager
Associate Professor of Medicine
Harvard Medical School
Boston
USA

Competing interests: None declared.

TABLE 1 Cilostazol 200 mg daily versus placebo (see text, pp 121, 122).

Ref	Duration (weeks)	Number of people				People self rated as worsened, unchanged, or unsure	Absolute claudication distance (m)	Initial claudication distance (m)
		Randomised	Protocol violation	Withdrawn				
16	24	466	35	64		47/205 (23%) v 68/226 (30%); RR 0.76 (95% CI 0.55 to 1.05)	350 v 300 (P < 0.001)	218 v 180 (P = 0.02)
17	16	298	59	27		53/119 (45%) v 78/120 (65%); RR 0.68 (95% CI 0.54 to 0.87)	333 v 281	NA
18	24	516	23	75		80/171 (47%) v 106/169 (63%); RR 0.75 (95% CI 0.61 to 0.91)	259 v 175 (P < 0.001)	138 v 96 (P < 0.001)
19	12	81	4	15		27/54 (50%) v 22/27 (81%); RR 0.61 (95% CI 0.45 to 0.85)	113 v 85 (P = 0.007)	232 v 152 (P = 0.002)

m, metres; NA, not available; ref, reference.

TABLE 2 Systematic reviews and a subsequent RCT of pentoxifylline versus placebo (see text, p 122).

Ref	Number of RCTs (people)	Initial claudication distance in metres (WMD)	Absolute claudication distance in metres (WMD)
11	13 (600)	21 (95% CI 0.7 to 41)	44 (95% CI 14 to 74)
16	1 (471)	22 (95% CI NA)	8 (95% CI NA)
21	11 (612)	29 (95% CI 13 to 46)	48 (95% CI 18 to 79)

NA, not available; ref, reference; WMD, weighted mean difference.

Search date December 2000

Clinical Evidence writers on primary prevention

Cardiovascular disorders

Key Messages

Exercise

- Observational studies have found that moderate to high physical activity reduces coronary heart disease (CHD) and stroke. They also found that sudden death after strenuous exercise was rare, more common in sedentary people, and did not outweigh the benefits.

Diet

- Observational studies have found that consumption of fruit and vegetables is associated with reduced ischaemic vascular disease.
- RCTs found no evidence that β carotene supplements are effective and have found that they may be harmful.
- We found insufficient evidence to support antioxidant supplements in healthy people.

Smoking

- Observational studies have found a strong association between smoking and overall mortality and ischaemic vascular disease.
- Several large cohort studies have found that the increased risk associated with smoking falls after stopping smoking.

SPECIFIC INTERVENTIONS

In people with raised blood pressure

- We found prospective evidence that lifestyle interventions reduce blood pressure but insufficient evidence that these interventions reduce mortality or morbidity.
- Systematic reviews have found good evidence that drug treatment reduces blood pressure.
- Trials of drug treatment have found a greater reduction in blood pressure compared with trials of lifestyle changes, although we found no head to head comparisons.
- Systematic reviews have found that the main determinant of benefit of treatment for hypertension is the pretreatment absolute cardiovascular disease risk.
- The evidence of beneficial effects on mortality and morbidity is strongest for diuretics, β blockers, and ACE inhibitors.
- We found no direct evidence on effects of lowering blood pressure beyond 140/80 mmHg.
- Systematic reviews have found that, in people over age 60 years with systolic blood pressures greater than 160 mmHg, lowering systolic blood pressure decreased total mortality and fatal and non-fatal cardiovascular events.

Antithrombotic drugs

- We found insufficient evidence to identify which asymptomatic individuals would benefit overall and which would be harmed by regular treatment with aspirin.
- One RCT found that the benefits and harms of oral anticoagulation among individuals without symptoms of cardiovascular disease were finely balanced and that net effects were uncertain.

Primary prevention

To lower cholesterol

- Systematic reviews have found that reducing cholesterol concentration in asymptomatic people lowers the rate of cardiovascular events but found no evidence that cholesterol reduction by any method reduces overall death rate in people at low baseline risk of cardiovascular events.

- Systematic reviews and RCTs have found that combined use of cholesterol lowering diet and lipid lowering drugs reduces cholesterol concentration more than lifestyle interventions alone.

DEFINITION Primary prevention in this context is the long term management of people at increased risk but with no evidence of cardiovascular disease. Clinically overt ischaemic vascular disease includes acute myocardial infarction (AMI), angina, stroke, and peripheral vascular disease. Many adults have no symptoms or obvious signs of vascular disease, even though they have atheroma and are at increased risk of ischaemic vascular events because of one or more risk factors (see aetiology below).

INCIDENCE/ In the USA, about 42% of all deaths are from vascular disease. AMI
PREVALENCE and its sequelae remain the most common single cause of death.

AETIOLOGY/ Identified major risk factors for ischaemic vascular disease include
RISK FACTORS increasing age, male sex, raised low density lipoprotein cholesterol, reduced high density lipoprotein cholesterol, raised blood pressure, smoking, diabetes, family history of cardiovascular disease, obesity, and sedentary lifestyle. For many of these risk factors, observational studies show a continuous gradient of increasing risk of cardio-vascular disease with increasing levels of the risk factor, with no obvious threshold level. Although by definition event rates are higher in high risk people, of all ischaemic vascular events that occur in the population, most occur in people with intermediate levels of absolute risk because there are many more of them than there are people at high risk; see appendix 1.[1]

PROGNOSIS About half of people who suffer an AMI die within 28 days, and two thirds of AMIs occur before the person reaches hospital.[2] The benefits of intervention in unselected people with no evidence of cardiovascular disease (primary prevention) are small because in such people the baseline risk is small. However, absolute risk of ischaemic vascular events varies dramatically, even among people with similar levels of blood pressure or cholesterol. Estimates of absolute risk can be based on simple risk equations or tables (see appendix 1).[3,4]

AIMS To reduce mortality and morbidity from cardiovascular disease, with minimum adverse effects.

OUTCOMES Incidence of fatal and non-fatal cardiovascular events (including coronary, cerebrovascular, renal, and eye disease, and heart fail-ure). Surrogate outcomes include changes in levels of individual risk factors, such as blood pressure.

METHODS *Clinical Evidence* search and appraisal December 2000.

QUESTION Does physical activity reduce the risk of vascular events in asymptomatic people?

Charles Foster and Michael Murphy

We found strong observational evidence that moderate to high levels of physical activity reduce the risk of non-fatal and fatal CHD and stroke. People who are physically active (those who undertake moderate levels of activity daily or almost daily) typically experience 30–50% reductions in relative risk of CHD compared with people who are sedentary, after adjustment for other risk factors. The absolute risk of sudden death after strenuous activity is small (although greatest in people who are habitually sedentary) and does not outweigh observed benefits.

Benefits: **Effects of physical activity on CHD:** We found no RCTs. Three systematic reviews (search date 1995,[5] and not stated[6,7]) evaluated observational studies and found increased risk of CHD in sedentary compared with active people. Since 1992, 17 large, well conducted prospective, non-randomised studies, with follow up periods ranging from 18 months to 29 years, have specifically examined the association between physical activity and risk of non-fatal or fatal CHD.[8-24] The studies found that risk declined with increasing levels of physical activity (for examples of activity levels see table 1, p 155) (AR for CHD death in people with sedentary lives [rare or no physical activity] 70 per 10 000 person years v 40 per 10 000 person years in people with the highest level of activity [> 3500 kcal per week], absolute benefit of high levels of physical activity 30 lives saved per 10 000 person years). **Effects of physical fitness on CHD:** We found no RCTs. One systematic review (search date not stated) identified seven large, well designed prospective, non-randomised studies of the effects of physical fitness on CHD.[25] All used reproducible measures of physical fitness. Five studies adjusted for other CHD risk factors. These found an increased risk of death from CHD in people with low levels of physical fitness compared with those with high levels (RR of death lowest quartile v highest quartile ranged from 1.2 to 4.0). Most studies reported only baseline measures of physical fitness, thus not accounting for changes in fitness. One recent large follow up study found lower risk among people who increased their fitness level (RR for CVD death compared with those whose level of fitness did not change 0.48, 95% CI 0.31 to 0.74).[26] **Effects of physical activity on stroke:** We found no RCTs and no systematic review of observational studies. We found 12 observational studies (published between 1990 and 1999), based on 3680 strokes among North American, Japanese, and European populations.[27-40] Most of these found that moderate activity was associated with reduced risk of stroke compared with inactivity (RR of stroke, moderate activity v inactivity about 0.5). One cohort study from Japan found that "heavy" physical activity reduced the risk of stroke compared with "moderate" activity (RR of stroke, "heavy" v "moderate" activity about 0.3; P < 0.05).[38] In most studies, the benefits were greater in older people and in men. Most studies were conducted in white men in late middle age, which potentially limits their applicability to other groups of people. The results usually persisted after adjustment for other known risk factors for stroke (blood pressure, blood lipids, body mass index, and smoking) and after exclusion of people with pre-existing diseases that might limit physical activity and increase risk of stroke. The more recent studies found maximum reduction in the risk of stroke with moderate as opposed to high levels of physical exercise levels.

Harms: No direct evidence of harm was reported in the studies described. We found two studies in people who had experienced non-fatal myocardial infarction, conducted in the USA and Germany. Each involved more than 1000 events and found that 4–7% of these events occurred within 1 hour of strenuous physical activity.[41-43] Strenuous activity was estimated to have raised the relative risk of AMI between two and sixfold in the hour after activity, with risks returning to baseline after that. However, the absolute risk remained low, variously estimated at six deaths per 100 000 middle aged men a year[44] or 0.3 to 2.7 events per 10 000 person hours of exercise.[45] Both studies found that the relative risk of AMI after strenuous activity was much higher in people who were habitually sedentary (RR 107, 95% CI 67 to 171) compared with the relative risk in those who engaged in heavy physical exertion on five or more occasions per week (RR 2.4, 95% CI 1.5 to 3.7).[41] Injury is likely to be the most common adverse event, but we found too few population data to quantify its risk.

Comment: Findings from these observational studies should be interpreted with caution. The studies varied in definitions of levels of activity and fitness. The level of activity or fitness experienced by each participant was not experimentally assigned by an investigator (as in an RCT) but resulted from self selection. Active (or fit) participants are likely to differ from inactive (or unfit) participants in other ways that also influence their risk of cardiovascular disease. Confounding of this type can be partially controlled by adjustment for other known risk factors (such as age, smoking status, and body mass index), but it is likely that some residual confounding will remain, which could overestimate the effect of exercise. The studies have found that the absolute risk of sudden death during or immediately after physical activity is small and does not outweigh the observed benefits.

QUESTION	What intensity and frequency of physical activity improves fitness?

Charles Foster and Michael Murphy

Small RCTs have found that at least moderate intensity exercise (equivalent to brisk walking) is necessary to improve fitness. We found insufficient evidence on the effects of short bouts of exercise several times a day compared with longer daily bouts.

Benefits: **Intensity:** We found no systematic review. Numerous small RCTs of varying quality have been conducted in different subpopulations. In general, these found that over a period of 6–12 months, low intensity activity programmes produced no measurable changes in maximum oxygen consumption (Vo_2max), whereas moderate intensity activity programmes (equivalent to brisk walking) typically produced improvements, of 20% in oxygen consumption in sedentary people. Table 1, p 155 gives the intensity of effort required for a range of physical activities. Two recent RCTs compared structured aerobic exercise (such as step classes and aerobics classes) with lifestyle activity programmes (such as regular walking and using stairs instead of elevators) among obese women[46] and sedentary men and women.[47] Both studies reported similar, significant changes in measures of cardiovascular fitness and blood pressure with each intervention, and these changes were sustained for at least 2 years after intervention. One prospective follow up study of women previously involved in a randomised trial of physical activity found that women who start a programme of regular walking maintain higher levels of physical activity 10 years after the intervention.[48] **Frequency:** We found no systematic review. One RCT (36 men) compared 8 weeks of a single daily session of 30 minutes of exercise versus three daily sessions of 10 minutes each.[49] It found no significant difference in fitness benefit between groups.

Harms: None reported.

Comment: None.

| QUESTION | What are the effects of dietary interventions on the risk of heart attack and stroke in asymptomatic people? |

Andy Ness

| OPTION | EATING MORE FRUIT AND VEGETABLES |

Cohort studies have found that eating more fruit and vegetables reduces the risk of heart attack and stroke. The size and nature of any real protective effect is uncertain.

Benefits: **Ischaemic heart disease:** We found no RCTs. We found three systematic reviews of observational studies.[50-52] With addition of recently published studies[53-60] to those reported in the first review,[50] a protective association was observed for ischaemic heart disease in 13 of 24 cohort studies. In the second review, the authors calculated a summary measure of the protective association of 15% between those above the 90th centile and those below the 10th centile for fruit and vegetable consumption.[51] In the third review the authors estimated that increased intake of fruit and vegetables of about 150 g a day was associated with a reduced risk of CHD of between 20–40%.[52] The validity of these estimates has been questioned. One large, high quality cohort study found that eating more vegetables was associated with decreased coronary mortality ($\geq$ 117 g vegetables per day v < 61 g vegetables per day RRR 34%, 95% CI 4% to 54%); for fruit, the association was more modest and not significant ($\geq$ 159 g fruit per day v < 75 g fruit per day RRR +23, 95% CI −12% to +46%).[61] **Stroke:** We found no RCTs but we found two systematic reviews examining the evidence from observational studies for stroke.[50,52] With addition of recently published studies[53,58,62-67] to those reported in the first review,[50] a protective association was observed in 10 of 16 cohort studies for stroke. In the second review the authors estimated that increased intake of fruit and vegetables of about 150 g a day was associated

Primary prevention

with a reduced risk of stroke of 0–25%.[52] The basis for this estimate is not clear. One large, high quality cohort study in US health professionals found that increased fruit and vegetable intake was associated with a decreased risk of ischaemic stroke (RRR per daily serving of fruit and vegetables 6%, 95% CI 1% to 10%; RRR in the fifth of the population eating the most fruit and vegetables v the fifth eating the least 31%, 95% CI 8% to 48%).[68]

Harms: None were identified.

Comment: Lack of trial evidence and deficiencies in the data available from observational studies mean that the size and nature of any real protective effect is uncertain.[69,70] The observed associations could be the result of confounding as people who eat more fruit and vegetables often come from higher socioeconomic groups and adopt other healthy lifestyles.[71]

OPTION   **ANTIOXIDANTS**

We found no evidence of benefit from β carotene supplements, and RCTs suggest that they may be harmful. Other antioxidant supplements may be beneficial, but we found insufficient trial evidence to support their use.

Benefits: **β Carotene:** We found one systematic review of prospective studies and RCTs (search date not stated, published in 1997), which did not pool data because of heterogeneity among studies.[72] Most prospective cohort studies of β carotene found a modest protective association with increased intake,[72-75] although several large trials of β carotene supplementation found no evidence of benefit.[75,76] **Vitamin C:** We found two systematic reviews,[72,77] which mostly included the same studies, and seven subsequent prospective studies.[57,63,67,69,78-80] Three of 14 cohort studies found a significant protective association between vitamin C and CHD, and two of 11 studies found a protective association between vitamin C and stroke. We found no large trials of vitamin C supplementation alone. Two large trials of multivitamin supplements have been carried out in Linxian, China.[72,81-83] One trial (that was included in the reviews) was carried out in 29 584 participants drawn from the general population who were randomised by using a factorial design to one of four arms: arm A–retinol (10 000 IU) and zinc (22.5 mg); arm B–riboflavin (5.2 mg) and niacin (40 mg); arm C–ascorbic acid (120 mg) and molybdenum (30 μg); arm D–carotene (15 mg), selenium (50 μg), and vitamin E (30 mg). After 6 years the trial found that the treatment assigned to people in arm D reduced all cause mortality and death due to stroke (RRR for death from any cause arm D v other arms 9%, 95% CI 1% to 16%). It found no reduction in stroke or all cause mortality among the other arms.[72] The other trial (subsequent to the reviews) included 3318 people with oesophageal dysplasia who were randomised to placebo or a multivitamin supplement that contained 14 vitamins and 12 minerals, including vitamin C (180 mg), vitamin E (60 IU [1 IU = 0.67 mg]), β carotene (15 mg), and selenium (50 μg). After 6 years it found that the supplement did not significantly reduce stroke or death from all causes (RRR for all cause mortality 7%, 95% CI –16% to +25%; RRR for stroke 33%, 95% CI –7% to

+63%).[81,82] **Vitamin E:** We found one systematic review and additional prospective studies.[72] Eight large cohort studies (5 of which were included in the review) have examined the association between vitamin E intake and ischaemic heart disease. Six found a significant protective association,[72,78,84] whereas two found no significant association.[57,85] In three studies the protective association was with dietary vitamin E.[72,82] In the others it was either wholly or mainly with vitamin E supplements.[72,85] In the review, the largest RCT of vitamin E alone versus placebo (in 29 133 Finnish smokers) found that vitamin E did not significantly reduce mortality compared with placebo (RRR for death 2%, 95% CI −9% to +5%) after 5–8 years. (See above for the results of the Linxian trials.)[72,81-83] Four cohort studies found no association between vitamin E intake and stroke.[67,79,80,86] **Antioxidant minerals:** We found little epidemiological evidence about the cardioprotective effect of copper, zinc, or manganese on the heart.[87] Cohort studies reported an increased risk of ischaemic heart disease in people with low blood selenium concentrations.[86] Most of these were carried out in Finland, a country with low intakes of antioxidants.[89] (See also the results of the Linxian trials.)[71,79-81] **Flavonoids:** We found no systematic review. We found five cohort studies,[65,89-92] three of which reported a reduced risk of ischaemic heart disease with increased flavonoid intake.[65,89,90] One of four observational studies reported a reduced risk of stroke with increased flavonoid intake.[65-67,86]

Harms: Several large trials found that β carotene supplements may increase cardiovascular mortality (pooled data from four RCTs, RRI for cardiovascular death 12%, 95% CI 4% to 22%).[75] Explanations for these results include use of the wrong isomer, the wrong dose, or a detrimental effect on other carotenoid levels.[93,94]

Comment: Trials of antioxidants such as β carotene and vitamin E have not produced any evidence of benefit. Routine use of antioxidant supplements is not justified by the currently available evidence. More trials of antioxidant supplementation are under way.[95]

<hr>

QUESTION **By how much does smoking cessation, or avoidance of starting smoking, reduce risk?**

Julian J Nicholas and Thomas Kottke

Observational studies have found that cigarette smoking is strongly related to overall mortality. We found evidence from both observational and randomised studies that cigarette smoking increases the risk of CHD and stroke. The evidence is strongest for stroke.

Benefits: Several large cohort studies examining the effects of smoking have been extensively reviewed by the US surgeon general[96] and the UK Royal College of Physicians.[97] The reviews concluded that cigarette smoking was causally related to disease and that smoking cessation substantially reduced the risk of cancer, respiratory disease, CHD, and stroke. **Death from all causes:** The longest prospective cohort study, in 34 439 male British doctors whose smoking habits were periodically assessed over 40 years (1951–1991), found a strong association between smoking and increased mortality. It found that smokers were about three times more likely to die in middle age (45–64 years) and twice as likely to die in older age (65–84 years) compared with lifelong non-smokers (95% CIs not given).[98] The prospective nurses' health study followed 117 001 middle aged female nurses for 12 years. It found that the total mortality in current smokers was nearly twice that in lifelong non-smokers (RR of death 1.87, 95% CI 1.65 to 2.13).[99] **CHD:** One review (published in 1990) identified 10 cohort studies, involving 20 million person years of observation.[96] All studies found a higher incidence of CHD among smokers (pooled RR of death from CHD compared with non-smokers 1.7, 95% CI not available).[96] People smoking more than 20 cigarettes a day were more likely to have a coronary event (RR 2.5, 95% CI not given).[97] Middle aged smokers were more likely to experience a first non-fatal AMI compared with people who had never smoked (RR in men 2.9, 95% CI 2.4 to 3.4; RR in women 3.6, 95% CI 3.0 to 4.4).[100,101] One RCT of advice encouraging smoking cessation in 1445 men aged 40–59 years found that more men given advice to stop smoking gave up cigarettes (mean absolute reduction in men continuing to smoke after advice v control 53%). The trial found no evidence that men given advice to stop had a significantly lower mortality from CHD (RRR 18%, 95% CI −18% to +43%).[102] The wide confidence intervals mean that there could have been anything from a 43% decrease to an 18% increase in rates of CHD death in men given advice to quit, regardless of whether they actually gave up smoking. **Stroke:** One systematic review (published in 1989) found 32 studies (17 cohort studies with concurrent or historical controls, 14 case control studies, and one hypertension intervention trial). It found good evidence that smoking was associated with an increased risk of stroke (RR of stroke in cigarette smokers v non-smokers 1.5, 95% CI 1.4 to 1.6).[103] Smoking was associated with an increased risk of cerebral infarction (RR 1.92, 95% CI 1.71 to 2.16) and subarachnoid haemorrhage (RR 2.93, 95% CI 2.48 to 3.46), but no increased risk of intracerebral haemorrhage (RR 0.74, 95% CI 0.56 to 0.98). The relative risk of stroke in smokers versus non-smokers was highest in those aged under 55 years (RR 2.9, 95% CI 2.40 to 3.59) and lowest in those aged over 74 years (RR 1.11, 95% CI 0.96 to 1.28).

Harms: We found no evidence that stopping smoking increases mortality in any subgroup of smokers.

Comment: We found no evidence of publication or other overt bias that may explain the observed association between smoking and stroke. There was a dose-response curve between the number of cigarettes smoked and the relative risk for stroke, consistent with a causal relation. The absolute risk reduction from stopping smoking will be highest for those with the highest absolute risk of vascular events.

QUESTION **How quickly do risks diminish when smokers stop smoking?**

Julian J Nicholas

Observational studies have found that the risk of death and cardiovascular events falls when people stop smoking. The risk can take many years to approach that of non-smokers, particularly in those with a history of heavy smoking.

Benefits: **Death from all causes:** In people who stopped smoking, observational studies found that death rates fell gradually to lie between those of lifelong smokers and people who had never smoked. Estimates for the time required for former smokers to bring their risk of death in line with people who had never smoked varied among studies but may be longer than 15 years.[104] Actuarial projections from one study among British doctors predicted that life expectancy would improve even among people who stopped smoking in later life (65 years and over).[98] **CHD:** Observational studies found that, in both male and female ex-smokers, the risk of coronary events rapidly declined to a level comparable with that of people who had never smoked after 2–3 years and was independent of the number of cigarettes smoked before quitting.[96] **Stroke:** The US surgeon general's review of observational studies found that the risk of stroke decreased in ex-smokers compared with smokers (RR of stroke, smokers v ex-smokers 1.2, 95% CI not available) but remained raised for 5–10 years after cessation compared with those who had never smoked (RR of stroke ex-smokers v never smokers 1.5, 95% CI not available).[96] One recent study in 7735 middle aged British men found that 5 years after smoking cessation the risk of stroke in previously light smokers (< 20 cigarettes per day) was identical to that of lifelong non-smokers, but the risk in previously heavy smokers (> 21 cigarettes per day) was still raised compared with lifelong non-smokers (RR of stroke, previously heavy smokers v never smokers 2.2, 95% CI 1.1 to 4.3).[105] One observational study in 117 001 middle aged female nurses also found a fall in risk on stopping smoking and found no difference between previously light and previously heavy smokers (RR in all former smokers 2–4 years after stopping smoking 1.17, 95% CI 0.49 to 2.23).[99]

Harms: We found no evidence that stopping smoking increases mortality in any subgroup of smokers.

Comment: For a review of the evidence on methods of changing smoking behaviour, see secondary prevention of ischaemic cardiac events, p 160.

QUESTION **What are the effects of lifestyle changes in asymptomatic people with primary hypertension?**

Cindy Mulrow

OPTION **PHYSICAL ACTIVITY**

One systematic review of RCTs has found that aerobic exercise reduces blood pressure (see table 2, p 156).

Benefits: We found no RCTs examining the effects of exercise on morbidity, mortality, or quality of life. One systematic review (search date 1996, 29 RCTs, 1533 sedentary adults with normal blood pressure, age 18–79 years) examined the effects on blood pressure of at least 4 weeks of regular aerobic exercise versus no exercise.[106] Exercise regimens included walking, jogging, cycling, or both, often lasting 45–60 minutes a session, for 3 days a week (mean exercise intensity about 60–70% of Vo_2max). Compared with non-exercising control groups, groups randomised to aerobic exercise reduced their systolic blood pressure by 4.7 mm Hg (95% CI 4.4 to 5.0 mm Hg) and diastolic blood pressure by 3.1 mm Hg (95% CI 3.0 to 3.3 mm Hg). Greater reductions were seen in people with higher initial blood pressures. Trials with interventions lasting longer than 6 months' duration in adults aged 45 years or over with hypertension found smaller mean reductions in blood pressure but with wide confidence intervals (systolic reduction 0.8 mm Hg, 95% CI 5.9 mm Hg reduction to 4.2 mm Hg increase).[107]

Harms: Musculoskeletal injuries may occur, but their frequency was not documented.

Comment: Many adults find aerobic exercise programmes difficult to sustain. The clinical significance of the observed reductions in blood pressure is uncertain. The type and amount of exercise most likely to result in benefits are unclear, with some recent studies showing some benefits with simple increases in lifestyle activity. One cohort study in 173 men with hypertension found that "regular heavy activity several times weekly" compared with no or limited spare time physical activity reduced all cause and cardiovascular mortality (all cause mortality RR 0.43, 95% CI 0.22 to 0.82; cardiovascular mortality RR 0.33, 95% CI 0.11 to 0.94).[108]

| OPTION | LOW FAT, HIGH FRUIT AND VEGETABLE DIET |

One RCT has found that a low fat, high fruit and vegetable diet modestly reduced blood pressure (see table 2, p 156).

Benefits: We found no systematic review and no RCTs examining the effects of low fat, high fruit and vegetable diet on morbidity or mortality in people with primary hypertension. For evidence from cohort studies in asymptomatic people in general see. One RCT (459 adults with systolic blood pressures of < 160 mm Hg and diastolic blood pressures of 80–90 mm Hg) compared effects on blood pressure of three diets (control diet low in both magnesium and potassium v fruit and vegetable diet high in both potassium and magnesium v combination of the fruit and vegetable diet with a low fat diet high in both calcium and protein).[109] After 8 weeks the fruit and vegetable diet reduced systolic and diastolic blood pressure compared with the control diet (mean change in systolic blood pressure −2.8 mm Hg, 97.5% CI −4.7 to −0.9 mm Hg; mean change in diastolic blood pressure −1.1 mm Hg, 97.5% CI −2.4 mm Hg to +0.3 mm Hg). The combination diet also reduced systolic and diastolic blood pressure compared with the control diet (mean change in systolic blood pressure −5.5 mm Hg, 97.5% CI −7.4 mm Hg to −3.7 mm Hg; mean change in diastolic blood pressure −3.0 mm Hg, 97.5% CI −4.3 to −1.6 mm Hg).

Harms: We found no direct evidence that a low fat, high fruit and vegetable diet is harmful.

Comment: The trial was of short duration and participants were supplied with food during the intervention period.[109] Other studies have found that long term maintenance of particular diets is difficult for many people, although low fat, high fruit and vegetable diets may have multiple benefits (see changing behaviour, p 38).

OPTION   REDUCED ALCOHOL CONSUMPTION

One systematic review of RCTs found inconclusive evidence regarding effects of alcohol reduction on blood pressure.

Benefits: We found no RCTs examining the effects of reducing alcohol consumption on morbidity or mortality. Over 60 population studies have reported associations between alcohol consumption and blood pressure; the relation was found to be generally linear, although several studies reported a threshold effect at about two to three standard drinks a day.[110] Any adverse effect of up to two drinks a day on blood pressure was found to be either small or non-existent. One systematic review of seven trials in 751 people with hypertension (mainly men) found that data were inconclusive on the benefits of reducing alcohol among moderate to heavy drinkers (25–50 drinks weekly).[111]

Harms: We found no direct evidence that reducing alcohol intake to as few as two drinks a day was harmful.

Comment: Most data were from observational studies. RCTs were small and lacked reliable information about adherence. Substantial reductions in alcohol use in both control and intervention groups were observed, with limited ability to detect differences between groups.

OPTION   SALT RESTRICTION

One systematic review of RCTs has found that salt restriction may lead to modest reductions in blood pressure, with more benefit in people older than 45 years than in younger people (see table 2, p 156).

Benefits: We found no RCT examining the effects of salt restriction on morbidity or mortality. We found one systematic review (search date 1997, 58 trials, 2161 people with hypertension, age 23–73 years)[112] and one subsequent RCT (875 men and women with hypertension, age 60–80 years, duration 30 months),[113] which examined the effects of salt restriction on blood pressure. Interventions were low salt diets, with or without weight reduction. People in the control groups took their usual diet. Changes in salt intake varied among trials in the systematic review; a mean reduction in sodium intake of 118 mmol (6.7 g) a day for 28 days led to reductions of 3.9 mm Hg (95% CI 3.0 to 4.8 mm Hg) in systolic blood pressure and 1.9 mm Hg (95% CI 1.3 to 2.5 mm Hg) in diastolic blood pressure.[112] The subsequent RCT in elderly people found that a mean decrease in salt intake of about 40 mmol (2.35 g) a day reduced systolic blood pressure by 2.6 mm Hg (95% CI 0.4 to 4.8 mm Hg) and diastolic blood pressure by 1.1 mm Hg (95% CI 0.3 mm Hg rise in diastolic to 2.5 mm Hg fall). An earlier systematic review (search date 1994) identified 28 RCTs in 1131 people with hypertension. It found that lesser reductions of 60 mmol per day led to smaller reductions in systolic/diastolic blood pressure of 2.2 mm Hg/0.5 mm Hg and found greater effects in trials, in which mean age was over 45 years (6.3/2.2 mm Hg).[114]

Harms: We found no direct evidence that low salt diets may increase morbidity or mortality. Epidemiological data conflict, with one observational study suggesting that very low salt intakes may be associated with increased incidence of myocardial infarction in middle aged men.[115]

Comment: Small trials tended to report larger reductions in systolic and diastolic blood pressure than larger trials. This is consistent with publication bias or less rigorous methodology in small trials.[114]

OPTION   SMOKING CESSATION

Epidemiological data clearly identify that smoking is a significant risk factor for cardiovascular disease (see question, p 135). We found no direct evidence that stopping smoking decreases blood pressure in people with hypertension.

Benefits: We found no direct evidence that stopping smoking reduces blood pressure in people with hypertension, although we found good evidence that, in general, smoking cessation reduces risk of cardiovascular disease (see question, p 135).

Harms: We found insufficient evidence in this context.

Comment: None.

OPTION   WEIGHT LOSS

One systematic review and additional RCTs have found that modest weight reductions of 3–9% of body weight are achievable in motivated middle aged and older adults, and may lead to modest reductions in blood pressure in obese people with hypertension. Many adults find it difficult to maintain weight loss (see table 2, p 156).

Benefits: We found no RCTs examining the effects of weight loss on morbidity and mortality. We found one systematic review (published in 1998, 18 RCTs, 2611 middle aged people, mean age 50 years, mean weight 85 kg, mean blood pressure 152/98 mm Hg, 55% men) and two subsequent RCTs[116,117] that examined the effects of weight loss on blood pressure.[118] In the systematic review, caloric intakes ranged from 450 to 1500 kcal a day; most diets led to weight reductions of 3–9% of body weight. Combined data from the six trials that did not vary antihypertensive regimens during the intervention period found that reducing weight reduced systolic and diastolic blood pressures (mean reduction in systolic pressure, weight loss v no weight loss 3 mm Hg, 95% CI 0.7 to 6.8 mm Hg; mean reduction in diastolic blood pressure 2.9 mm Hg diastolic, 95% CI 0.1 to 5.7 mm Hg). Trials that allowed adjustment of antihypertensive regimens found that lower doses and fewer antihypertensive drugs were needed in the weight reduction groups compared with control groups. The two subsequent RCTs found that sustained weight reduction of 2–4 kg significantly reduced systolic blood pressure at 1–3 years by about 1 mmHg.[116,117]

Harms: We found no direct evidence that intentional gradual weight loss of less than 10% of body weight is harmful in obese adults with hypertension.

Comment: None.

OPTION   POTASSIUM SUPPLEMENTATION

One systematic review of RCTs has found that a daily potassium supplementation of about 60 mmol (2 g, which is about the amount contained in 5 bananas) is feasible for many adults and reduces blood pressure a little (see table 3, p 156).

Benefits: We found no RCTs examining the effects of potassium supplementation on morbidity or mortality. One systematic review (search date 1995, 21 RCTs, 1560 adults with hypertension, age 19–79 years) compared the effects on blood pressure of potassium supplements (60–100 mmol potassium chloride daily) versus placebo or no supplement.[119] It found that, compared with the control interventions, potassium supplements reduced systolic and diastolic blood pressures (mean decrease in systolic blood pressure with potassium supplements 4.4 mm Hg systolic, 95% CI 2.2 to 6.6 mm Hg; mean decrease in diastolic blood pressure 2.5 mm Hg diastolic, 95% CI 0.1 to 4.9 mm Hg).

Harms: We found no direct evidence of harm in people without kidney failure and in people not taking drugs that increase serum potassium concentration. Gastrointestinal adverse effects such as belching, flatulence, diarrhoea, or abdominal discomfort occurred in 2–10% of people.[119]

Comment: None.

OPTION   FISH OIL SUPPLEMENTATION

One systematic review of RCTs has found that fish oil supplementation in large doses of 3 g a day modestly lowers blood pressure (see table 3, p 156).

Benefits: We found no RCTs examining the effects of fish oil supplementation on morbidity or mortality. One systematic review (search date not stated, 7 brief RCTs, 339 people with hypertension — mainly middle aged white men, mean age 50 years) compared effects on blood pressure of fish oil (usually 3 g daily as capsules) versus no supplements or "placebo".[120] The contents of placebo capsules varied among trials. Some used oil mixtures containing omega-3 polyunsaturated fatty acids, some without. The review found that fish oil supplements reduced blood pressure compared with control interventions (mean decrease in blood pressure in treatment group v control group 4.5 mm Hg systolic, 95% CI 1.2 to 7.8 mm Hg, and 2.5 mm Hg diastolic, 95% CI 0.6 to 4.4 mm Hg).

Harms: Belching, bad breath, fishy taste, and abdominal pain occurred in about a third of people taking high doses of fish oil.[120]

Comment: The trials were of short duration and used high doses of fish oil. Such high intake may be difficult to maintain. We found no evidence of beneficial effect on blood pressure at lower intakes.

Cardiovascular disorders

OPTION   CALCIUM SUPPLEMENTATION

We found insufficient evidence on the effects of calcium supplementation specifically in people with hypertension. One systematic review of RCTs in people both with and without hypertension found that calcium supplementation may reduce systolic blood pressure by small amounts (see table 3, p 156).

Benefits: We found no RCTs examining the effects of calcium supplementation on morbidity or mortality. One systematic review (search date 1994, 42 RCTs, 4560 middle aged adults) compared the effects on blood pressure of calcium supplementation (500–2000 mg daily) versus placebo or no supplements.[121] It found that calcium supplements reduced blood pressure by a small amount (mean systolic blood pressure reduction, supplement v control 1.4 mm Hg, 95% CI 0.7 to 2.2 mm Hg; mean diastolic reduction 0.8 mm Hg, 95% CI 0.2 to 1.4 mm Hg).

Harms: Adverse gastrointestinal effects, such as abdominal pain, were generally mild and varied among particular preparations.

Comment: Data relating specifically to people with hypertension are limited by few studies with small sample sizes and short durations.

OPTION   MAGNESIUM SUPPLEMENTATION

We found limited and conflicting evidence on the effect of magnesium supplementation on blood pressure in people with hypertension and normal magnesium concentrations.

Benefits: We found no RCTs examining the effects of magnesium supplementation on morbidity or mortality. A few small, short term RCTs found mixed results on effects on blood pressure reduction (see table 3, p 156).

Harms: We found insufficient evidence.

Comment: None.

QUESTION   **What are the effects of drug treatment in primary hypertension?**

Cindy Mulrow

OPTION   ANTIHYPERTENSIVE DRUGS VERSUS PLACEBO

Many systematic reviews of RCTs have found that drug treatment decreases the risk of fatal and non-fatal stroke, cardiac events, and total mortality in specific populations of people. The biggest benefit is seen in people with highest baseline risk of cardiovascular disease.

Benefits: We found many systematic reviews. One review (search date 1997, 17 RCTs with morbidity and mortality outcomes, duration > 1 year, 37 000 people) found that antihypertensive drugs versus placebo produced variable reductions of systolic/diastolic blood pressure that averaged around 12–16/5–10 mm Hg.[122] It found evidence of benefit in total death rate, cardiovascular death rate, stroke, major coronary events, and congestive cardiac failure, but the absolute results depended on age and the severity of the hypertension (see below). The biggest benefit was seen in those with the highest baseline risk. The trials mainly compared placebo versus diuretics (usually thiazides with the addition of amiloride or triamterene) and versus β blockers (usually atenolol or metoprolol) in a stepped care approach. One systematic review (search date 1999, 8 RCTs, 15 693 people) found that, in people over 60 years old with systolic hypertension, treatment of systolic pressures greater than 160 mm Hg decreased total mortality and fatal and non-fatal cardiovascular events. Absolute benefits were greater in men than women, in people aged over 70, and in those with prior cardio-vascular events or wider pulse pressure. The relative hazard rates associated with a 10 mm Hg higher initial systolic blood pressure were 1.26 (P = 0.0001) for total mortality, 1.22 (P = 0.02) for stroke, but only 1.07 (P = 0.37) for coronary events. Active treatment reduced total mortality (RR 0.87, 95% CI 0.78 to 0.98, P = 0.02).[123] **Target diastolic blood pressure:** We found one RCT (18 790 people, mean age 62 years, diastolic blood pressures between 100–115 mm Hg), which aimed to evaluate the effects on cardiovascular risk of target diastolic blood pressures of 90, 85, and 80 mm Hg.[124] However, mean achieved diastolic blood pressures were 85, 83, and 81 mm Hg, which limited power to detect differences among groups. There were no significant differences in major cardiovascular events among the three groups.

Harms: **Mortality and major morbidity:** One systematic review of RCTs comparing diuretics and β blockers versus placebo found no increase in non-cardiovascular mortality in treated people.[122] One systematic review (9 case control and 3 cohort studies) found that long term diuretic use may be associated with an increased risk of renal cell carcinoma (OR in case control studies 1.55, 95% CI 1.4 to 1.7).[125] Absolute risks cannot be calculated from these studies, but renal cell carcinoma is rare, so the absolute risk increase of any real effect would be correspondingly small. Renal cell carcinoma can cause hypertension; this fact may have confounded the results of these studies. **Quality of life and tolerability:** One systematic review and several recent trials found that quality of life was not adversely affected and may be improved in those who remain on treatment.[126,127]

Comment: Trials included people who were healthier than the general popula-tion, with lower rates of cardiovascular risk factors, cardiovascular disease, and comorbidity. People with higher cardiovascular risk can expect greater short term absolute risk reduction than seen in the trials, whereas people with major competing risks such as terminal cancer or end stage Alzheimer's disease can expect smaller risk reduction. In the systematic review,[122] five of the trials were in middle aged adults with mild to moderate hypertension. Seven of the trials were in people older than 60 years. On average, every 1000 person years of treatment in older adults prevented five strokes (95% CI 2 to 8), three coronary events (95% CI 1 to 4), and four cardiovascular deaths (95% CI 1 to 8). Drug treatment in middle aged adults prevented one stroke (95% CI 0 to 2) for every 1000 person years of treatment and did not significantly affect coronary events or mortality.

OPTION   **COMPARING ANTIHYPERTENSIVE DRUG TREATMENTS**

Two systematic reviews have found that initial treatment with diuretics, ACE inhibitors, or β blockers reduces mortality and morbidity, with minimal adverse effects. RCTs found no significant morbidity or mortality differences among these agents. We found limited evidence from one systematic review of RCTs that diuretics, β blockers, and ACE inhibitors reduced coronary heart disease and heart failure more than calcium channel antagonists. One RCT has found that a thiazide diuretic is superior to an α blocker in reducing cardiovascular events, particularly congestive heart failure.

Benefits:
β Blockers versus diuretics: One systematic review (search date 1995, > 48 000 people) identified RCTs comparing effects of high and low dose diuretics versus β blockers.[128] A second systematic review (search date 1998) was limited to 10 RCTs in 16 164 elderly people.[129] These reviews did not summarise direct comparisons of diuretics versus β blockers but compared results of trials that used diuretics as first line agents versus results of trials that used β blockers as first line agents. The reviews found no significant difference between diuretics and β blockers for lowering blood pressure. They found that diuretics reduced coronary events, but found no evidence that β blockers reduced coronary events. **β Blockers versus ACE inhibitors:** One single blind RCT (10 985 people, aged 25–66 years) found that an ACE inhibitor (captopril) was no more effective than conventional treatment (diuretics or β blockers) in reducing cardiovascular morbidity or mortality. Captopril increased the risk of stroke compared with β blockers (125 people would need to be treated with ACE inhibitor rather than β blocker for one extra stroke to occur, 95% CI 69 to 651 people). However, the methods of the trial may limit the validity of results (see comment below).[130] **Comparison of β blockers, diuretics, ACE inhibitors, and calcium channel antagonists:** One unblinded RCT (6600 people, aged 70–84 years) compared diuretics, β blockers, or both, versus calcium channel antagonists (felodipine or isradipine) versus ACE inhibitors (enalapril or lisinopril). It found no significant difference in blood pressure control or cardiovascular morbidity or mortality.[131] One systematic review (search date 2000, 8 RCTs) compared different antihypertensive regimens, and found no significant differences in outcome among people initially treated with β blockers, diuretics, or ACE inhibitors.[132] However, it found that β blockers or diuretics decreased coronary events compared with calcium channel antagonists, and increased stroke rate, although there was no significant difference for all cause mortality (OR for mortality, β blockers or diuretics v calcium antagonists 1.01, 95% CI 0.92 to 1.11). ACE inhibitors did not significantly alter all cause mortality or stroke rate compared with calcium channel antagonists, but decreased coronary events (OR for ACE inhibitor v calcium antagonist 1.03, 95% CI 0.91 to 1.18 for all cause mortality; 1.02, 95% CI 0.85 to 1.21 for stroke; 0.81,

95% CI 0.68 to 0.97 for coronary events).[132] **Comparison of α blockers and diuretics:** A double blind RCT (335 high risk people with hypertension) found no differences in coronary heart disease outcomes between doxazosin, an α blocker, compared with chlortalidone. However, doxazosin compared with chlortalidone increased the total number of cardiovascular events (4 year rate 25% v 22%; HR 1.25, 95% CI 1.17 to 1.33) and, in particular, increased congestive heart failure (4 year rate 8% v 4%; HR 2.04, 95% CI 1.79 to 2.32).[133] **Drug treatment in people with diabetes:** See cardiovascular disease in diabetes, p 17.

Harms: **Quality of life and tolerability:** In the three long term, double blind comparisons of low dose diuretics, β blockers, ACE inhibitors, and calcium channel blockers, tolerability and overall quality of life indicators tended to be more favourable for diuretics and β blockers than for newer drugs.[134-136] One systematic review (search date 1998) of RCTs comparing thiazides versus β blockers found that thiazides were associated with fewer withdrawals because of adverse effects (RR 0.69, 95% CI 0.63 to 0.76).[137] Adverse effects are agent specific. The recent unblinded RCT comparing diuretics, β blockers, calcium channel antagonists, and ACE inhibitors found that after 5 years of follow up, 26% of people receiving felodipine or isradipine reported ankle oedema, 30% receiving enalapril or lisonopril reported cough, and 9% receiving diuretics and/or β blockers reported cold hands and feet.[131] **Major harm controversies:** Case control, cohort, and randomised studies suggest that short and intermediate acting dihydropyridine calcium channel blockers, such as nifedipine and isradipine, may increase cardiovascular morbidity and mortality.[138]

Comment: Results of the large ACE inhibitor trial reported above warrant cautious interpretation because a flaw in the randomisation process resulted in unbalanced groups.[130]

QUESTION **What are the effects of lowering cholesterol concentration in asymptomatic people?**

Michael Pignone

Systematic reviews have found that, in people with a high baseline risk, cholesterol reduction reduces non-fatal myocardial infarction (see cholesterol reduction under secondary prevention of ischaemic cardiac events, p 171). RCTs have found that benefit is related to an individual's baseline risk of cardiovascular events and to the degree of cholesterol lowering rather than to the individual's absolute cholesterol concentration (see figure 1, p 159).

Benefits: We found many reviews of the effects of cholesterol lowering on cardiovascular event rates, CHD mortality, and total mortality in people with no previous history of cardiovascular disease. Most concluded that cholesterol reduction lowered cardiovascular events but that there was insufficient evidence that cholesterol reduction lowers overall mortality when used in people with no existing cardiovascular symptoms (primary prevention).[144-148] **Statins:** We found four systematic reviews that considered the effect of

Primary prevention

HMG-CoA reductase inhibitors (statins) versus placebo on clinical outcomes in people given long term ($\geq$ 6 months) treatment.[144-148] All included the two large primary prevention trials using statins (13 200 people). All found similar results. After 4–6 years of treatment for primary prevention, statins compared with placebo did not significantly reduce all cause mortality (OR 0.87, 95% CI 0.71 to 1.06) or CHD mortality (OR 0.73, 95% CI 0.51 to 1.05), but did reduce major coronary events (OR 0.66, 95% CI 0.57 to 0.76) and cardiovascular mortality (OR 0.68, 95% CI 0.50 to 0.93).[149] The absolute risk reduction for CHD events, CHD mortality, and total mortality varied with the baseline risk in the placebo group of each trial (see figure 1, p 159).[147] **Other treatments:** We found no systematic review specifically in people with low baseline risk (< 0.5% annual risk of CHD events). We found two systematic reviews that looked at statins and non-statin treatments together versus placebo or no treatment, specifically for primary prevention. Both found similar results. The most recent review found four RCTs (2 with statins, one with fibrates, and one with colestyramine, 21 087 people).[147] It found that cholesterol reduction therapy versus placebo significantly reduced CHD events and CHD mortality, but found no significant effect on overall mortality (OR for therapy v placebo; 0.70, 95% CI 0.62 to 0.79 for CHD events; 0.71, 95% CI 0.56 to 0.91 for CHD mortality; 0.94, 95% CI 0.81 to 1.09 for overall mortality). **Low fat diet:** See changing behaviour, p 48.

Harms: Specific harms of statins are discussed under secondary prevention of ischaemic cardiac events, p 173.

Comment: The CHD event rate in the placebo group of the two large primary prevention trials using statins was 0.6%[139] and 1.5 %[143] a year. If the 17% relative reduction in total mortality observed in the higher risk West of Scotland trial is real, then about 110 high risk people without known CHD would need to be treated for 5 years to save one life. We found no RCTs evaluating the effect of statins in asymptomatic people aged over 75 years. Several large studies are under way.[150] We found one systematic review (search date 1996, 59 RCTs, 173 160 people receiving drug treatments, dietary intervention, or ileal bypass), which did not differentiate primary and secondary prevention and included RCTs of any cholesterol lowering intervention, irrespective of duration, as long as mortality data were reported.[151] Overall, baseline risk was similar in people allocated to all interventions. Among non-surgical treatments, the review found that only statins reduced CHD mortality (RR v control: 0.69, 95% CI 0.59 to 0.80 for statins; 0.44, 95% CI 0.18 to 1.07 for n–3 fatty acids; 0.98, 95% CI 0.78 to 1.24 for fibrates; 0.71, 95% CI 0.51 to 0.99 for resins; 1.04, 95% CI 0.93 to 1.17 for hormones; 0.95, 95% CI 0.83 to 1.10 for niacin; 0.91, 95% CI 0.82 to 1.01 for diet), and that only statins and n–3 fatty acids reduced all cause mortality (RR v control: 0.79, 95% CI 0.71 to 0.89 for statins; 0.68, 95% CI 0.53 to 0.88 for n–3 fatty acids; 1.06, 95% CI 0.78 to 1.46 for fibrates; 0.85, 95% CI 0.66 to 1.08 for resins; 1.09, 95% CI 1.00 to 1.20 for hormones; 0.96, 95% CI 0.86 to 1.08 for niacin; 0.97, 95% CI 0.81 to 1.15 for diet).

Cathie Sudlow

OPTION **ANTIPLATELET TREATMENT**

We found the role of antiplatelet treatment in individuals without symptoms of cardiovascular disease to be uncertain. We found insufficient evidence from RCTs to identify which individuals would benefit overall and which would be harmed by regular treatment with aspirin (see table 4, p 157 and table 5, p 158)

Benefits: We found two systematic reviews[155,156] and one subsequent RCT.[157] We have included this trial in our own meta-analysis, which pools data from the five large RCTs that we have found to date, comparing aspirin versus control in a total of about 55 000 low risk individuals with or without identifiable risk factors (see table 4, p 157 and table 5, p 158).[124,152-154,157] The first systematic review of RCTs of antiplatelet treatment (search date 1990) included about 30 000 people.[155] Most were involved in two large trials of aspirin versus control among male doctors in the UK (aspirin dose 500 mg daily) and the USA (aspirin dose 325 mg every other day).[152,153] We found three RCTs published after the review, in asymptomatic individuals with identifiable risk factors for vascular events. All three had a factorial design. Results are summarised (see table 4, p 157 and table 5, p 158). The first compared aspirin (75 mg daily) versus placebo, and low intensity warfarin (target international normalised ratio [INR] 1.5) versus placebo in 5000 middle-aged men with CHD score in the top 20–25% of the population distribution.[154] The second RCT compared aspirin (75 mg daily) versus placebo in three groups with different intensities of blood pressure reduction in a total of about 19 000 people with hypertension, most of whom had no history of vascular disease.[124] The third RCT compared aspirin (100 mg daily) versus placebo, and vitamin E versus placebo in about 4500 people aged > 50 years, recruited from general practices. Participants had at least one major cardiovascular risk factor (hypertension, hypercholesterolaemia, diabetes, obesity, family history of premature myocardial infarction, or age ⩾ 65 years).[157] Our meta-analysis also included these three RCTs, and found that, overall, aspirin reduced myocardial infarction, slightly reduced vascular events (ARR 1/1000 people per year), but had an uncertain effect on stroke (see table 4, p 157). The second systematic review (published 2000) found similar results, but did not include the most recently published RCT.[157] It included one RCT (among about 3000 individuals with diabetes), who were at substantially higher risk of vascular events (about 4% per year) than the low risk individuals in the primary prevention trials included in our meta-analysis (see table 4, p 157).

Harms: Serious, potentially life threatening bleeding is the most important adverse effect of antiplatelet treatment. Intracranial bleeds are uncommon, but they are often fatal and usually cause substantial disability in survivors. Major extracranial bleeds occur mainly in the gastrointestinal tract and may require hospital admission or blood transfusion but do not generally result in permanent disability and are rarely fatal. Table 5 shows the approximate excess annual rates for intracranial and major extracranial bleeds (see table 5, p 158).

Comment: Individuals in primary prevention trials were at much lower risk of vascular events (average 1% per year in the control group) than the high risk people with clinical manifestations of cardiovascular disease that were included in the first overview (average 9% per year in the control group).[155] The absolute benefit of aspirin was therefore small and, as it was of similar magnitude to the risks of bleeding, the net effects were statistically uncertain. The size and direction of the effects of aspirin in particular individuals may well depend on specific factors, such as age, blood pressure, smoking status, or history of diabetes mellitus. At present there is insufficient information to identify which individuals would benefit overall and which would be harmed by regular treatment with aspirin. Futher information will soon be available from a detailed overview of individual participant data from the completed primary prevention trials (Baigent C, personal communication, 2001); from the Women's Health Study, comparing aspirin 100 mg daily versus placebo among 40 000 healthy postmenopausal women;[158] and from the Aspirin in Asymptomatic Atherosclerosis trial, comparing low dose aspirin versus placebo among 3 300 middle-aged participants with asymptomatic atherosclerosis, identified by an ankle brachial pressure index of ≥ 0.9 (Fowkes G, personal communication, 2000).

OPTION   **ANTICOAGULANT TREATMENT**

We found evidence from one RCT that the benefits and risks of low intensity oral anticoagulation among individuals without evidence of cardiovascular disease are finely balanced, and the net effects are uncertain.

Benefits: We found no systematic review. We found one RCT assessing anticoagulation (with a low target INR of 1.5) among people without evidence of cardiovascular disease.[154] It found that the proportional effects of warfarin were similar among people allocated aspirin or placebo, and overall warfarin non-significantly reduced the odds of a vascular event over about 6.5 years compared with placebo (253 events in 2762 people allocated to warfarin, AR 9.2% v 288 events in 2737 people allocated to placebo, AR 10.5%; mean ARR warfarin v placebo about 2 events per 1000 individuals per year; reduction in odds of vascular event warfarin v placebo 14%, 95% CI −2% to +28%). Compared with placebo, warfarin reduced the rate of all ischaemic heart disease by 21% (95% CI 4% to 35%), but had no significant effect on the rate of stroke (increase in AR 15%, 95% CI −22% to +68%) or other causes of vascular death.

Harms: Allocation to warfarin was associated with a non-significant excess of about 0.4 intracranial bleeds per 1000 individuals a year (14/ 2762 [0.5%] warfarin v 7/2737 [0.3%] placebo) and a non-significant excess of extracranial bleeds of about 0.5 per 1000 individuals a year (21/2545 [0.8%] warfarin v 12/2540 [0.5%] placebo).

Comment: As is the case for aspirin, the benefits and risks of low intensity oral anticoagulation among people without evidence of cardiovascular disease are finely balanced. The number of individuals randomised to date is only about 10% of the number included in primary prevention trials of aspirin (see p 147), and so the reliable identification of those who may benefit from such treatment will require further large scale randomised evidence.

REFERENCES

1. Heller RF, Chinn S, Pedoe HD, Rose G. How well can we predict coronary heart disease? Findings of the United Kingdom heart disease prevention project. *BMJ* 1984;288:1409–1411.

2. Tunstall-Pedoe H, Morrison C, Woodward M, Fitzpatrick B, Watt G. Sex differences in myocardial infarction and coronary deaths in the Scottish MONICA population of Glasgow 1985 to 1991: presentation, diagnosis, treatment, and 28-day case fatality of 3991 events in men and 1551 events in women. *Circulation* 1996;93: 1981–1992.

3. Anderson KV, Odell PM, Wilson PWF, Kannel WB. Cardiovascular disease risk profiles. *Am Heart J* 1991;121:293–298.

4. National Health Committee. Guidelines for the management of mildly raised blood pressure in New Zealand. Wellington Ministry of Health, 1993. http://www.nzgg.org.nz/library/gl_complete/bloodpressure/table1.cfm

5. Powell KE, Thompson PD, Caspersen CJ, Kendrick JS. Physical activity and the incidence of coronary heart disease. *Ann Rev Public Health* 1987;8: 253–287. Search date 1995; primary sources computerised searches of personal files, *J Chronic Dis* 1983–1985 and *Am J Epidemiol* 1984–1985.

6. Berlin JA, Colditz GA. A meta-analysis of physical activity in the prevention of coronary heart disease. *Am J Epidemiol* 1990;132:612–628. Search date not stated; primary sources review articles and Medline.

7. Eaton CB. Relation of physical activity and cardiovascular fitness to coronary heart disease. Part I: A meta-analysis of the independent relation of physical activity and coronary heart disease. *J Am Board Fam Pract* 1992;5:31–42. Search date not stated; primary source Medline.

8. Fraser GE, Strahan TM, Sabate J, Beeson WL, Kissinger D. Effects of traditional coronary risk factors on rates of incident coronary events in a low-risk population: the Adventist health study. *Circulation* 1992;86:406–413.

9. Lindsted KD, Tonstad S, Kuzma JW. Self-report of physical activity and patterns of mortality in Seventh-Day Adventist men. *J Clin Epidemiol* 1991;44:355–364.

10. Folsom AR, Arnett DK, Hutchinson RG, Liao F, Clegg LX, Cooper LS. Physical activity and incidence of coronary heart disease in middle-aged women and men. *Med Sci Sports Exerc* 1997;29:901–909.

11. Jensen G, Nyboe J, Appleyard M, Schnohr P. Risk factors for acute myocardial infarction in Copenhagen, II: Smoking, alcohol intake, physical activity, obesity, oral contraception, diabetes, lipids, and blood pressure. *Eur Heart J* 1991;12: 298–308.

12. Simonsick EM, Lafferty ME, Phillips CL, et al. Risk due to inactivity in physically capable older adults. *Am J Public Health* 1993;83:1443–1450.

13. Haapanen N, Miilunpalo S, Vuori I, Oja P, Pasanen M. Association of leisure time physical activity with the risk of coronary heart disease, hypertension and diabetes in middle-aged men and women. *Int J Epidemiol* 1997;26:739–747.

14. Sherman SE, D'Agostino RB, Cobb JL, Kannel WB. Does exercise reduce mortality rates in the elderly? Experience from the Framingham heart study. *Am Heart J* 1994;128:965–672.

15. Rodriguez BL, Curb JD, Burchfiel CM, et al. Physical activity and 23-year incidence of coronary heart disease morbidity and mortality among middle-aged men: the Honolulu heart program. *Circulation* 1994;89:2540–2544.

16. Eaton CB, Medalie JH, Flocke SA, Zyzanski SJ, Yaari S, Goldbourt U. Self-reported physical activity predicts long-term coronary heart disease and all-cause mortalities: 21-year follow-up of the Israeli ischemic heart disease study. *Arch Fam Med* 1995;4:323–329.

17. Stender M, Hense HW, Doring A, Keil U. Physical activity at work and cardiovascular disease risk: results from the MONICA Augsburg study. *Int J Epidemiol* 1993;22:644–650.

18. Leon AS, Myers MJ, Connett J. Leisure time physical activity and the 16-year risks of mortality from coronary heart disease and all-causes in the multiple risk factor intervention trial (MRFIT). *Int J Sports Med* 1997;18(suppl 3):208–315.

19. Rosolova H, Simon J, Sefrna F. Impact of cardiovascular risk factors on morbidity and mortality in Czech middle-aged men: Pilsen longitudinal study. *Cardiology* 1994;85:61–68.

20. Luoto R, Prattala R, Uutela A, Puska P. Impact of unhealthy behaviors on cardiovascular mortality in Finland, 1978–1993. *Prev Med* 1998;27: 93–100.

21. Woo J, Ho SC, Yuen YK, Yu LM, Lau J. Cardiovascular risk factors and 18-month mortality and morbidity in an elderly Chinese population aged 70 years and over. *Gerontology* 1998;44: 51–55.

22. Gartside PS, Wang P, Glueck CJ. Prospective assessment of coronary heart disease risk factors: The NHANES I epidemiologic follow-up study (NHEFS) 16-year follow-up. *J Am Coll Nutr* 1998; 17:263–269.

23. Dorn JP, Cerny FJ, Epstein LH, Naughton J, et al. Work and leisure time physical activity and mortality in men and women from a general population sample. *Ann Epidemiol* 1999;9: 366–373.

24. Hakim AA, Curb JD, Petrovitch H, et al. Effects of walking on coronary heart disease in elderly men: the Honolulu heart program. *Circulation* 1999; 100:9–13.

25. Eaton CB. Relation of physical activity and cardiovascular fitness to coronary heart disease, part II: cardiovascular fitness and the safety and efficacy of physical activity prescription. *J Am Board Fam Pract* 1992;5:157–165. Search date not stated; primary sources Medline and hand searches.

26. Blair SN, Kohl HW 3rd, Barlow CE, Paffenbarger RS Jr, Gibbons LW, Macera CA. Changes in physical fitness and all-cause mortality: a prospective study of healthy and unhealthy men. *JAMA* 1995;273:1093–1098.

27. Sacco RL, Gan R, Boden-Albala B, et al. Leisure-time physical activity and ischemic stroke risk: the Northern Manhattan stroke study. *Stroke* 1998; 29:380–387.

Primary prevention

28. Shinton R. Lifelong exposures and the potential for stroke prevention: the contribution of cigarette smoking, exercise, and body fat. *J Epidemiol Community Health* 1997;51:138–143.

29. Gillum RF, Mussolino ME, Ingram DD. Physical activity and stroke incidence in women and men. The NHANES I epidemiologic follow-up study. *Am J Epidemiol* 1996;143:860–869.

30. Kiely DK, Wolf PA, Cupples LA, Beiser AS, Kannel WB. Physical activity and stroke risk: the Framingham study [correction appears in *Am J Epidemiol* 1995;141:178]. *Am J Epidemiol* 1994; 140:608–620.

31. Abbott RD, Rodriguez BL, Burchfiel CM, Curb JD. Physical activity in older middle-aged men and reduced risk of stroke: the Honolulu heart program. *Am J Epidemiol* 1994;139:881–893.

32. Haheim LL, Holme I, Hjermann I, Leren P. Risk factors of stroke incidence and mortality: a 12-year follow-up of the Oslo study. *Stroke* 1993; 24:1484–1489.

33. Wannamethee G, Shaper AG. Physical activity and stroke in British middle aged men. *BMJ* 1992; 304:597–601.

34. Menotti A, Keys A, Blackburn H, et al. Twenty-year stroke mortality and prediction in twelve cohorts of the seven countries study. *Int J Epidemiol* 1990; 19:309–315.

35. Lindenstrom E, Boysen G, Nyboe J. Risk factors for stroke in Copenhagen, Denmark. I. Lifestyle factors. *Neuroepidemiology* 1993;12:43–50.

36. Lindenstrom E, Boysen G, Nyboe J. Lifestyle factors and risk of cerebrovascular disease in women: the Copenhagen City heart study. *Stroke* 1993;24:1468–1472.

37. Folsom AR, Prineas RJ, Kaye SA, Munger RG. Incidence of hypertension and stroke in relation to body fat distribution and other risk factors in older women. *Stroke* 1990;21:701–706.

38. Nakayama T, Date C, Yokoyama T, Yoshiike N, Yamaguchi M, Tanaka H. A 15.5-year follow-up study of stroke in a Japanese provincial city: the Shibata study. *Stroke* 1997;28:45–52.

39. Lee IM, Hennekens CH, Berger K, Buring JE, Manson JE. Exercise and risk of stroke in male physicians. *Stroke* 1999;30:1–6.

40. Evenson KR, Rosamond WD, Cai J, et al. Physical activity and ischemic stroke risk: the atherosclerosis in communities study. *Stroke* 1999;30:1333–1339.

41. Mittleman MA, Maclure M, Tofler GH, Sherwood JB, Goldberg RJ, Muller JE. Triggering of acute myocardial infarction by heavy physical exertion. Protection against triggering by regular exertion: determinants of myocardial infarction onset study investigators. *N Engl J Med* 1993;329:1677–1683.

42. Willich SN, Lewis M, Lowel H, Arntz HR, Schubert F, Schroder R. Physical exertion as a trigger of acute myocardial infarction: triggers and mechanisms of myocardial infarction study group. *N Engl J Med* 1993;329:1684–1690.

43. Pate RR, Pratt M, Blair SN, et al. Physical activity and public health. A recommendation from the Centers for Disease Control and Prevention and the American College of Sports Medicine. *JAMA* 1995;273:402–407.

44. Thompson PD. The cardiovascular complications of vigorous physical activity. *Arch Intern Med* 1996;156:2297–2302.

45. Oberman A. Exercise and the primary prevention of cardiovascular disease. *Am J Cardiol* 1985;55: 10–20.

46. Andersen RE, Wadden TA, Bartlett SJ, Zemel B, Verde TJ, Franckowiak SC. Effects of lifestyle activity vs structured aerobic exercise in obese women: a randomized trial. *JAMA* 1999;281: 335–340.

47. Dunn AL, Marcus BH, Kampert JB, Garcia ME, Kohl HW, Blair SN. Comparison of lifestyle and structured interventions to increase physical activity and cardiorespiratory fitness: a randomized trial. *JAMA* 1999;281:327–434.

48. Pereira MA, Kriska AM, Day RD, Cauley JA, LaPorte RE, Kuller LH. A randomized walking trial in postmenopausal women: effects on physical activity and health 10 years later. *Arch Intern Med* 1998;158:1695–1701.

49. DeBusk RF, Stenestrand U, Sheehan M, Haskell WL. Training effects of long versus short bouts of exercise in healthy subjects. *Am J Cardiol* 1990; 65:1010–1013.

50. Ness AR, Powles JW. Fruit and vegetables and cardiovascular disease: a review. *Int J Epidemiol* 1997;26:1–13. Search date 1995; primary sources Medline, Embase, and hand searches of personal bibliographies, books, reviews, and citations in located reports.

51. Law MR, Morris JK. By how much does fruit and vegetable consumption reduce the risk of ischaemic heart disease? *Eur J Clin Nutr* 1998; 52:549–556. Search date not stated; primary sources Medline, Science Citation Index, and hand searches of review articles.

52. Klerk M, Jansen MCJF, van't Veer P, Kok FJ. *Fruits and vegetables in chronic disease prevention*. Wageningen: Grafisch Bedrijf Ponsen and Looijen, 1998. Search date 1998; primary sources Medline, Current Contents, and Toxline.

53. Key TJA, Thorogood M, Appleby PN, Burr ML. Dietary habits and mortality in 11 000 vegetarians and health conscious people: results of a 17 year follow up. *BMJ* 1996;313:775–779.

54. Pietinen P, Rimm EB, Korhonen P, et al. Intake of dietary fibre and risk of coronary heart disease in a cohort of Finnish men. *Circulation* 1996;94: 2720–2727.

55. Mann JI, Appleby PN, Key TJA, Thorogood M. Dietary determinants of ischaemic heart disease in health conscious individuals. *Heart* 1997;78: 450–455.

56. Geleijnse M. Consumptie van groente en fruit en het risico op myocardinfarct 1997. Basisrapportage. Rotterdam: Erasmus Universiteit (cited in appendix XIII of review by Klerk).

57. Todd S, Woodward M, Tunstall-Pedoe H, Bolton-Smith C. Dietary antioxidant vitamins and fiber in the etiology of cardiovascular disease and all-cause mortality: results from the Scottish heart health study. *Am J Epidemiol* 1999;150: 1073–1080.

58. Bazzano L, Ogden LG, Vupputuri S, Loria C, Myers L, Whelton PK. Fruit and vegetable intake reduces cardiovascular mortality: results from the NHANES I epidemiologic follow-up study (NHEFS). 40th Annual Conference Cardiovascular Epidemiology and Prevention [abstract]. *Circulation* 2000;8–8.

59. Lui S, Manson JE, Cole SR, Willett WC, Buring JE. Fruit and vegetable intake and risk of cardiovascular disease. 40th Annual Conference Cardiovascular Epidemiology and Prevention [abstract]. *Circulation* 2000;30–31.

60. Lui S, Manson JE, Lee I-M, et al. Fruit and vegetable intake and risk of cardiovascular disease: the Women's Health Study. *Am J Clin Nutr* 2000;72:922–928.

61. Knekt P, Reunanen A, Jarvinen R, Heliovaara M, Aromaa A. Antioxidant vitamin intake and coronary mortality in a longitudinal population study. *Am J Epidemiol* 1994;139:1180–1189.

62. Keli SO, Hertog MGL, Feskens EJM, Kromhout D. Dietary flavonoids, antioxidant vitamins, and incidence of stroke. *Arch Intern Med* 1996;156: 637–642.

63. Daviglus ML, Orencia AJ, Dyer AR, et al. Dietary vitamin C, beta-carotene and 30-year risk of stroke: results from the Western Electric study. *Neuroepidemiology* 1997;16:69–77.

64. Ascherio A, Rimm EB, Hernan MA, et al. Prospective study of potassium intake and risk of stroke among US men. *Can J Cardiol* 1997;13: 44B.

65. Yochum L, Kushi LH, Meyer K, Folsom AR. Dietary flavonoid intake and risk of cardiovascular disease in postmenopausal women. *Am J Epidemiol* 1999; 149:943–949.

66. Knekt P, Isotupa S, Rissanen H, et al. Quercetin intake and the incidence of cerebrovascular disease. *Eur J Clin Nutr* 2000;54:415–417.

67. Hirvonen T, Virtamo J, Korhonen P, Albanes D, Pietinen P. Intake of flavonoids, carotenoids, vitamin C and E, and risk of stroke in male smokers. *Stroke* 2000;31:2301–2306.

68. Joshipura KJ, Ascherio A, Manson JE, et al. Fruit and vegetable intake in relation to risk of ischemic stroke. *JAMA* 1999;282:1233–1239.

69. Ness AR, Powles JW. Does eating fruit and vegetables protect against heart attack and stroke? *Chem Indus* 1996;792–794.

70. Ness AR, Powles JW. Dietary habits and mortality in vegetarians and health conscious people: several uncertainties exist. *BMJ* 1997;314:148.

71. Serdula MK, Byers T, Mokhad AH, Simoes E, Mendleim JM, Coates RJ. The association between fruit and vegetable intake and chronic disease risk factors. *Epidemiology* 1996;7: 161–165.

72. Lonn EM, Yusuf S. Is there a role for antioxidant vitamins in the prevention of cardiovascular disease? An update on epidemiological and clinical trials data. *Can J Cardiol* 1997;13: 957–965. Search date not stated; primary sources Medline, science citation index, handsearching.

73. Jha P, Flather M, Lonn E, Farkouh M, Yusuf S. The antioxidant vitamins and cardiovascular disease: a critical review of epidemiologic and clinical trial data. *Ann Intern Med* 1995;123:860–872.

74. Roxrode KM, Manson JE. Antioxidants and coronary heart disease: observational studies. *J Cardiovasc Risk* 1996;3:363–367.

75. Egger M, Schneider M, Davey Smith G. Spurious precision? Meta-analysis of observational studies. *BMJ* 1998;316:140–144.

76. Gaziano JM. Randomized trials of dietary antioxidants in cardiovascular disease prevention and treatment. *J Cardiovasc Risk* 1996;3: 368–371.

77. Ness AR, Powles JW, Khaw KT. Vitamin C and cardiovascular disease — a systematic review. *J Cardiovasc Risk* 1997;3:513–521. Search date 1996; primary sources Medline, Embase, and hand searches of personal bibliographies, books, reviews and citations in located reports.

78. Klipstein-Grobusch K, Geleijnse JM, den Breeijen JH, et al. Dietary antioxidants and risk of myocardial infarction in the elderly: the Rotterdam study. *Am J Clin Nutr* 1999;69:261–266.

79. Ascherio A, Rimm EB, Hernan M, et al. Relation of consumption of vitamin E, vitamin C, and carotenoids to risk for stroke among men in the United States. *Ann Intern Med* 1999;130: 963–970.

80. Yochum L, Folsom AR, Kushi LH. Intake of antioxidant vitamins and risk of death from stroke in postmenopausal women. *Am J Clin Nutr* 2000; 72:476–483.

81. Li J, Taylor PR, Li B, et al. Nutrition intervention trials in Linxian, China: multiple vitamin/mineral supplementation, cancer incidence, and disease-specific mortality among adults with esophageal dysplasia. *J Natl Cancer Inst* 1993;85: 1492–1498.

82. Mark SD, Wang W, Fraumeni JF, et al. Lowered risks of hypertension and cerebrovascular disease after vitamin/mineral supplementation. *Am J Epidemiol* 1996;143:658–664.

83. Mark SD, Wang W, Fraumeni JFJ, et al. Do nutritional supplements lower the risk of stroke or hypertension? *Epidemiology* 1998;9:9–15.

84. Losonczy KG, Harris TB, Havlik RJ. Vitamin E and vitamin C supplement use and risk of all-cause and coronary mortality in older persons: the established populations for epidemiologic studies of the elderly. *Am J Clin Nutr* 1996;64:190–196.

85. Sahyoun NR, Jacques PF, Russell RM. Carotenoids, vitamin C and E, and mortality in an elderly population. *Am J Epidemiol* 1996;144: 501–511.

86. Keli SO, Hertog MGL, Feskens EJM, Kromhout D. Dietary flavonoids, antioxidant vitamins, and incidence of stroke. *Arch Intern Med* 1996;156: 637–642.

87. Houtman JP. Trace elements and cardiovascular disease. *J Cardiovasc Risk* 1996;3:18–25.

88. Nève J. Selenium as a risk factor for cardiovascular disease. *J Cardiovasc Risk* 1996;3: 42–47.

89. Hertog MGL, Feskens EJM, Hollman PCH, Katan MB, Kromhout D. Dietary antioxidant flavonoids and risk of coronary heart disease: the Zutphen elderly study. *Lancet* 1993;342:1007–1011.

90. Knekt P, Jarvinen R, Reunanen A, Maatela J. Flavonoid intake and coronary mortality in Finland: a cohort study. *BMJ* 1996;312:478–481.

91. Rimm EB, Katan MB, Ascherio A, Stampfer MJ, Willett WC. Relation between intake of flavonoids and risk for coronary heart disease in male health professionals. *Ann Intern Med* 1996;125: 384–389.

92. Hertog MGL, Sweetnam PM, Fehily AM. Antioxidant flavonols and ischemic heart disease in a Welsh population of men: the Caerphilly study. *Am J Clin Nutr* 1997;65:1489–1494.

93. Doering WV. Antioxidant vitamins, cancer, and cardiovascular disease. *N Engl J Med* 1996;335: 1065.

94. Pietrzik K. Antioxidant vitamins, cancer, and cardiovascular disease. *N Engl J Med* 1996;335: 1065–1066.

95. Hennekens CH, Gaziano JM, Manson JE, Buring JE. Antioxidant vitamin cardiovascular disease hypothesis is still promising, but still unproven: the need for randomised trials. *Am J Clin Nutr* 1995; 62(suppl):1377–1380.

96. US Department of Health and Human Services. *The health benefits of smoking cessation: a report of the Surgeon General*. Rockville, Maryland: US Department of Health and Human Services, Public Health Service, Centers for Disease Control, 1990. DHHS Publication (CDC) 90–8416.

97. Royal College of Physicians. *Smoking and health now*. London: Pitman Medical and Scientific Publishing, 1971.

98. Doll R, Peto R, Wheatley K, Gray R, Sutherland I. Mortality in relation to smoking: 40 years' observations on male British doctors. *BMJ* 1994; 309:901–911.

99. Kawachi I, Colditz GA, Stampfer MJ, et al. Smoking cessation in relation to total mortality rates in women: a prospective cohort study. *Ann Intern Med* 1993;119:992–1000.

100. Rosenberg L, Kaufman DW, Helmrich SP, Shapiro S. The risk of myocardial infarction after quitting smoking in men under 55 years of age. *N Engl J Med* 1985;313:1511–1514.

101. Rosenberg L, Palmer JR, Shapiro S. Decline in the risk of myocardial infarction among women who stop smoking. *N Engl J Med* 1990;322: 213–217.

102. Rose G, Hamilton PJ, Colwell L, Shipley MJ. A randomised controlled trial of anti-smoking advice: 10-year results. *J Epidemiol Community Health* 1982;36:102–108.

103. Shinton R, Beevers G. Meta-analysis of relation between cigarette smoking and stroke. *BMJ* 1989;298:789–794. Search date 1988; primary source index references from three studies on cigarette smoking and stroke on medicine 1965–1988.

104. Rogot E, Murray JL. Smoking and causes of death among US veterans: 16 years of observation. *Public Health Rep* 1980;95:213–222.

105. Wannamethee SG, Shaper AG, Ebrahim S. History of parental death from stroke or heart trouble and the risk of stroke in middle-aged men. *Stroke* 1996;27:1492–1498.

106. Halbert JA, Silagy CA, Finucane P, Withers RT, Hamdorf PA. The effectiveness of exercise training in lowering blood pressure: a meta-analysis of randomised controlled trials of 4 weeks or longer. *J Hum Hypertens* 1997;11: 641–649. Search date 1996; primary sources Medline, Embase, Science Citation Index.

107. Ebrahim S, Davey Smith G. Lowering blood pressure: a systematic review of sustained non-pharmacological interventions. *J Public Health Med* 1998;20:441–448. Search date 1995; primary source Medline.

108. Engstom G, Hedblad B, Janzon L. Hypertensive men who exercise regularly have lower rate of cardiovascular mortality. *J Hypertens* 1999;17: 737–742.

109. Appel LJ, Moore TJ, Obarzanek E, et al. A clinical trial of the effects of dietary patterns on blood pressure. *N Engl J Med* 1997;336:1117–1124.

110. Beilin LJ, Puddey IB, Burke V. Alcohol and hypertension: kill or cure? *J Hum Hypertens* 1996;10(suppl 2):1–5.

111. Campbell NRC, Ashley MJ, Carruthers SG, et al. Recommendations on alcohol consumption. *Can Med Assoc J* 1999;(suppl 9):13–20. Search date 1996; primary source Medline.

112. Graudal NA, Galloe AM, Garred P. Effects of sodium restriction on blood pressure, renin, aldosterone, catecholamines, cholesterols, and triglyceride. *JAMA* 1998;279:1383–1391. Search date 1997; primary source Medline.

113. Whelton PK, Appel LJ, Espelland MA, et al. Sodium reduction and weight loss in the treatment of hypertension in older persons: a randomized controlled trial of non pharmacologic interventions in the elderly (TONE). *JAMA* 1998; 279:839–846.

114. Midgley JP, Matthew AG, Greenwood CMT, Logan AG. Effect of reduced dietary sodium on blood pressure. *JAMA* 1996;275:1590–1597. Search date 1994; primary sources Medline, Current Contents.

115. Alderman MH, Madhavan S, Cohen H, Sealey JE, Laragh JH. Low urinary sodium associated with greater risk of myocardial infarction among treated hypertensive men. *Hypertension* 1995; 25:1144–1152.

116. Stevens VJ, Obarzanek E, Cook NR, et al. Long-term weight loss and changes in blood pressure: results of the trials of hypertension prevention, phase 11. *Ann Intern Med* 2001;134:1–11.

117. Metz JA, Stern JS, Kris-Etherton P, et al. A randomized trial of improved weight loss with a prepared meal plan in overweight and obese patients. *Arch Intern Med* 2000;160: 2150–2158.

118. Brand MB, Mulrow CD, Chiquette E, et al. Weight-reducing diets for control of hypertension in adults. In: The Cochrane Library, Issue 4, 1998 Oxford: Update Software. Search date 1997; primary source Cochrane Library, Medline.

119. Whelton PK, He J, Cutler JA, et al. Effects of oral potassium on blood pressure: meta-analysis of randomized controlled clinical trials. *JAMA* 1997; 277:1624–1632. Search date 1995; primary source Medline.

120. Morris MC, Sacks F, Rosner B. Does fish oil lower blood pressure? A meta-analysis of controlled clinical trials. *Circulation* 1993;88:523–533. Search date not given; primary source Index Medicus.

121. Griffith LE, Guyatt GH, Cook RJ, et al. The influence of dietary and nondietary calcium supplementation on blood pressure. *Am J Hypertens* 1999;12:84–92. Search date 1994; primary sources Medline, Embase.

122. Gueyffier F, Froment A, Gouton M. New meta-analysis of treatment trials of hypertension: improving the estimate of therapeutic benefit. *J Hum Hypertens* 1996;10:1–8. Search date 1997; primary source Medline.

123. Staessen JA, Gasowski J, Wang JG, et al. Risks of untreated and treated isolated systolic hypertension in the elderly: meta-analysis of outcome trials. *Lancet* 2000;355:865–872. Search date 1999; primary sources other systematic reviews and reports from collaborative trialists.

124. Hansson L, Zanchetti AZ, Carruthers SG, et al. Effects of intensive blood pressure lowering and low-dose aspirin in patients with hypertension: principal results of the hypertension optimal treatment (HOT) trial. *Lancet* 1998;351: 1755–1762.

125. Grossman E, Messerli FH, Goldbourt U. Does diuretic therapy increase the risk of renal cell carcinoma? *Am J Cardiol* 1999;83:1090–1093. Search dates 1966 to 1998; primary sources Medline.

126. Beto JA, Bansal VK. Quality of life in treatment of hypertension: a meta-analysis of clinical trials. *Am J Hypertens* 1992;5:125–133. Search date 1990; primary sources Medline, ERIC.

127. Croog SH, Levine S, Testa MA. The effects of antihypertensive therapy on quality of life. *N Engl J Med* 1986;314:1657–1664.

128. Psaty BM, Smith NS, Siscovick DS, et al. Health outcomes associated with antihypertensive therapies used as first line agents: a systematic review and meta-analysis. *JAMA* 1997;277: 739–745. Search date 1995; primary source Medline.

129. Messerli FH, Grossman E, Goldbourt. Are beta blockers efficacious as first-line therapy for hypertension in the elderly? A systematic review. *JAMA* 1998;279:1903–1907. Search date 1998; primary source Medline.

130. Hansson L, Lindholm LH, Niskanen L, et al. Effect of angiotensin-converting-enzyme inhibition compared with conventional therapy on cardiovascular morbidity and mortality in hypertension: the captopril prevention project (CAPP) randomised trial. *Lancet* 1999;353: 611–616.

131. Hansson L, Lindholm L, Ekbom T, et al. Randomised trial of old and new antihypertensive drugs in elderly patients: cardiovascular mortality and morbidity the Swedish trial in old patients with hypertension-2 study. *Lancet* 1999;354: 1751–1756.

132. Blood Pressure Lowering Treatment Trialists' Collaboration. Effects of ACE inhibitors, calcium antagonists, and other blood-pressure-lowering

drugs: results of prospectively designed overviews of trials. *Lancet* 2000;356: 1955–1964. Search date July 2000; primary sources WHO-International Society of Hypertension registry of randomised trials; trials were sought that had not published or presented their results before July 1995.

133. The ALLHAT Officers and Coordinators for the ALLHAT Collaborative Research Group. Major cardiovascular events in hypertensive patients randomized to doxazosin vs chlorthalidone: the antihypertensive and lipid-lowering treatment to prevent heart attack trial (ALLHAT). *JAMA* 2000; 283:1967–1975.

134. Neaton JD, Grimm RH, Prineas RJ, et al. Treatment of mild hypertension study: final results. *JAMA* 1993;270:713–724.

135. Materson BJ, Reda DJ, Cushman WC, et al. Single drug therapy for hypertension in men. *N Engl J Med* 1993;328:914–921.

136. Philipp T, Anlauf M, Distler A, Holzgreve H, Michaelis J, Wellek S. Randomised, double blind, multicentre comparison of hydrochlorothiazide, atenolol, nitrendipine, and enalapril in antihypertensive treatment: results of the HANE study. *BMJ* 1997;315:154–159.

137. Wright JM, Lee CH, Chambers CK. Systematic review of antihypertensive therapies: does the evidence assist in choosing a first line drug? *Can Med Assoc J* 1999;161:25–32. Search date 1998; primary sources Medline 1996 to 1997, Cochrane Library to 1998.

138. Cutler JA. Calcium channel blockers for hypertension — uncertainty continues. *N Engl J Med* 1998;338:679–680.

139. Downs JR, Clearfield M, Weis S, et al. Primary prevention of acute coronary events with lovastatin in men and women with average cholesterol levels: results of the AFCAPS/ TexCAPS. *JAMA* 1998;279:1615–1622.

140. Scandinavian Simvastatin Survival Study Group. Randomized trial of cholesterol lowering in 4444 patients with coronary heart disease: the Scandinavian simvastatin survival study (4S). *Lancet* 1995;344:1383–1389.

141. Long-term Intervention with Pravastatin in Ischemic Disease (LIPID) Study Program. Prevention of cardiovascular events and death with pravastatin in patients with coronary heart disease and a broad range of initial cholesterol levels. *N Engl J Med* 1998;339:1349–1357.

142. Sacks FM, Pfeffer MA, Moye LA, et al, for the Cholesterol and Recurrent Events Trial Investigators. Effect of pravastatin on coronary events after myocardial infarction in patients with average cholesterol levels. *N Engl J Med* 1996; 335:1001–1009.

143. Shepherd J, Cobbe SM, Ford I, et al, for the West of Scotland Coronary Prevention Study Group. Prevention of coronary heart disease with pravastatin in men with hypercholesterolemia. *N Engl J Med* 1995;333:1301–1307.

144. Katerndahl DA, Lawler WR. Variability in meta-analytic results concerning the value of cholesterol reduction in coronary heart disease: a meta-meta-analysis. *Am J Epidemiol* 1999; 149:429–441. Search date 1995; primary sources Medline and meta-analysis bibliographies.

145. Froom J, Froom P, Benjamin M, Benjamin BJ. Measurement and management of hyperlipidemia for the primary prevention of coronary heart disease. *J Am Board Fam Pract* 1998;11:12–22.

146. Ebrahim S, Davey Smith G, McCabe CCC, et al. What role for statins? A review and economic model. *Health Technology Assessment* 1999;3:

19;1–91. Search dates 1997; primary sources Medline, Cochrane Controlled Trials Register, and personal contact with investigators working in the field of cholesterol lowering.

147. Pignone M, Phillips C, Mulrow C. Use of lipid lowering drugs for primary prevention of coronary heart disease: meta-analysis of randomised trials. *BMJ* 2000;321(7267):983–986. Search date 1999; primary sources Medline, Cochrane Library, and hand searches of bibliographies of systematic reviews and clinical practice guidelines.

148. Cucherat M, Lievre M, Gueyffier F. Clinical benefits of cholesterol lowering treatments. Meta-analysis of randomized therapeutic trials. *Presse Med* 2000 May 13;29:965–976. Search date and primary sources not stated.

149. LaRosa JC, He J, Vupputuri S. Effect of statins on risk of coronary disease: a meta-analysis of randomized controlled trials. *JAMA* 1999;282: 2340–2346. Search date 1998; primary sources Medline, bibliographies and authors' reference files.

150. Carlsson CM, Carnes M, McBride PE, Stein JH. Managing dyslipidaemia in older adults. *J Am Geriatr Society* 1999;47:1458–1465.

151. Bucher HC, Griffith LE, Guyatt G. Systematic review on the risk and benefit of different cholesterol-lowering interventions. *Arterioscler Thromb Vasc Biol* 1999:19;187–195. Search date October 1996; primary sources Medline, Embase, and hand searches of bibliographies.

152. Peto R, Gray R, Collins R, et al. Randomised trial of prophylactic daily aspirin in British male doctors. *BMJ* 1988;296:313–316.

153. Steering Committee of the Physicians' Health Study Research Group. Final report on the aspirin component of the ongoing physicians' health study. *N Engl J Med* 1989;321:129–135.

154. Medical Research Council's General Practice Research Framework. Thrombosis prevention trial: randomised trial of low-intensity anticoagulation with warfarin and low dose aspirin in the primary prevention of ischaemic heart disease in men at increased risk. *Lancet* 1998;351:233–241.

155. Antiplatelet Trialists' Collaboration. Collaborative overview of randomised trials of antiplatelet therapy — I: prevention of death, myocardial infarction, and stroke by prolonged antiplatelet therapy in various categories of patients. *BMJ* 1994;308:81–106. Search date 1990; primary sources Medline, Current Contents, hand searches of reference lists of trials and review articles, journal abstracts and meeting proceedings, trial register of the International Committee on Thrombosis and Haemostasis, and personal contacts with colleagues and antiplatelet manufacturers.

156. Hart RG, Halperin JL, McBride R, Benavente O, Man-Son-Hing M, Kronmal RA. Aspirin for the primary prevention of stroke and other major vascular events. Meta-analysis and hypotheses. *Arch Neurol* 2000;57:326–332. Search date 1998; primary sources unspecified computerised medical databases 1980 to 1998, Cochrane Collaboration registry 1998, and hand searched references of Antiplatelet Trialists' Collaboration publications.

157. Collaborative group of the Primary Prevention Project (PPP). Low-dose aspirin and vitamin E in people at cardiovascular risk: a randomised trial in general practice. *Lancet* 2001;357:89–95.

158. Buring JE, Hennekens CH for the Women's Health Study Group. Women's health study: summary of the study design. *J Myocard Ischemia* 1992;4:27–29.

Cardiovascular disorders

Michael Murphy
Director, ICRF General Practice Research
Group

Charles Foster
British Heart Foundation Scientist

Cathie Sudlow
Specialist Registrar in Neurology

Department of Neurology
Derriford Hospital
Plymouth
UK

Julian Nicholas
Resident Physician
Mayo Clinic
Rochester, MN
USA

Cindy Mulrow
Professor of Medicine
University of Texas
Health Science Center
San Antonio, TX
USA

Andy Ness
Senior Lecturer in Epidemiology
University of Bristol
Bristol
UK

Michael Pignone
Assistant Professor of Medicine
Division of General Internal Medicine
University of North Carolina
Chapel Hill, NC
USA

Competing interests: CM has participated in multicentre
research trials evaluating antihypertensive agents that
were funded by industry; other authors, none declared.

TABLE 1	Examples of common physical activities by intensity of effort required in multiples of the resting rate of oxygen consumption during physical activity. Based on table from Pate et al (see text, pp 131, 133).[43]

Activity type	Light activity (< 3.0 METs)	Moderate activity (3.0–6.0 METs)	Vigorous activity (> 6.0 METs)
Walking	Slowly (1–2 mph)	Briskly (3–4 mph)	Briskly uphill or with a load
Swimming	Treading slowly	Moderate effort	Fast treading or swimming
Cycling	–	For pleasure or transport (≤ 10 mph)	Fast or racing (> 10 mph)
Golf	Power cart	Pulling cart or carrying clubs	–
Boating	Power boat	Canoeing leisurely	Canoeing rapidly (> 4 mph)
Home care	Carpet sweeping	General cleaning	Moving furniture
Mowing lawn	Riding mower	Power mower	Hand mower
Home repair	Carpentry	Painting	–

mph, miles per hour; METs, work metabolic rate/resting metabolic rate; 1 MET represents the rate of oxygen consumption of a seated adult at rest.

TABLE 2 Effectiveness of lifestyle interventions for lowering blood pressure in people with primary hypertension: results of RCTs (see text, pp 138–140).

Intervention	Mean decrease in syst/diast BP (mmHg)	Number of RCTs (people)	Participants	Duration (weeks)	Mean change in targeted factor
Exercise	5/3	29 (1533)	80% male, age 28–72	> 4	50 mins aerobic 3 x a week
Low fat high fruit and vegetable diet	5.5/3*	1 (459)	50% male, mean age 44	8	
Weight loss	3/3	18 (2611)	55% male, mean age 50	2–52	3–9% of body weight
Salt restriction	4/2	58 (2161)	Mean age 49	1–52	118 mmol/day
	2/0.5	28 (1131)	Mean age 47	4	60 mmol/day

*Data presented for 459 people with systolic BP below 160 mmHg and diastolic BP 80–95 mmHg; for the subgroup of 133 people with systolic BP ≥ 160 mmHg and diastolic BP 80–95 mmHg; for the subgroup of 133 people with systolic BP ≥ 140 mmHg or diastolic BP ≥ 90 mmHg, the mean decrease of BP was 11.4/5.5; syst/diast BP, systolic/diastolic blood pressure.

TABLE 3 Effectiveness of dietary supplementation for lowering blood pressure in people with primary hypertension: results of RCTs (see text, pp 141–143).

Intervention	Decrease in syst/diast BP (mmHg)	Number of RCTs (people)	Participants	Duration	Change in targeted factor
Potassium supplement	4.4/2.5	21 (1560)	Age 19–79	1–24 weeks	60–100 mmol/day
Fish oil supplement	4.5/2.5	7 (339)	Mean age 50	Mean 8 weeks	3 g/day or more
Calcium supplement	2/0	12 (383)	Not clear	8 weeks median	800–1500 mg/day

TABLE 4   Effects of antiplatelet treatment (mainly aspirin) on vascular events (non-fatal myocardial infarction, non-fatal stroke, or vascular death) in RCTs among individuals without evidence of cardiovascular disease (see text, p 147).

Trials (duration)	Annual risk of vascular event (control)	Vascular events Antiplatelet, Control, and Odds ratio* (CI†)	Avoided events (1000 person years)	Myocardial infarction Antiplatelet, Control, and Odds ratio* (CI†)	Stroke Antiplatelet, Control, and Odds ratio* (CI†)
UK doctors[152] (70 months)	1.5%	288/3429, 280/3420‡, 1.03 (0.6 to 2.3)	−0.4	169/3429, 176/3420‡, 0.96 (0.7 to 1.4)	91/3429, 78/3420‡, 1.16 (0.7 to 1.9)
US physicians[153] (60 months)	0.7%	321/11037, 387/11034, 0.82 (0.7 to 1.0)	1.2	139/11037, 239/11034, 0.58 (0.5 to 0.8)	119/11 037, 98/11 034, 1.22 (0.9 to 1.7)
TPT[154] (76 months)	1.8%	239/2545, 270/2540, 0.87 (0.7 to 1.1)	2.0	154/2545, 190/2540, 0.80 (0.7 to 1.1)	47/2545, 48/2540, 0.98 (0.6 to 1.7)
HOT[124] (46 months)	1.0%	315/9399, 368/9391, 0.85 (0.7 to 1.0)	1.5	82/9399, 127/9391, 0.65 (0.5 to 0.9)	146/9399, 148/9391, 0.99 (0.7 to 1.3)
PPP[157] (44 months)	0.8%	45/2226, 64/2269, 0.71 (0.4 to 1.2)	2.2	19/2226, 28/2269, 0.69 (0.3 to 1.5)	16/2226, 24/2269, 0.68 (0.3 to 1.6)
All trials (56 months)	1.0%	1208/28 636 (4.2%), 1369/28 654 (4.8%), 0.86§ (0.8 to 0.9)	1.2	563/28 636 (2.0%), 760/28 654 (2.4%), 0.71§ (0.7 to 0.8)	419/28 636 (1.5%), 396/28 654 (1.4%), 1.05§ (0.9 to 1.2)

Data from individual trial publications and from the APT overview (1994).[155] The effects of aspirin were similar in the absence or presence of warfarin, so the data presented are not stratified by warfarin allocation. * Odds ratios calculated using the "observed minus expected" method;[155] † 99% CI for individual trials 95% CI for "All trials"; ‡ Number of patients in control group was 1710 (randomisation ratio 2 : 1); numerator and denominator multiplied by 2 to calculate totals for absolute differences between antiplatelet and control group event rates; actual numbers of events used to calculate odds ratios and confidence intervals; ¶ Weighted by study size; § Heterogeneity of odds ratios between 5 trials not significant (P > 0.05).

TABLE 5 Effects of aspirin on intracranial bleeds and major extracranial bleeds in RCTs among individuals without evidence of cardiovascular disease (see text, pp 147, 148).

Trials	Antiplatelet	Control	Summary odds ratio* (95% CI)	Excess bleeds per 1000 patients treated per year
Intracranial bleeds				
UK doctors[152]	13/3429	12/3420†		
US physicians[153]	23/11037	12/11034		
TPT[156]	12/2545	6/2540		
HOT[124]	14/9399	15/9391		
PPP[157]	2/2226	3/2269		
All trials	64/28 636 (0.22%)	48/28654 (0.17%)	1.4 (0.9 to 2.0)	0.1 (P = 0.1)
Major extracranial bleeds				
UK Doctors[152]	21/3429	20/3420†		
US Physicians[153]	48/1 037	28/11 034		
TPT[156]	20/2545	13/2540		
HOT[124]	122/9399	63/9391		
All trials	211/26 410 (0.8%)	134/28 095 (0.5%)	1.7 (1.4 to 2.1)	0.7 (P < 0.00001)

Data from individual trial publications. * Odds ratios calculated using the "observed minus expected" method.[155]
† Number of patients in control group was 1710 (randomisation ratio 2 : 1); numerator and denominator multiplied by 2 to calculate totals for absolute differences between antiplatelet and control group event rates; actual numbers of events used to calculate odds ratios and confidence intervals.

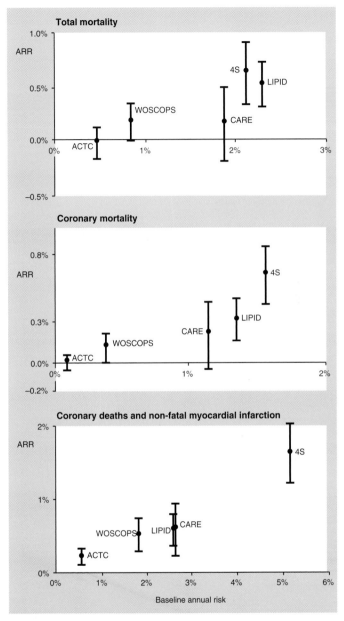

FIGURE 1 **Effects of cholesterol lowering: relation between the ARR (for annual total mortality, coronary heart disease mortality, coronary deaths, and non-fatal myocardial infarction) and the baseline risk of those events in the placebo group for 5 large statin trials (ACTC = AFCAPS/TexCAPS,[139] 4S,[140] LIPID,[141] CARE,[142] WOSCOPS[143]) (see text, pp 145, 146).**

Search date November 2000

Clinical Evidence writers on secondary prevention of ischaemic cardiac events

Key Messages

Antithrombotic treatment

- One collaborative overview and subsequent RCTs have found that antiplatelet treatment reduces the risk of serious vascular events, and suggests that aspirin 75 mg daily is as effective as higher doses. We found no clear evidence that any other antiplatelet regimen is definitely superior to medium dose aspirin (75–325 mg daily) in the prevention of vascular events. One systematic review has found that clopidogrel is a safe and effective alternative to aspirin.

- One systematic review has found that anticoagulants produce a similar reduction in the risk of serious vascular events to that produced by aspirin. However, aspirin versus oral anticoagulants causes fewer haemorrhages. The systematic review has found no clear evidence that the addition of oral anticoagulants to aspirin produced additional benefit.

Other drug treatments

- Systematic reviews have found that:
  - β Blockers reduce all cause mortality, coronary mortality, recurrent non-fatal myocardial infarction (MI), and sudden death in people after MI.
  - In people who have had an MI with or without left ventricular dysfunction, angiotensin converting enzyme (ACE) inhibitors reduce rates of death, hospitalisation for congestive heart failure, and recurrent non-fatal MI.
  - Using class I antiarrhythmic agents after MI increases the risk of cardiovascular mortality and sudden death.
  - Amiodarone reduces the risk of sudden death and marginally reduces overall mortality in people at high risk of death after MI. We found limited evidence that sotalol may be harmful rather than beneficial in people after MI.
  - Calcium channel blockers do not reduce mortality in people after MI or with chronic coronary heart disease. Diltiazem and verapamil may reduce rates of reinfarction and refractory angina in people after MI who do not have heart failure.

- One large well designed RCT of hormone replacement therapy (HRT) versus placebo found no reduction of major cardiovascular events in postmenopausal women with established coronary artery disease, despite strong evidence from RCTs that HRT improves some cardiovascular risk factors.

Cholesterol reduction

- One systematic review has found that lowering cholesterol with statins substantially reduces the risk of cardiovascular mortality and morbidity with no evidence of an increase in non-cardiovascular mortality.

Blood pressure reduction

- We found no direct evidence of the effects of lowering blood pressure in people with established coronary heart disease. Observational studies and extrapolation from trials of blood pressure reduction in people with no history of ischaemic cardiac events support the lowering of blood pressure in those with concomitant risk factors that put them at higher risk. The evidence for benefit is strongest for β blockers.

Non-drug treatments

- The role of vitamin E, β carotene, and vitamin C remains unclear.

Cardiovascular disorders

Secondary prevention of ischaemic cardiac events

- RCTs found that advising people with coronary artery disease to eat more fish (particularly fatty fish) or more fruit and vegetables, bread, pasta, potatoes, olive oil, and rapeseed margarine (a more Mediterranean diet) may result in a substantial survival benefit. We found no strong evidence from RCTs of a beneficial effect of low fat or high fibre diets on major non-fatal coronary heart disease events or coronary heart disease mortality.

- Systematic reviews have found that cardiac rehabilitation improves coronary risk factors and reduces the risk of major cardiac events in people after MI. The role of exercise alone in reducing the risk of adverse cardiovascular outcomes is not clear.

- We found no RCTs of the effects of smoking cessation on cardiovascular events in people with coronary heart disease. Epidemiological studies have found that people with coronary heart disease who stop smoking rapidly reduce their risk of recurrent coronary events or death. The use of nicotine patches seems safe in people with coronary heart disease.

- One systematic review of mainly poor quality RCTs found that psychological and stress management may decrease rates of MI or cardiac death in people with coronary heart disease.

Surgical treatments

- RCTs performed up to the mid 1980s have found that, compared with medical treatment, coronary artery bypass grafting (CABG) carries a greater risk of death in the first year but reduces the risk of death from coronary artery disease at 5 and 10 years. Greatest benefit occurrs in people with more severe disease (multivessel disease, left ventricular dysfunction, or MI). We found no evidence of increased protection against subsequent MI. One more recent RCT, using modern techniques and with optimal background medical treatment, has found even greater superiority of surgical revascularisation over non-invasive treatment.

- RCTs have found that, in comparison with percutaneous transluminal coronary angioplasty (PTA), intracoronary stents affords superior acute and long term clinical and angiographic results.

DEFINITION	Secondary prevention in this context is the long term management of people with a prior acute MI, and of people at high risk of ischaemic cardiac events for other reasons, such as a history of angina or coronary surgical procedures.
INCIDENCE/ PREVALENCE	Coronary artery disease is the leading cause of death in developed countries and is becoming a major cause of mortality and morbidity in developing countries. There are pronounced international, regional, and temporal differences in death rates. In the USA, the prevalence of overt coronary artery disease approaches 4%.[1]
AETIOLOGY/ RISK FACTORS	Most ischaemic cardiac events are associated with atheromatous plaques that can cause acute obstruction of coronary vessels. Atheroma is more likely in elderly people, in those with established coronary artery disease, and in those with risk factors (such as smoking, hypertension, high cholesterol, diabetes mellitus).
PROGNOSIS	Almost half of those who suffer an acute MI die before they reach hospital. Of those hospitalised, 7–15% die in hospital and another 7–15% die during the following year. People who survive the acute stage of MI fall into three prognostic groups, based on their baseline risk (see table 1, p 190):[2-4] high (20% of all survivors), moderate

(55%), and low (25%) risk. Long term prognosis depends on the degree of left ventricular dysfunction, the presence of residual ischaemia, and the extent of any electrical instability. Further risk stratification procedures include evaluation of left ventricular function (by echocardiography or nuclear ventriculography) and of myocardial ischaemia (by non-invasive stress testing).[4-8] Those with low left ventricular ejection fraction, ischaemia, or poor functional status may be evaluated further by cardiac catheterisation.[9]

AIMS	To improve long term survival and quality of life; to prevent (recurrent) MI, unstable angina, left ventricular dysfunction, heart failure, and sudden cardiac death; and to restore and maintain normal activities.
OUTCOMES	Mortality (total, cardiovascular, coronary, sudden death, non-cardiovascular); morbidity (MI, severe angina, and stroke); or quality of life.
METHODS	*Clinical Evidence* search and appraisal November 2000.

QUESTION   **What are the effects of antithrombotic treatment?**

Cathie Sudlow

OPTION   **ANTIPLATELET TREATMENT**

One collaborative overview has found that prolonged antiplatelet treatment reduces the risk of serious vascular events in people at high risk of ischaemic cardiac events. Along with subsequent RCTs, it found that, for prolonged use, aspirin 75 mg daily is as effective as higher doses. We found no clear evidence that any other antiplatelet regimen is superior to medium dose aspirin (i.e. 75–325 mg daily) to prevent vascular events, although one RCT has found that clopidogrel appears to be a safe and effective alternative.

Benefits: **Antiplatelet treatment versus control:** One collaborative overview (search date not stated) found that a month or more of antiplatelet treatment significantly reduced the odds of a vascular event (non-fatal MI, non-fatal stroke, or vascular death) by about a quarter compared with control, among about 70 000 people at high risk of occlusive arterial disease (odds reduction 27%, 95% CI 24% to 30%).[10] Most of these people were at high risk of ischaemic cardiac events, and some people (including those with a history of MI, those with stable angina, and those who had undergone coronary revascularisation procedures) were at particularly high risk. Among the 20 000 people with a prior MI, antiplatelet treatment prevented 18 non-fatal recurrent MIs, six non-fatal strokes, and 13 vascular deaths per 1000 people treated for about 2 years. The review also found that antiplatelet treatment reduced all cause mortality (see figure 1, p 191). **Different daily doses of aspirin:** About two thirds of the RCTs in the overview involved an aspirin regimen, and medium dose aspirin (75–325 mg daily) was the most widely tested of these. Indirect comparisons found that daily doses of less than 160 mg (mostly 75–150 mg), 160–325 mg, and 500–1500 mg prevented similar proportions of vascular events among high risk people, whereas direct comparisons also showed that daily aspirin doses of 75–325 mg or 500–1500 mg were similarly effective.[10] One additional recent RCT (almost 3000 people at high risk of cardiovascular events) directly compared lower doses of aspirin (81 mg or 325 mg daily) versus higher doses (650 mg or 1300 mg daily). It found that lower doses produced a slightly lower rate of stroke, MI, or death than higher doses (AR 6.2% with lower doses v AR 8.4 % with higher doses; P = 0.03).[11] The review found only limited evidence for the effectiveness of daily doses of aspirin of less than 160 mg. One subsequent RCT (2000 people with stable angina) compared aspirin 75 mg daily with placebo.[12] It found that a daily dose of aspirin 75 mg reduced the composite outcome of MI or sudden death compared with placebo (RRR 34%, 95% CI 24% to 49%).

Alternative antiplatelet regimens to aspirin: The 1994 review found no evidence that any antiplatelet regimen was more effective than medium dose aspirin alone in the prevention of vascular events.[10] One systematic review of randomised trials (search date 1999), comparing either ticlopidine or clopidogrel with aspirin, found four trials among 22 656 people at high risk of vascular disease (including 6000 presenting with recent MI).[13] Most of these people were included in a large trial of clopidogrel (75 mg daily) versus aspirin (325 mg daily).[14] Compared with aspirin, the thienopyridines reduced the odds of a vascular event by 9% (OR 0.91, 95% CI 0.84 to 0.98; P = 0.01), but there was substantial uncertainty about the size of any additional benefit (11 events prevented per 1000 people treated for about 2 years [95% CI 2 to 19 events]).[13]

Harms:

Bleeding is the most important adverse effect of antiplatelet treatment. The 1994 overview found that the excess risk of intracranial bleeding with antiplatelet treatment was small (at most 1 or 2 bleeds per 1000 people per year) in trials of long term treatment.[10] Antiplatelet treatment produced a small but significant excess of non-fatal major extracranial bleeds (3 bleeds per 1000 people), but there was no clear excess of fatal extracranial bleeds.[10] In one RCT directly comparing two different doses of aspirin, 1200 mg daily was associated with more gastrointestinal bleeding than 325 mg daily,[15] although we found no good evidence for a variation in gastrointestinal bleeding risk in the range 75–325 mg daily. The systematic review of randomised trials of the thienopyridine derivatives versus aspirin found that the thienopyridines produced significantly less gastrointestinal haemorrhage and upper gastrointestinal upset than aspirin. However, they increased the odds of skin rash and of diarrhoea: ticlopidine by about twofold and clopidogrel by about a third. Ticlopidine (but not clopidogrel) increased the odds of neutropenia.[13] Observational studies have also found that ticlopidine is associated with thrombocytopenia and thrombotic thrombocytopenic purpura.[16,17] However, we found no clear evidence of an excess of haematological adverse side effects with clopidogrel.[18,19] The results of two RCTs (about 1700 people undergoing coronary artery stenting) of clopidogrel plus aspirin versus ticlopidine plus aspirin suggested clopidogrel to be superior to ticlopidine in terms of safety and tolerability.[20,21]

Comment: Among people at high risk of cardiac events, the large absolute reductions in serious vascular events far outweighed any absolute risks.

OPTION   **ORAL ANTICOAGULANTS IN THE ABSENCE OF ANTIPLATELET TREATMENT**

One systematic review has found that high or moderate intensity oral anticoagulants given alone reduce the risk of serious vascular events in people with coronary artery disease, but were associated with substantial risks of bleeding. Oral anticoagulants require regular monitoring for intensity of anticoagulant effect.

Benefits: One systematic overview (search date 1999) of the effects of oral anticoagulation in people with coronary artery disease found 16 trials of high intensity anticoagulation (international normalised ratio [INR] > 2.8 — see glossary, p 185) versus control in 10 056 people, and four trials of moderate intensity anticoagulation (INR 2–3) versus control in 1365 people. Antiplatelet therapy was not routinely given in any of these 20 trials. The review found that high intensity anti-coagulation reduced the odds of the combined outcome of death, MI, or stroke compared with control (odds reduction 43%, 95% CI 37% to 49%; about 98 events avoided per 1000 people treated). Compared with control, moderate intensity anticoagulation reduced these odds by a somewhat smaller, non-significant amount.[22] In direct comparisons of high or moderate intensity oral anticoagulation with aspirin, the effects on death, MI, or stroke were similar (OR 1.04, 95% CI 0.80 to 1.34).[22]

Harms: Compared with control, high intensity anticoagulation increased the odds of major (mainly extracranial) bleeding about sixfold (OR 6.0, 95% CI 4.4 to 8.2; absolute increase of 39 events per 1000 people treated), and moderate intensity anticoagulation also increased the odds of major bleeding about eightfold (OR 7.7, 95% CI 3.3 to 17.6).[22] Compared with aspirin, high or moderate intensity oral anticoagulation increased the odds of major bleeding more than twofold (OR 2.4, 95% CI 1.6 to 3.6).[22]

Comment: Oral anticoagulants provide substantial protection against vascular events in the absence of antiplatelet therapy, but the risks of serious bleeding are higher than for antiplatelet treatment and regular monitoring is required. Medium dose aspirin provides similar protection, but is safer and easier to use; see antiplatelet treatment below.

OPTION   **ORAL ANTICOAGULANTS IN ADDITION TO ANTIPLATELET TREATMENT**

One systematic review found no evidence that the addition of low intensity oral anticoagulation (target INR < 1.5) to aspirin produces additional benefit. The effects of adding a more intensive anticoagulant regimen (target INR 2–3) are uncertain.

Benefits: One systematic overview (search date 1999) found six RCTs that examined the effects of adding an oral anticoagulant regimen to aspirin in 8915 people with coronary artery disease. Three of these trials assessed the addition of a low intensity (target INR < 1.5) regimen to aspirin in a total of 8435 people, and found no significant reduction in the odds of death, MI, or stroke (OR 0.91, 95% CI 0.79 to 1.06).[22] Trials assessing the addition of a moderate intensity (INR 2–3) oral anticoagulant regimen to aspirin were too small (480 people) to produce reliable estimates of efficacy and safety.[22]

Harms: Too few major bleeds have been recorded in RCTs to quantify reliably the effects of adding oral anticoagulants to aspirin. The review found a non-significant excess of major bleeds produced by the addition of low intensity oral anticoagulation to aspirin (OR 1.29, 95% CI 0.96 to 1.75), as well as by the addition of more intense anticoagulation (OR 1.88, 95% CI 0.59 to 6.00).[22]

Comment: The issue of whether adding a moderately intense oral anticoagulant regimen to aspirin provides additional net benefit to people at high risk of ischaemic cardiac events is being assessed in several ongoing RCTs.

QUESTION   **What are the effects of other drug treatments?**

Eva Lonn

OPTION   β BLOCKERS

We found strong evidence from systematic reviews of RCTs that β blockers reduce the risk of all cause mortality, coronary mortality, recurrent non-fatal MI, and sudden death in people after MI. Most benefit was seen in those at highest risk of death after an MI (> 50 years old; previous MI, angina pectoris, hypertension, or treatment with digitalis; transient mechanical or electrical failure; higher heart rate at study entry). About a quarter of people suffered adverse effects.

Benefits: **Survival and reinfarction:** One systematic review (search date 1993, 26 RCTs, over 24 000 people) compared oral β blockers versus placebo within days or weeks of an acute MI (late intervention trials) and continued for between 6 weeks to 3 years. Most RCTs followed participants for 1 year. The review found improved survival in people given β blockers (RRR 23%, 95% CI 14% to 30%).[23] One prior systematic review (search date not stated, 24 RCTs) found that long term use of β blockers versus placebo after MI reduced total mortality (RRR about 20%; NNT 48), sudden death (RRR about 30%; NNT 63), and non-fatal reinfarction (RRR about 25%; NNT 56).[24] **Anginal symptoms:** We found no good RCTs evaluating the antianginal effects of β blockers in people after MI. One trial found atenolol more effective than placebo in people with chronic stable effort angina or silent ischaemia.[25] **Different types of β blockers:** The earlier review found no differences between β blockers with and without cardioselectivity or membrane stabilising properties, but it raised concerns about the lack of efficacy of β blockers with intrinsic sympathomimetic activity in long term management after MI.[24] One RCT (607 people after MI) found that acebutolol, a β blocker with moderate partial agonist activity, decreased 1 year mortality compared with placebo (AR of death:

11% with placebo, 6% with acebutolol; RRR 48%, 95% CI 9% to 71%).[26] **Effects in different subgroups:** One systematic review (search date 1983, 9 RCTs) compared β blockers versus placebo started more than 24 hours after onset of symptoms of acute MI and continued for 9–24 months.[27] Pooled analysis of individual data (13 679 people) found that the benefits of β blockers versus placebo on mortality seemed comparable in men and women. The highest absolute benefit from β blockers was found in subgroups with the highest baseline risks (that is, those with the highest mortality on placebo): those over 50 years of age; those with a history of previous MI, angina pectoris, hypertension, or treatment with digitalis; those with transient signs or symptoms of mechanical or electrical failure in the early phases of MI; and those with a higher heart rate at study entry. Low risk subgroups had smaller mean absolute benefit.

Harms: Adverse effects include shortness of breath, bronchospasm, brady-cardia, hypotension, heart block, cold hands and feet, diarrhoea, fatigue, reduced sexual activity, depression, nightmares, faintness, insomnia, blacking out, and hallucinations. Rates vary in different studies. One RCT reported an absolute risk increase for any adverse effect on propranolol compared with placebo of 24% (95% CI not available). Serious adverse effects were uncommon and only a small proportion of people withdrew as a result.[28]

Comment: Continued benefit has been reported from the use of β blockers up to 6 years after MI (ARR for mortality 5.9%, 95% CI not available; P = 0.003; RRR 18%). However, the study was not blinded after 33 months.

OPTION   **ANGIOTENSIN CONVERTING ENZYME (ACE) INHIBITORS**

In people who have had an MI and have left ventricular dysfunction, there is strong evidence from a systematic review of RCTs that ACE inhibitors versus placebo reduce rates of death, hospitalisation for congestive heart failure, and recurrent non-fatal MI. The effects of ACE inhibitors in people who have had an MI but do not have left ventricular dysfunction have not yet been adequately evaluated.

Benefits: **In people with low left ventricular ejection fraction:** One sys-tematic review (search date not stated, 3 RCTs)[29] compared ACE inhibitors (captopril, ramipril, or trandolapril) versus placebo started 3–16 days after acute MI and continued for 15–42 months. It analysed individual data from 5966 people with a recent MI and with clinical manifestations of congestive heart failure or moderate left ventricular dysfunction (left ventricular ejection fraction ≥ 35–40%). ACE inhibitors versus placebo significantly reduced rates of death (RRR 26%, 95% CI 17% to 34%; NNT 17 people treated for about 2 years to prevent 1 death), hospitalisation for congestive heart failure (RRR 27%, 95% CI 15% to 37%; NNT 28), and recurrent non-fatal MI (RRR 20%, 95% CI 6% to 31%; NNT 43). **In people without impaired ventricular function or evidence of congestive heart failure:** We found no systematic review but found one large RCT (9297 people at high risk of cardiovascular events), which found that the ACE inhibitor ramipril (10 mg/day) versus placebo reduced the composite primary outcome of cardio-vascular death, stroke, or MI over an average of 4.7 years (RRR for composite outcome: 22%, NNT 26; RRR for cardiovascular death: 26%, NNT 50; RRR for MI: 20%, NNT 42; RRR for stroke: 32%, NNT 67; RRR for death from all causes: 16%, NNT 56). The RCT found that ramipril reduced the need for revascularisation proce-dures and reduced heart failure related outcomes (need for revas-cularisation: RRR 15%, no CI provided; heart failure related out-comes: RRR 23%, no CI provided). Ramipril versus placebo produced benefit in subgroups examined, including women and men; people aged over and under 65 years; those with and without a history of coronary artery disease; hypertension; diabetes; periph-eral vascular disease; cerebrovascular disease; and those with and without microalbuminuria at study entry.[30] **In people with diabetes:** See antihypertensive treatment under cardiovascular disease in dia-betes, p 20.

Harms: The major adverse effects reported in these trials were cough (ARI versus placebo of 5–10%), dizziness, hypotension (5–10%), renal failure (< 3%), hyperkalaemia (< 3%), angina, syncope, diarrhoea (2%), and, for captopril, alteration in taste (2% of captopril users).[29]

Comment: There are several other ongoing large RCTs evaluating the use of ACE inhibitors in people without clinical manifestations of heart failure and with no or with mild impairment in left ventricular systolic function. These include one trial of trandolapril in 8000 people with coronary artery disease, and one trial of perindopril in 10 500 people with stable coronary artery disease.[32]

| OPTION | CLASS I ANTIARRHYTHMIC AGENTS (QUINIDINE, PROCAINAMIDE, DISOPYRIMIDE, ENCAINIDE, FLECAINIDE, MORACIZINE) |

One systematic review of RCTs has found that the use of class I antiarrhythmic agents after MI increases the risk of cardiovascular mortality and sudden death.

Benefits: None (see harms below).

Harms: One systematic review (search date 1993, 51 RCTs, 23 229 people) compared class I antiarrhythmic drugs versus placebo; given acutely and later in the management of MI.[23] The review found that the antiarrhythmic agents increased mortality (AR of death 5.6% v 5.0% with placebo; OR 1.14, 95% CI 1.01 to 1.28). One RCT (1498 people with MI and asymptomatic or mildly symp-tomatic ventricular arrhythmia) found that encainide or flecainide versus placebo increased the risk of death or cardiac arrest after 10 months (RR 2.38, 95% CI 1.59 to 3.57; NNH 17).[33]

Comment: The evidence implies that class I antiarrhythmics should not be used in people after MI or with significant coronary artery disease.

CLASS III ANTIARRHYTHMIC AGENTS (AMIODARONE, SOTALOL)

Two systematic reviews of RCTs have found that amiodarone versus placebo reduces the risk of sudden death and marginally reduces mortality in people at high risk of death after MI. Limited evidence on the effects of sotalol suggests that it may be harmful rather than beneficial in this setting.

Benefits: We found two systematic reviews.[34,35] The first systematic review (search date not stated, individual data from 6553 high risk people in 13 RCTs) compared amiodarone versus control treatments. Participants were selected with a recent MI and a high risk of death from cardiac arrhythmia (based on low left ventricular ejection fraction, frequent ventricular premature depolarisations or non-sustained ventricular tachycardia, but no history of sustained symptomatic ventricular tachycardia or ventricular fibrillation); 78% from eight RCTs had a recent MI, and 22% from five RCTs had congestive heart failure.[34] Most trials were placebo controlled with a mean follow up of about 1.5 years. The people with congestive heart failure were symptomatic but stable and did not have a recent MI, although in most cases the heart failure was ischaemic in origin. All RCTs used a loading dose of amiodarone (400 mg/day for 28 days or 800 mg/day for 14 days) followed by a maintenance dose (200–400 mg/day). Amiodarone versus placebo significantly reduced total mortality (ARs 10.9% per year with amiodarone v 12.3% per year with placebo; RRR 13%, 95% CI 1% to 22%; NNT 71 per year to avoid 1 additional death), and rates of sudden cardiac death (RRR 29%, 95% CI 15% to 41%; NNT 59). Amiodarone had similar effects in the post MI and congestive heart failure studies. The second systematic review (search date 1997, 5864 people with MI, congestive heart failure, left ventricular dysfunction, or cardiac arrest) found similar results.[35]

Harms: Adverse events leading to discontinuation of amiodarone were hypothyroidism (expressed per 100 person years: 7.0 v 1.1 on placebo; OR 7.3), hyperthyroidism (1.4 v 0.5; OR 2.5), peripheral neuropathy (0.5 v 0.2; OR 2.8), lung infiltrates (1.6 v 0.5; OR 3.1), bradycardia (2.4 v 0.8; OR 2.6), and liver dysfunction (1.0 v 0.4; OR 2.7).[34]

Comment: The reviews' conclusions are probably specific to amiodarone.[34,35] One RCT found increased mortality with the class III antiarrhythmic agent sotalol compared with placebo in 3121 people with MI and left ventricular dysfunction (ARs for death 5% v 3.1%; RR 1.65, 95% CI 1.15 to 2.36). The trial was terminated prematurely after less than 1 year of follow up.[36] The two largest RCTs of amiodarone after MI found a favourable interaction between β blockers and amiodarone, with additional reduction in cardiac mortality.[37,38]

CALCIUM CHANNEL BLOCKERS

One systematic review of RCTs found no benefit from calcium channel blockers in people after MI or with chronic coronary heart disease. Diltiazem and verapamil may reduce rates of reinfarction and refractory angina in people after MI who do not have heart failure.

Secondary prevention of ischaemic cardiac events

Benefits: One systematic review (search date 1993, 24 RCTs) compared calcium channel blockers (including dihydropyridines, diltiazem, and verapamil) versus placebo administered early or late during the course of acute MI or unstable angina and continued in the intermediate or long term.[23] Two of the RCTs used angiographic regression of coronary stenosis as an outcome in people with stable coronary heart disease treated with calcium channel blockers. The review found no significant difference in the absolute risk of death compared with placebo (AR 9.7% v 9.3%; ARI on calcium channel blockers compared with placebo 0.4%, 95% CI −0.4% to +1.2%; OR 1.04, 95% CI 0.95 to 1.14). **Diltiazem and verapamil:** The review found no significant effect compared with placebo (OR 0.95, 95% CI 0.82 to 1.09).[23] Three RCTs comparing diltiazem or verapamil versus placebo found decreased rates of recurrent infarction and refractory angina with active treatment but only for those people without signs or symptoms of heart failure. For those with clinical manifestations of heart failure, the trends were towards harm.[39-41] **Dihydropyridines:** The review found no significant effect compared with placebo (OR 1.16, 95% CI 0.99 to 1.35). Several individual RCTs of dihydropyridines found increased mortality, particularly when these agents were started early in the course of acute MI and in the absence of β blockers.

Harms: Adverse effects reported of verapamil and diltiazem include atrioventricular block, atrial bradycardia, new onset heart failure, hypotension, dizziness, oedema, rash, constipation, and pruritus.

Comment: Newer generation dihydropyridines, such as amlodipine and felodipine, have not been well studied in people after MI but have been found to be safe in people with heart failure, including heart failure of ischaemic origin.

OPTION	HORMONE REPLACEMENT THERAPY

We found no clear evidence from RCTs that HRT reduces major cardiovascular events in postmenopausal women with established coronary artery disease, despite strong evidence from RCTs that HRT improves some cardiovascular risk factors.

Benefits: **Combined oestrogen and progestins:** We found no systematic review. One large RCT (2763 postmenopausal women with coronary heart disease) found that conjugated equine oestrogen (0.625 mg/day) plus medroxyprogesterone acetate (2.5 mg/day) versus placebo for an average of 4.1 years produced no significant difference in the risk of non-fatal MI plus deaths caused by coronary heart disease (172/1380 [12.5%] with HRT v 176/1383 [12.7%] with placebo; ARR +0.2%, 95% CI −2.2% to +2.7%; RRR +1%, 95% CI −2.2% to +2.0%).[42] It also found no significant difference in secondary cardiovascular outcomes (coronary revascularisation, unstable angina, congestive heart failure, resuscitated cardiac arrest, stroke or transient ischaemic attack, and peripheral arterial disease) or in all cause mortality. **Oestrogen alone:** We found no good RCTs of oestrogen alone (without progestins) in the secondary prevention of coronary heart disease in postmenopausal women.

One RCT found that high dose oestrogen (5 mg conjugated equine oestrogen/day) increased the risk of MI and thromboembolic events in men with pre-existing coronary heart disease.[43]

Harms: Pooled estimates from observational studies found an increased risk of endometrial cancer (RR > 8) and of breast cancer (RR 1.25 to 1.46) when oestrogen was used for over 8 years. In most observational studies, the addition of progestins prevented endometrial cancer but not breast cancer. The risk of venous thromboembolism, including pulmonary embolism and deep vein thrombosis, was three to four times higher with HRT than without. However, because the incidence of venous thromboembolism is low in postmenopausal women, the absolute increase in risk was only about one to two additional cases of venous thromboembolism in 5000 users a year.[44] In the RCT described above,[42] more women in the HRT than in the placebo group experienced venous thromboembolism (34/1380 v 12/1383; OR 2.65, 95% CI 1.48 to 4.75) and gall bladder disease (84/1380 v 62/1383; OR 1.38, 95% CI 0.99 to 1.92).

Comment: Many observational studies have found reduced rates of clinical events caused by coronary heart disease in postmenopausal women using HRT, especially in women with pre-existing coronary heart disease. Hormone users experienced 35–80% fewer recurrent events than non-users.[45,46] Meanwhile, several RCTs have found that HRT improves cardiovascular risk factors.[47] It is not known whether studies longer than 4 years would show a benefit.

QUESTION What are the effects of cholesterol reduction?

Michael Pignone

Systematic reviews and large subsequent RCTs have found that lowering cholesterol in people at high risk of ischaemic coronary events substantially reduces the risk of overall mortality, cardiovascular mortality, and non-fatal cardiovascular events. One systematic review of primary and secondary prevention trials has found that statins constitute the single most effective type of treatment for reducing cholesterol and reducing cardiovascular risk. The absolute benefits increased as baseline risk increased, but were not additionally influenced by the individual's absolute cholesterol concentration. We found no direct evidence for effects in people aged over 75 years, or for effects of combined treatments to reduce cholesterol and other cardiovascular risk factors.

Benefits: **Statins:** We found one systematic review (search date 1998, 5 RCTs, 30 817 people) that compared long term (≥ 4 years) treatment with statins versus placebo.[48] Combining the three secondary prevention trials, the review found that statins reduced coronary heart disease mortality, cardiovascular mortality, and all cause mortality compared with control over a mean of 5.4 years (coronary heart disease mortality: OR 0.71, 95% CI 0.63 to 0.80; cardiovascular mortality: OR 0.73, 95% CI 0.66 to 0.82; all cause mortality: OR 0.77, 95% CI 0.70 to 0.85). Combining primary and secondary prevention, it found that statins compared with control reduced major coronary events (RRR 31%, 95% CI 26% to 35%; ARR 3.6%, 95% CI 2.9% to 4.3%; NNT 28, 95% CI 23 to 34) and all cause mortality (RRR 21%, 95% CI 14% to 28%; ARR 16%, 95% CI 11% to 22%; NNT 61, 95% CI 45 to 95). Absolute risk reduction increased as baseline risk increased in primary prevention (see figure 1 in primary prevention, p 159). Differences between the baseline cholesterol concentration seemed to play no role in determining the results of the trials, in the ranges studied to date. **Effects of statins in different groups of people:** Combining results from primary and secondary prevention trials, the review found that, compared with placebo, statins reduced coronary events by a similar proportional amount in men (reduction in OR 31%, 95% CI 26% to 35%; ARR 3.7%, 95% CI 2.9% to 4.4%), in women (reduction in OR 29%, 95% CI 31% to 42%; ARR 3.3%, 95% CI 1.3% to 5.2%), in people under 65 years (reduction in OR 31%, 95% CI 24% to 36%; ARR 3.2%, 95% CI 2.4% to 4.0%), and in people over 65 years (reduction in OR 32%, 95% CI 23% to 39%; ARR 4.4%, 95% CI 3.0% to 5.8%). The reduction of coronary heart disease events in women involved more non-fatal and fewer fatal events than in men. One large RCT found no significant increase in mortality with statins versus placebo for the subgroup of women, but the confidence interval was wide (RR 1.16, 95% CI 0.68 to 1.99).[48] Other RCTs have not yet reported mortality results for women. **Intensity of statin treatment:** We found one RCT (1351 people with a history of saphenous vein coronary artery bypass graft) that compared aggressive reduction of cholesterol with lovastatin and, if necessary, colestyramine (aiming for target low density lipoprotein cholesterol 1.6–2.2 mmol/l [60–85 mg/dl]) with more moderate reduction (target low density lipoprotein cholesterol 3.4–3.7 mmol/l [130–140 mg/dl]) with the same drugs. The trial found that aggressive treatment reduced the risk of needing repeat revascularisation at 4 years (6.5% with aggressive treatment v 9.2% with moderate treatment, P = 0.03).[49] After an additional 3 years, aggressive treatment reduced the risk of revascularisation and cardiovascular death compared with moderate treatment (AR of revascularisation 19% with aggressive treatment v 27% with moderate treatment, P = 0.0006; AR for cardiovascular death 7.4% with aggressive treatment v 11.3% with moderate treatment, P = 0.03).[50] **Fibrates:** We found one systematic review[51] and two additional RCTs.[52,53] The systematic review (search date 1999, 4 RCTs) compared fibrates versus placebo in people with known coronary heart disease. The review identified one RCT (2531 men with coronary heart disease and a level of high density lipoprotein cholesterol below 1 mmol/l) that found gemfibrozil versus placebo reduced the composite outcome of non-fatal MI plus death from coronary heart disease after a median of 5.1 years (AR 219/1264 [17%] for gemfibrozil v 275/1267 [22%] for placebo; ARR 4.4%, 95% CI 1.4% to 7%; RRR 20%, 95% CI 6% to 32%; NNT 23, 95% CI 14 to 73). The review identified three trials comparing clofibrate versus placebo, which found no consistent difference between groups. The two additional RCTs[52,53] both compared bezafibrate versus placebo. The larger RCT (3090 people selected with previous MI or stable angina, high density lipoprotein cholesterol < 45 mg/dl, and low density lipoprotein cholesterol < 180 mg/dl) found that bezafibrate versus placebo did not significantly reduce all cause mortality or the composite end point of MI plus sudden death (AR for MI or sudden death 13.6% with bezafibrate v 15.0% with placebo; cumulative ARR at 6.2 years 7.3%, P = 0.24).[52] The smaller RCT (92 young male survivors of MI) found that bezafibrate versus placebo significantly reduced the combined outcome of death, reinfarction, plus revascularisation (26% with bezafibrate v 7% with placebo, P = 0.019).[53] **Other treatments:** We found one systematic review (search date 1996, 59 RCTs, 173 160 people), which did not differentiate primary and secondary prevention, and included RCTs of any cholesterol lowering intervention, irrespective of duration, as long as mortality data were reported. It included drug treatments (statins, n–3 fatty acids, fibrates, resins, hormones, or niacin), dietary intervention alone, or surgery (ileal bypass) alone.[54] Overall, baseline risk was similar among all intervention groups. Among non-surgical treatments, the review found that only statins reduced coronary heart disease mortality, and that only statins and n–3 fatty acids reduced all cause mortality (RR of coronary heart disease mortality, treatment v control 0.69, 95% CI 0.59 to 0.80 for statins; 0.44, 95% CI 0.18 to 1.07 for n–3 fatty acids; 0.98, 95% CI 0.78 to 1.24 for fibrates; 0.71, 95% CI 0.51 to 0.99 for resins; 1.04, 95% CI 0.93 to 1.17 for hormones; 0.95, 95% CI 0.83 to 1.10 for niacin; 0.91, 95% CI 0.82 to 1.01 for diet. RR of all cause mortality, treatment v control 0.79, 95% CI 0.71 to 0.89 for statins; 0.68, 95% CI 0.53 to 0.88 for n–3 fatty acids; 1.06, 95% CI 0.78 to 1.46 for fibrates; 0.85, 95% CI 0.66 to 1.08 for resins; 1.09, 95% CI 1.00 to 1.20 for hormones; 0.96, 95% CI 0.86 to 1.08 for niacin; 0.97, 95% CI 0.81 to 1.15 for diet). **Cholesterol lowering versus angioplasty:** We found no systematic review. One RCT found that aggressive lipid lowering treatment was as effective as PTA for reducing ischaemic events, although anginal symptoms were reduced more by PTA (see PTA versus medical treatment, p 181).

Harms: Total non-cardiovascular events, total and tissue specific cancers, and accident and violent deaths have been reported in statin trials. However, the systematic review of long term statin trials found no significant difference between statins and placebo in terms of non-cardiovascular mortality, cancer incidence, asymptomatic elevation of creatinine kinase (> 10 times upper reference limit), or elevation of transaminases (> 3 times upper reference limit) during a mean of 5.4 years of treatment (OR of event, statin v placebo 0.93, 95% CI 0.81 to 1.07 for non-cardiovascular mortality; 0.99, 95% CI 0.90 to 1.08 for cancer; 1.25, 95% CI 0.83 to 1.89 for creatinine kinase rise; 1.13, 95% CI 0.95 to 1.33 for transaminase rise).[48] We found no evidence of additional harm associated with cholesterol lowering in elderly people, or in people following acute MI.

Comment: The evidence indicates that, in a wide range of clinical contexts, the relative risk reduction depends on the size of the fall in cholesterol and is not otherwise dependent on the method by which cholesterol is lowered. The absolute benefit over several years of lowering cholesterol will therefore be greatest in people with the highest baseline risk of an ischaemic cardiac event. Even if the relative risk reduction attenuates at older age, the absolute reduction risk for ischaemic cardiac events may be higher in elderly people than in younger individuals. However, long term benefit for cholesterol lowering has not yet been directly shown in those older than 75 years. Additional information may be provided by the Heart Protection Study (20 000 participants, completion 2000, simvastatin),[55] the Women's Health Initiative (48 000 participants, completion 2007, diet, up to age 79 years),[56] and the Antihypertensive and Lipid Lowering Treatment to Prevent Heart Disease Trial (10 000 participants, completion 2002, pravastatin, no upper age limit).[57] It is not known whether cholesterol reduction will provide benefit for those with initial cholesterol concentrations lower than those selected in the published trials. We found no evidence to indicate whether starting statin treatment immediately after acute infarction provides additional benefits. We found no large direct comparisons of cholesterol modifying drugs; it remains unclear whether any one drug has advantages over others in subgroups of high risk people with particular lipid abnormalities. Because the main aim of treatment is to reduce absolute risk (rather than to reduce the cholesterol to any particular concentration), treatments aimed at lowering cholesterol need evaluating for effectiveness in comparison and in combination with other possible risk factor interventions in each individual.

QUESTION   **What are the effects of blood pressure reduction?**

Eva Lonn

We found no direct evidence of the effects of blood pressure lowering in people with established coronary heart disease. Observational studies, and extrapolation of primary prevention trials of blood pressure reduction, support the lowering of blood pressure in those at high risk of ischaemic coronary events. The evidence for benefit is strongest for β blockers, although not specifically in people with raised blood pressure. The target blood pressure in these people is not clear.

Benefits: We found no systematic review and no RCTs designed specifically to examine blood pressure reduction in those with established coronary heart disease. Prospective epidemiological studies have established that blood pressure continues to be a risk factor for cardiovascular events in people who have already experienced MI. Prospective follow up of 5362 men who reported prior MI during screening for one large RCT found no detectable association between systolic blood pressure and coronary heart disease mortality, and increased coronary heart disease mortality for those with lowest diastolic blood pressure in the first 2 years of follow up.[58] After 15 years there were highly significant linear associations between both systolic and diastolic blood pressure and increased risk of coronary heart disease mortality (stronger relation for systolic blood pressure), with apparent benefit for men with blood pressure maintained at levels lower than the arbitrarily defined "normal" levels. Experimental evidence of benefit from lowering of blood pressure in those with coronary heart disease requires extrapolation from primary prevention trials, because trials of antihypertensive treatment in elderly people[59-61] are likely to have included people with preclinical coronary heart disease. Mortality benefit has been established for β blockers after MI (see option, p 166), for vera-pamil and diltiazem after MI in those without heart failure (see calcium channel blockers, p 169), and for ACE inhibitors after MI, especially in those with heart failure (see ACE inhibitors, p 167).

Harms: Some observational studies have found increased mortality among those with low diastolic blood pressure.[62] Trials in elderly people of blood pressure lowering for hypertension or while treating heart failure[63] found no evidence of a J shaped relation between blood pressure and death.

Comment: Without specific studies comparing different antihypertensive treat-ments, the available evidence is strongest for a beneficial effect of β blockers when treating survivors of an MI who have raised blood pressure. We found no specific evidence about the target level of blood pressure.

QUESTION   **What are the effects of non-drug treatments?**

Andy Ness and Eva Lonn

OPTION   **DIETARY INTERVENTIONS**

RCTs have found that advising people with coronary heart disease to eat more fish (particularly oily fish), more fruit and vegetables, bread, pasta, potatoes, olive oil, and rapeseed margarine (a more Mediterranean diet) may result in a substantial survival benefit. We found no strong evidence from RCTs for a beneficial effect of low fat or high fibre diets on major non-fatal coronary heart disease events or coronary heart disease mortality.

Benefits: **Low fat diets:** One systematic review (search date not stated) found no evidence that allocation to a low fat diet reduced mortality from coronary heart disease in people after MI (RR 0.94, 95% CI 0.84 to 1.06).[64] One large RCT (2033 middle aged men with a recent MI) compared three dietary options: fat advice (to eat less fat); fibre advice (to eat more cereal fibre); and fish advice (to eat at least two portions of fatty fish a week).[65] Advice to reduce fat was complicated and, though fat intake reduced only slightly in the fat advice group, fruit and vegetable intake increased by about 40 g a day.[66] However, there was no clear reduction in mortality (unad-justed RR at 2 years for death from any cause 0.97, 95% CI 0.75 to 1.27). **High fibre diets:** In the trial, people advised to eat more fibre doubled their intake, but survival was non-significantly worse (unadjusted RR at 2 years for death from any cause 1.23, 95% CI 0.95 to 1.60). **High fish diets:** In the trial, those advised to eat more fish ate three times as much fish, although about 14% could not tolerate the fish and were given fish oil capsules. Those given fish advice were significantly less likely to die within 2 years (RRR 29%, 95% CI 7% to 46%; NNT 30). In a second trial, 11 324 people who had survived a recent MI were randomised to receive 1 g daily of n-3 PUFA (fish oil) or no fish oil. Those given fish oil were less likely to die within 3.5 years (RRR 0.14, 95% CI 0.03 to 0.24).[67] **Mediterranean diet:** One RCT (605 middle aged people with a recent MI) compared advice to eat a Mediterranean diet

Secondary prevention of ischaemic cardiac events

(more bread, more vegetables, more fruit, more fish, and less meat, and to replace butter and cream with rapeseed margarine) versus usual dietary advice.[68] There were several dietary differences between the groups. Fruit intake, for example, was about 50 g/day higher in the intervention group than the control group. After 27 months the trial was stopped prematurely because of better outcomes in the intervention group. There were 20 deaths in the control group and eight in the intervention group (adjusted RRR of death 70%, 95% CI 18% to 89%; NNT 25 over 2 years).

Harms: No major adverse effects have been reported.

Comment: Diets low in saturated fat and cholesterol can lead to 10–15% reductions in cholesterol concentrations in highly controlled settings, such as in metabolic wards.[69] In people in the community, the effects are more modest: 3–5% reductions in cholesterol concentrations in general population studies and 9% reductions in people after MI.[64,70-72] Several RCTs of intensive dietary intervention in conjunction with multifactorial risk reduction treatment found decreased progression of anatomic extent of coronary heart disease on angiography.[73] A trial of advice to eat more fruit and vegetables in men with angina is under way (M Burr, personal communication). **Effect on cardiovascular risk factors:** Other studies have investigated the effects of dietary interventions on cardiovascular risk factors rather than the effect on cardiovascular morbidity and mortality. One systematic review (search date 1992) suggested that garlic may reduce cholesterol by about 10%.[74] Some trials in this review had methodological flaws. More recent reports (published in 1998) found no effects of garlic powder or garlic oil on cholesterol concentrations.[75,76] One systematic review (search date 1991) reported modest reductions in cholesterol levels of 2–5% from oats and psyllium enriched cereals (high fibre diets), although we found no evidence that high fibre diets reduce mortality in people with coronary heart disease.[73] One systematic review of soy protein also reported modest reductions in cholesterol concentrations.[77]

OPTION	ANTIOXIDANT VITAMINS (VITAMIN E, β CAROTENE, VITAMIN C)

The role of vitamin E, β carotene, and vitamin C in the long term management of people at high risk for ischaemic cardiac events remains unclear.

Benefits: We found no systematic review of RCTs. **Vitamin E and β carotene:** Four large RCTs have looked at vitamin E in people with coronary artery disease.[67,78-80] The first RCT (2002 people with angiographically proven ischaemic heart disease)[78] used a high dose of vitamin E (400 IU or 800 IU) and follow up was brief (median 510 days). The RCT found that vitamin E reduced non-fatal coronary events (RRR 77%, 95% CI 53% to 89%), but also found a nonsignificant increase in coronary death (RRI +18%, 95% CI −0.4% to +127%), and all cause mortality. The second RCT (29 133 male Finnish smokers) compared β carotene and vitamin E supplements with placebo. The dose of vitamin E (50 mg/day) was smaller than that used in the first trial. In the subgroup analysis of data from the 1862 men with prior MI, the trial found that vitamin E reduced non-fatal MI (RRR 38%, 95% CI 4% to 59%), but non-significantly increased coronary death (RRI +33%, 95% CI −14% to +105%).[79] There were significantly more deaths from coronary heart disease on β carotene than placebo. The third RCT (11 324 people)[67] used a factorial design to compare vitamin E (300 mg) daily versus no vitamin E (as well as fish oil versus no fish oil). After 3.5 years there was a small and non-significant reduction in the risk of cardio-vascular death and deaths from all causes in those who received vitamin E compared with those who did not (RRR all cause mortality 0.92%, 95% CI 0.82% to 1.04%). There was no significant change in the rate of non-fatal coronary events in those who received vitamin E (RRI 4%, 95% CI −12% to +22%).[67] The fourth RCT (9541 people at high cardiovascular risk, 80% with prior clinical coronary artery disease, remainder with other atherosclerotic disease or diabetes with ≥ 1 additional cardiovascular risk factor) compared natural source vitamin E (D-alpha tocopherol acetate) 400 IU/day versus placebo and followed participants for an average of 4.7 years.[80] It found no significant differences in any cardio-vascular outcomes between vitamin E and placebo (AR for major fatal or non-fatal cardiovascular event 16.2% with vitamin E v 15.5% with placebo, P = NS; AR for cardiovascular death 7.2% with vitamin E v 6.9% with placebo, P = NS; AR for non-fatal MI 11.2% v 11.0% with placebo, P = NS; AR for stroke 4.4% with vitamin E v 3.8% with placebo, P = NS; AR for death from any cause 11.2% with vitamin E v 11.2% with placebo, P = NS). Pooled analysis from all four of these major RCTs found no evidence that vitamin E altered cardiovascular events and all cause mortality compared with placebo when given for 1.3–4.5 years. One additional smaller RCT (196 people on haemodialysis, aged 40–75 years) compared high dose vitamin E (800 IU/day) versus placebo.[81] After a median of 519 days, it found that vitamin E reduced the rate of combined cardiovascular end points but found no significant effect for all cause mortality (RRR for cardiovascular end points, vitamin E v placebo 46%, 95% CI 11% to 77%; mortality, vitamin E v placebo RRI 9%, 95% CI RRR 30% to RRI 70%).[81]

Vitamin C: We found three small RCTs comparing vitamin C with placebo. The first RCT (538 people admitted to an acute geriatric unit) compared vitamin C (200 mg daily) versus placebo for 6 months.[82] The second RCT (297 elderly people with low vitamin C levels) compared vitamin C (150 mg daily for 12 weeks, then 50 mg daily) versus placebo for 2 years.[83] The third RCT (199 elderly people) compared vitamin C (200 mg daily) versus placebo for 6 months.[84] The three RCTs were small and brief, and their combined results provide no evidence of any substantial early benefit of vitamin C supplementation (RRI for mortality for vitamin v placebo +8%, 95% CI −7% to +26%).

Harms: Two of the trials of vitamin E found non-significant increases in the risk of coronary death (see benefits above).[78,79] Four large RCTs of β carotene supplementation in primary prevention found no cardio-vascular benefits, and two of the trials raised concerns about increased mortality (RRI for cardiovascular death, β carotene v placebo 12%, 95% CI 4% to 22%) and cancer rates.[85]

Comment: One systematic review of epidemiological studies found consistent associations between increased dietary or supplemental intake of

Secondary prevention of ischaemic cardiac events

vitamin E, or both, and lower cardiovascular risk and less consistent associations for β carotene and vitamin C.[85] Most observational studies of antioxidants have excluded people with pre-existing disease.[86,87] The results of the trial in people on haemodialysis raises the possibility that high dose vitamin E supplementation may be beneficial in those at high absolute risk of coronary events.[81] Further trials in such groups are required to confirm or refute this finding.

OPTION **CARDIAC REHABILITATION INCLUDING EXERCISE**

Systematic reviews of RCTs have found that cardiac rehabilitation improves coronary risk factors and reduces the risk of major cardiac events in people after MI. The role of exercise alone in reducing the risk of adverse cardiovascular outcomes is not clear.

Benefits:
Cardiac rehabilitation: Three systematic reviews identified RCTs of cardiac rehabilitation, including exercise in people after MI.[88-90] Rehabilitation included medical evaluation, prescribed exercise, cardiac risk factor modification, education, and counselling. The reviews found 20–25% reductions in cardiovascular deaths in the treatment groups. One review (22 RCTs, 4554 people with a recent MI) found, after a mean of 3 years, significant reductions in total mortality (RRR 20%, no CI given), cardiovascular mortality (RRR 22%, no CI given), and fatal reinfarction (RRR 25%, no CI given), but no significant difference in non-fatal reinfarction.[89] **Exercise alone:** One more recent qualitative systematic review (search date not stated) found that rehabilitation with exercise alone had little effect on rates of non-fatal MI or overall mortality but a small beneficial effect on angina.[91]

Harms:
No study documented an increased risk of reinfarction or other adverse cardiovascular outcomes for exercise rehabilitation compared with control. Rates of adverse cardiovascular outcomes (syncope, arrhythmia, MI, or sudden death) were low (2–3/ 100 000 person hours) in supervised rehabilitation programmes, and rates of fatal cardiac events during or immediately after exercise training were reported in two older surveys as ranging from one in 116 400 to one in 784 000 person hours.[91]

Comment:
The three reviews included RCTs performed before the widespread use of thrombolytic agents and β blockers after MI. Most participants were men under 70 years of age. Other interventions aimed at risk factor modification were often provided in the intervention groups (including nutritional education, counselling in behavioural modification, and, in some trials, lipid lowering medications). We found no strong evidence that exercise training and cardiac rehabilitation programmes increased the proportion of people returning to work after MI.

OPTION	SMOKING CESSATION

We found no RCTs of the effects of smoking cessation on cardiovascular events in people with coronary heart disease. Moderate evidence from epidemiological studies indicates that people with coronary heart disease who stop smoking rapidly reduce their risk of recurrent coronary events or death. The use of nicotine patches seems safe in people with coronary heart disease.

Benefits:
We found no RCTs evaluating the effects of smoking cessation on coronary mortality and morbidity. Many observational studies found that people with coronary heart disease who stop smoking rapidly reduce their risk of cardiac death and MI (RRR about 50% for recurrent coronary events or premature death compared with continuing smokers)[92] (see smoking cessation under primary prevention, p 135). The studies found that about half of the benefits occur in the first year of stopping smoking, followed by a more gradual decrease in risk, reaching the risk of never smokers after several years of abstinence.[92] Among people with peripheral arterial disease and stroke, smoking cessation has been shown in observational studies to be associated with improved exercise tolerance, decreased risk of amputation, improved survival, and reduced risk of recurrent stroke.

Harms:
Two recent RCTs found no evidence that nicotine replacement using transdermal patches in people with stable coronary heart disease increased cardiovascular events.[93,94]

Comment:
One RCT compared the impact of firm and detailed advice to stop smoking in 125 survivors of acute MI versus conventional advice in 85 people.[95] Allocation to the intervention or control group was determined by day of admission. At follow up over 1 year after admission, 62% of the intervention group and 28% of the control group were non-smokers. Mortality and morbidity were not reported.

OPTION	PSYCHOLOGICAL AND STRESS MANAGEMENT INTERVENTIONS

One systematic review of mainly poor quality RCTs found that psychological and stress management may decrease rates of MI or cardiac death in people with coronary heart disease.

Benefits:
One systematic review (search date not stated, 23 RCTs, 3180 people with coronary artery disease) compared a diverse range of psychosocial treatments (2024 people) versus usual treatment (1156 people).[96] Mortality results were available in only 12 RCTs. Psychosocial interventions versus control interventions significantly reduced mortality (RRR for death 41%; OR survival 1.70, 95% CI 1.09 to 2.64) and non-fatal events in the first 2 years of follow up after MI (RRR 46%; OR for no event 1.84, 95% CI 1.12 to 2.99).[96]

Harms:
No specific harms were reported.

Comment:
These results should be interpreted with caution because of the methodological limitations of the individual RCTs and the use of a diverse range of interventions (relaxation, stress management, counselling). The RCTs were generally small, with short follow up,

and used non-uniform outcome measures. Methods of conceal-
ment allocation were not assessed. The authors of the review
acknowledged the strong possibility of publication bias but made no
attempt to quantify it. The results were inconsistent across trials.[97]
Several observational studies have found that depression and social
isolation (lack of social and emotional support) are independent
predictors of mortality and non-fatal coronary heart disease events
in people after MI.[98]

QUESTION   **What are the effects of surgical treatments?**

Charanjit Rihal

OPTION   CORONARY ARTERY BYPASS GRAFTING (CABG) VERSUS MEDICAL TREATMENT

RCTs performed up to the mid 1980s have found that, in comparison with medical treatment, CABG carried a greater risk of death in the first year but reduced the risk of death from coronary artery disease at 5 and 10 years. Greatest benefit occurred in people with more severe disease (multivessel disease, left ventricular dysfunction, or MI). There was no evidence of increased protection against subsequent MI. A more recent RCT, using modern techniques and with optimal background medical treatment, found even greater superiority of revascularisation.

Benefits:
One systematic review (search date not stated, 7 RCTs, individual results from 2649 people with coronary heart disease) compared CABG with medical treatment.[99] Most participants were middle aged men with multivessel disease but good left ventricular function who were enrolled from 1972 to 1984 (97% were male; 82% 41–60 years old; 80% with ejection fraction > 50%; 60% with prior MI; and 83% with two or three vessel disease).[99] Participants assigned to CABG also received medical treatment, and 40% initially assigned to medical treatment underwent CABG in the following 10 years. One subsequent RCT (558 people with asymptomatic ischaemia with positive exercise test or ambulatory electrocardiogram) compared medical treatment versus revascularisation (CABG or PTA).[100] **Mortality and MI:** The systematic review found that CABG versus medical treatment reduced mortality at 5 years (intention to treat analysis: RRR 39%, 95% CI 23% to 52%), 7 years (RRR 32%, 95% CI 17% to 44%), and 10 years (RRR 17%, 95% CI 2% to 30%).[99] In the subsequent RCT, mortality at 2 years was significantly lower after routine revascularisation (AR of death 1.1% v 6.6% and 4.4% in the two medical groups, P < 0.02).[100] No impact of CABG on subsequent infarction was found either in individual trials or in the systematic review, possibly because those assigned to surgery had increased rates of infarction in the perioperative period (see harms below). In the RCT, revascularisation reduced rates of death or MI compared with medical treatment (AR of MI or death 4.7% with revascularisation v 8.8% and 12.1% with medical treatment, P < 0.04).[100] **Other non-fatal end points:** Most trials did not prospectively collect data on re-admission rates, recurrent angina, or quality of life. **Effects in different people:** The systematic review found that the relative benefits were similar in participants with different baseline risk (OR for death 0.61 if left

ventricular function normal and 0.59 if abnormal). The absolute benefit of CABG was greatest in people with an abnormal ejection fraction, because the baseline risk of death was twice as high in this group (ejection fraction > 50%: ARR of death over 5 years 5%; ejection fraction < 50%: ARR 10%). Both absolute and relative mortality benefits were higher in people with a greater number of diseased coronary arteries, especially those with three vessel disease (OR of death 0.58, P < 0.001), and those with left main coronary artery disease (OR 0.32, P = 0.004) or any involvement of the left anterior descending coronary artery (OR 0.58), even if only one or two vessels were involved.[99]

Harms: **Perioperative complications:** In the systematic review, of the 1240 participants who underwent CABG, 40 (3.2%) died and 7.1% had documented non-fatal MI within 30 days of the procedure. At 1 year, the estimated incidence of death or MI was 11.6% with CABG and 8% with medical treatment (RRI 45%, 95% CI 18% to 103%).[99] The diagnosis of MI after CABG is difficult, and its true incidence may be higher. In the recent RCT, those assigned to routine revascularisation had significantly lower rates of death or MI after 2 years (AR for death 1.1% v 6.6% and 4.4% for the 2 medical groups, P < 0.02; AR for death or MI 4.7% v 12.1% and 8.8% in the 2 medical groups, P < 0.04).[100]

Comment: The results of the systematic review may not be generaliseable to current practice. Participants were 65 years or younger, but over half of CABG procedures are now performed on people over 65 years. Almost all participants were male. High risk people, such as those with severe angina and left main coronary artery stenosis, were under represented. Internal thoracic artery grafts were used in less than 5% of participants. Lipid lowering agents (particularly statins) and aspirin were used infrequently (aspirin used in 3% of participants at enrolment). Only about half of participants were taking β blockers. The systematic review may underestimate the real benefits of CABG in comparison with medical treatment alone becuase medical and surgical treatment for coronary artery disease were not mutually exclusive; by 5 years, 25% of people receiving medical treatment had undergone CABG surgery and by 10 years, 41% had undergone CABG surgery. The underestimate of effect would be greatest among people at high risk. People with previous CABG have not been studied in RCTs, although they now represent a growing proportion of those undergoing CABG.

OPTION **CORONARY PERCUTANEOUS TRANSLUMINAL ANGIOPLASTY (PTA) VERSUS MEDICAL TREATMENT FOR STABLE CORONARY ARTERY DISEASE**

One systematic review has found that in people with stable coronary artery disease, in comparison with medical treatment, coronary PTA is more effective for alleviating angina pectoris and improving exercise tolerance, but is associated with a higher rate of CABG. The review found no evidence that PTA reduces mortality, MI, or need for later angioplasty. RCTs have found that PTA is associated with increased risk of emergency CABG and of MI during and soon after the procedure.

Benefits: We found one systematic review (search date 1998, 6 RCTs, 1904 people with stable coronary artery disease) comparing balloon

Secondary prevention of ischaemic cardiac events

angioplasty versus balloon PTA.[101] Follow up varied from 6–57 months. **Mortality, MI, angina, and subsequent intervention:** The review found that PTA significantly reduced the rate of angina, but increased the rate of CABG compared with medical treatment (RR for angina: PTA v medical treatment 0.70, 95% CI 0.50 to 0.98; RR for CABG: PTA v medical treatment 1.59, 95% CI 1.09 to 2.32). The review found no significant difference between PTA and medical treatment for death (RR 1.32, 95% CI 0.65 to 2.70), for MI (RR 1.42, 95% CI 0.90 to 2.25), or in the need for later PTA (RR 1.29, 95% CI 0.72 to 3.36). The review found significant heterogeneity among trials. **Quality of life:** The largest RCT identified by the review (1018 people) found that PTA improved physical functioning, vitality, and general health compared with medical treatment at 3 months and 1 year (measured with SF-36 instrument at 1 year: 33% of people treated with PTA rated their health as "much improved" v 22% with medical therapy, P = 0.008), but found no significant difference at 3 years. The improvements were related to breathlessness, angina, and treadmill tolerance. High transfer (27%) from the medical to PTA group may partly explain the lack of difference between groups at 3 years.[102] **Effects in different people:** One of the RCTs in the systematic review found that antianginal benefit from PTA was limited to people with moderate to severe (grade 2 or worse) angina (20% lower incidence of angina and 1 minute longer treadmill exercise times compared with medical treatment).[103] People with mild symptoms at enrolment derived no significant improvement in symptoms.

Harms: Procedural death and MI, as well as repeat procedures for restenosis, are the main hazards of PTA. Four RCTs included in the review reported complications of PTA. In the first RCT, two (1.9%) emergency CABG operations and five (4.8%) MIs occurred at the time of the procedure. By 6 months, the PTA group had higher rates of CABG surgery (7% v 0%) and non-protocol PTA (15.2% v 10.3%).[104,105] In the second RCT, the higher rate of death or MI with PTA was attributable to one death and seven procedure related MIs.[103] The third RCT found a procedure related CABG rate and MI rate of 2.8% each, and the fourth found rates of 2% for CABG and 3% for MI.[101]

Comment: We found good evidence that PTA treats the symptoms of angina pectoris, but we found no evidence that it reduces the overall incidence of death or MI in people with stable angina. This may be because of the risk of complications during and soon after the procedure, and because most PTAs are performed for single vessel disease.

OPTION **CORONARY PTA VERSUS CABG FOR MULTIVESSEL DISEASE**

One systematic review has found that, in low to medium risk people, PTA versus CABG has no significant effect on mortality, the risk of MI, and the quality of life. PTA is less invasive but increases the number of repeat procedures. The relevant RCTs were too small to exclude a 20–30%

difference in mortality. The largest RCT has found that CABG versus PTA improves long term survival in people with diabetes who are treated with oral hypoglycaemic drugs or insulin and have multivessel coronary disease.

Benefits: We found two systematic reviews (search date not stated, 8 RCTs, 3371 people)[106,107] and one subsequent RCT.[108] **Angina pectoris:** One systematic review[105] found that the prevalence of moderate to severe angina pectoris (grade 2 or worse) was significantly higher after PTA than after CABG at 1 year (RR 1.6, 95% CI 1.3 to 1.9). After 3 years this difference had decreased as rates of repeat revascularisation increased in the people allocated to PTA (RR 1.2, 95% CI 1.0 to 1.5). **Mortality:** The systematic review[106] found no significant difference in all cause mortality between groups (AR 7.3% after PTA v 6.8%; OR 1.09, 95% CI 0.88 to 1.35).[106] The smaller subsequent RCT (392 people) found no significant difference between CABG and PTA after 8 years of follow up, although the trial was too small to exclude a clinically important difference (AR for survival 83% with CABG v 79% with PTA, P = 0.40).[108] **Death or MI:** In all RCTs, the combined end point of death or MI was not significantly different between groups (AR 13.8% v 13.4%; OR 1.05, 95% CI 0.89 to 1.23).[107] The largest of these RCTs found that CABG versus PTA had no significant effect on death or MI after a mean follow up of 7.7 years (alive and no MI: 75.3% with CABG v 73.5% with PTA, P = 0.46).[109] **Repeat procedures:** In all RCTs, the need for repeat procedures was significantly higher in people allocated to PTA (AR 44% with PTA v 6.0% with CABG; OR 7.9, 95% CI 6.9 to 9.0).[110] **Quality of life:** Both PTA and CABG groups had significant improvements in quality of life measures and return to employment, but no difference was found between the PTA and CABG groups over 3–5 years of follow up.[111,112]

Harms: See harms of PTA versus medical treatment, p 182. CABG is more invasive than PTA, but PTA is associated with a greater need for repeat procedures.

Comment: **In people with diabetes:** Subgroup analysis of the largest RCT (1829 people) found that in people with diabetes (353 people), CABG reduced all cause mortality more than PTA both after 5 years (AR of death 19.4% with CABG v 34.5% with PTA; P = 0.003)[110] and after 7 years (AR of death with CABG 23.6% v 44.3% with PTA; P = 0.0011).[109] Such a difference was not observed among non-diabetics or any other subgroup (AR of death in people without diabetes 13.6% with CABG v 13.2% with PTA, P = 0.72).[109] **In all participants:** Although no major differences in death or MI were observed in the nine RCTs,[106,108] these trials enrolled people at relatively low risk of cardiac events. It is therefore premature to conclude that PTA and CABG are equivalent for all people with multivessel disease. Fewer than 20% of participants had left ventricular dysfunction, almost 70% had one or two vessel disease, and observed mortality was only 2.6% for the first year, and 1.1% a year thereafter. Participants enrolled in the largest trial more closely approximated to moderate risk people, but this was caused primarily by the higher proportion of participants with diabetes mellitus.[110] Even in that trial nearly 60% of participants had two vessel coronary artery disease. Finally, even though nine trials were included in the meta-analysis, the total enrolment of 5200 falls short of what would be needed to show mortality differences of 20–30% among people at low and moderate risk. Large mortality differences between the two procedures (40–50%) are unlikely. **Multivessel stenting versus multivessel CABG:** One RCT (unpublished as of December 2000) has compared multivessel CABG versus multivessel PTA in 1205 people with an ejection fraction greater than 30% (the ARTS Investigators, personal communication, 1999).

OPTION	CORONARY PTA VERSUS INTRACORONARY STENTS

RCTs have found that, in comparison with coronary PTA, intracoronary stents afford superior acute and long term clinical and angiographic results.

Benefits: We found no systematic review. **For disease of native coronary arteries:** We found four RCTs comparing elective stenting with PTA.[112-115] At 12 months, intracoronary stents significantly reduced the risk of recurrent angina (13% v 30%, P = 0.04) but not of death, MI, or need for CABG.[109] At 6 months, all four RCTs found a lower prevalence of angiographic restenosis (31% v 42%, P = 0.046; 22% v 32%, P = 0.02; 17% v 40%, P = 0.02; 18.2% v 24.9%, P = 0.055), and a lower rate of repeat PTA (13.5% v 23.3%; RR 0.58, 95% CI 0.40 to 0.85).[112-115] After 2 years of follow up, the fourth trial found that stenting reduced all clinical cardiac events compared with PTA (AR for death, MI, repeat PTA, or CABG 19.8% with stent v 27.5% with PTA, P = 0.048). The difference was accounted for almost entirely by lower rates of repeat target lesion revascularisation in the stent group (AR 17.2% with stent v 25.5% with PTA, P = 0.02).[115] **For saphenous vein graft lesions in people with prior CABG:** We found one RCT (220 people) comparing elective stents with standard balloon angioplasty.[114] Acute angiographic results were better with stents than balloon angioplasty. At 6 months, there was no significant difference in rates of restenosis (37% v 46%, P = 0.24), but the overall incidence of death, MI, CABG, or repeat PTA was lower in the stent group (27% v 42%, P = 0.03). **For treatment of chronic total occlusions:** Chronic occlusions of the coronary arteries are particularly prone to restenosis and reocclusion following PTA. We found three RCTs comparing PTA alone with PTA followed by insertion of stents.[116-118] One RCT (119 people with chronic total occlusion) found that stenting compared with PTA reduced angina (angina free at 6 months: 57% of stent group v 24% of PTA only group, 95% CI not available, P < 0.001) and angiographic restenosis (> 50% stenosis on follow up angiography: 74% with PTA v 32% with stent, P < 0.001). Repeat procedures were undertaken less often among people with a stent than among people receiving PTA (22% v 42%, P = 0.025).[117] In the second RCT (110 people) those treated with stents experienced less ischaemia (14% v 46%, P = 0.002), had less restenosis (32% v 68%, P < 0.001), and underwent fewer repeat procedures (5.3% v 22%, P = 0.038) by 9 months.[118] The third RCT (110 people) found that, at angiographic follow up after 4 months, those with stents experienced less restenosis (26% v 62%, P = 0.01), less reocclusion (2% v 1%, P = 0.05), and fewer repeat PTAs (24% v 55%, P = 0.05). No deaths or CABG operations occurred in either group. The incidence of MI was low in both groups (0% stent v 2% PTA, P = NS).[119] **For treatment of restenosis after initial PTA:** We found one RCT (383 people) of coronary stenting versus balloon angioplasty for treatment of restenosis. During 6 months of follow up, the stent group experienced fewer recurrent restenoses (18% v 32%, P = 0.03) and repeat procedures (10% v 27%, P = 0.001). Survival free of MI or repeat revascularisation was 84% in the stent group and 72% in the PTA group (P = 0.04).[120]

Harms: Initially, aggressive combination antithrombotic and anticoagulant regimens were used because of a high incidence of stent thrombosis and MI. These regimens led to a high incidence of arterial access site bleeding.[108] More recently, improved stent techniques and use of aspirin and ticlopidine have reduced both stent thrombosis and arterial access site bleeding.[115,120] Currently, the risk of stent thrombosis is less than 1%.[114,121,122] Haemorrhage (particularly femoral artery bleeding) was more frequent after stenting than PTA alone,[116] but occurred in less than 3% following stenting when antiplatelet drugs were used without long term anticoagulants.

Comment: It is unclear whether stenting influences the relative benefits and harms of percutaneous procedures compared with CABG.

GLOSSARY

International normalised ratio (INR) A value derived from a standardised laboratory test that measures the effect of an anticoagulant. The laboratory materials used in the test are calibrated against internationally accepted standard reference preparations, so that variability between laboratories and different reagents is minimised. Normal blood has an INR of 1. Therapeutic anticoagulation often aims to achieve an INR value of 2–3.5.

REFERENCES

1. Greaves EJ, Gillum BS. 1994 Summary: national hospital discharge survey. Advance data from Vital and Health Statistics, no. 278. Hyattsville, Maryland: National Center for Health Statistics, 1996.

2. Shaw LJ, Peterson ED, Kesler K, Hasselblad V, Califf RM. A meta-analysis of predischarge risk stratification after acute myocardial infarction with stress electrocardiographic, myocardial perfusion, and ventricular function imaging. Am J Cardiol 1996;78:1327–1337. Search date 1995; primary sources Medline, and hand search of bibliographies of review articles.

3. Kudenchuk PJ, Maynard C, Martin JS, et al. Comparison, presentation, treatment and outcome of acute myocardial infarction in men versus women (the myocardial infarction triage and intervention registry). Am J Cardiol 1996;78: 9–14.

4. The Task Force on the Management of Acute Myocardial Infarction of the European Society of Cardiology. Acute myocardial infarction: pre-hospital and in-hospital management. Eur Heart J 1996;17:43–63.

5. Peterson ED, Shaw LJ, Califf RM. Clinical guideline: part II. Risk stratification after myocardial infarction. Ann Intern Med 1997;126: 561–582.

6. The Multicenter Postinfarction Research Group. Risk stratification and survival after myocardial infarction. N Engl J Med 1983;309:331–336.

7. American College of Cardiology/American Heart Association Task Force on Practice Guidelines (Committee on Exercise Testing). ACC/AHA guidelines for exercise testing. J Am Coll Cardiol 1997;30:260–315.

8. Fallen E, Cairns J, Dafoe W, et al. Management of the postmyocardial infarction patient: a consensus report – revision of the 1991 CCS guidelines. Can J Cardiol 1995;11:477–486.

9. Madsen JK, Grande P, Saunamaki, et al. Danish multicenter randomized study of invasive versus conservative treatment in patients with inducible ischemia after thrombolysis in acute myocardial infarction (DANAMI). Circulation 1997;96: 748–755.

10. Antiplatelet Trialists' Collaboration. Collaborative overview of randomised trials of antiplatelet therapy – I: prevention of death, myocardial infarction, and stroke by prolonged antiplatelet therapy in various categories of patients. BMJ 1994;308:81–106. Search date March 1990; primary source Medline; Current Contents; hand search of journals, reference lists and conference proceedings; authors of trials and drug manufacturers.

11. Taylor DW, Barnett HJM, Haynes RB, et al, for the ASA and Carotid Endarterectomy (ACE) Trial Collaborators. Low-dose and high-dose acetylsalicylic acid for patients undergoing carotid endarterectomy: a randomised controlled trial. Lancet 1999;353:2179–2184.

12. Juul-Möller S, Edvardsson N, Jahnmatz B, Rosen A, Sorenson S, Omblus R, for the Swedish Angina Pectoris Aspirin Trial (SAPAT) Group. Double-blind trial of aspirin in primary prevention

of myocardial infarction in patients with stable chronic angina pectoris. *Lancet* 1992;340: 1421–1425.

13. Hankey GJ, Sudlow CLM, Dunbabin DW. Thienopyridine derivatives (ticlopidine, clopidogrel) versus aspirin for preventing stroke and other serious vascular events in high vascular risk patients. In: The Cochrane Library, Issue 2, 2000. Oxford: Update Software. Search date March/July 1999; primary sources Medline; Embase; Cochrane Stroke Group Register March 1999; Antithrombotics Trialists' database; authors of trials; and drug manufacturers.

14. CAPRIE Steering Committee. A randomised, blinded, trial of clopidogrel versus aspirin in patients at risk of ischaemic events. *Lancet* 1996; 348:1329–1339.

15. Farrell B, Godwin J, Richards S, Warlow C. The United Kingdom transient ischaemic attack (UK-TIA) aspirin trial: final results. *J Neurol Neurosurg Psychiatry* 1991;54:1044–1054.

16. Moloney BA. An analysis of the side effects of ticlopidine. In: Hass WK, Easton JD, eds. *Ticlopidine, Platelets and Vascular Disease*. New York: Springer, 1993:117–139.

17. Bennett CL, Davidson CJ, Raisch DW, Weinberg PD, Bennett RH, Feldman MD. Thrombotic thrombocytopenic purpura associated with ticlopidine in the setting of coronary artery stents and stroke prevention. *Arch Int Med* 1999;159: 2524–2528.

18. Bennett CL, Connors JM, Carwile JM, et al. Thrombotic thrombocytopenic purpura associated with clopidogrel. *N Engl J Med* 2000;342: 1773–1777.

19. Hankey GJ. Clopidogrel and thrombotic thrombocytopenic purpura. *Lancet* 2000;356: 269–270.

20. Müller C, Büttner HJ, Petersen J, Roskamm H. A randomized comparison of clopidogrel and aspirin versus ticlopidine and aspirin after the placement of coronary-artery stents. *Circulation* 2000;101: 590–593.

21. Bertrand ME, Rupprecht H-J, Urban P, Gershlick AH, for the CLASSICS Investigators. Double-blind study of the safety of clopidogrel with and without a loading dose in combination with aspirin compared with ticlopidine in combination with aspirin after coronary stenting. The Clopidogrel Aspirin Stent International Cooperative Study (CLASSICS). *Circulation* 2000;102:624–629.

22. Anand SS, Yusuf S. Oral anticoagulant therapy in patients with coronary artery disease: a meta-analysis. *JAMA* 1999;282:2058–2067. Search date July 1999; primary sources Medline, Embase, Current Contents, hand searches of reference lists, experts, pharmaceutical companies.

23. Teo KK, Yusuf S, Furberg CD. Effects of prophylactic antiarrhythmic drug therapy in acute myocardial infarction. *JAMA* 1993;270: 1589–1595. Search date 1993; primary sources Medline; hand search of reference lists; details of unpublished trials sought from pharmaceutical industry/other investigators.

24. Yusuf S, Peto R, Lewis J, Collins R, Sleight P. Beta blockade during and after myocardial infarction: An overview of the randomized trials. *Prog Cardiovasc Dis* 1985;27:335–371. No details of search date or primary sources given.

25. Pepine CJ, Cohn PF, Deedwania PC, et al for the ASIST Study Group. Effects of treatment on outcome in mildly symptomatic patients with ischemia during daily life: the atenolol silent ischemia study (ASIST). *Circulation* 1994;90: 762–768.

26. Boissel J-P, Leizerovicz A, Picolet H, et al, for the APSI Investigators. Secondary prevention after high-risk acute myocardial infarction with low-dose acebutolol. *Am J Cardiol* 1990;66:251–260.

27. The Beta-Blocker Pooling Project Research Group. The beta-blocker pooling project (BBPP): subgroup findings from randomized trials in post infarction patients. *Eur Heart J* 1988;9:8–16. Search date placebo controlled trials published by December 1983; details of primary sources not given.

28. Beta-blocker Heart Attack Trial Research Group. A randomized trial of propranolol in patients with acute myocardial infarction: I. Mortality results. *JAMA* 1982;247:1707–1714.

29. Flather M, Kober L, Pfeffer MA, et al. Meta-analysis of individual patient data from trials of long-term ACE-inhibitor treatment after acute myocardial infarction (SAVE, AIRE, and TRACE studies). *Circulation* 1997;96(suppl 1;abs 3957): I–706. No details of search date or primary sources given.

30. The Heart Outcomes Prevention Evaluation (HOPE) Investigators. Effects of an angiotensin-converting enzyme inhibitor, ramipril, on cardiovascular events in high-risk patients. *N Engl J Med* 2000; 342;145–153.

31. Heart Outcomes Prevention Evaluation (HOPE) Investigators. Effects of ramipril on cardiovascular and microvascular outcomes on people with diabetes mellitus: results of the hope study and MICRO-HOPE substudy. *Lancet* 2000;355: 253–259.

32. Yusuf S, Lonn E. Anti-ischaemic effects of ACE inhibitors: review of current clinical evidence and ongoing clinical trials. *Eur Heart J* 1998;19(suppl J):J36–44.

33. Echt DS, Liebson PR, Mitchell LB, et al. Mortality and morbidity in patients receiving encainide, flecainide, or placebo. *N Engl J Med* 1991;324: 781–788.

34. Amiodarone Trials Meta-Analysis Investigators. Effect of prophylactic amiodarone on mortality after acute myocardial infarction and in congestive heart failure: meta-analysis of individual data from 6500 patients in randomised trials. *Lancet* 1997; 350:1417–1424. No details of search date or primary sources given.

35. Sim I, McDonald KM, Lavori PW, Norbutas CM, Hlatky MA. Quantitative overview of randomized trials of amiodarone to prevent sudden cardiac death. *Circulation* 1997;96:2823–2829. Search date 1997; primary sources Medline, and Biosis.

36. Waldo AL, Camm AJ, de Ruyter H, et al, for the SWORD Investigators. Effect of d-sotalol on mortality in patients with left ventricular dysfunction after recent and remote myocardial infarction. *Lancet* 1996;348:7–12.

37. Cairns JA, Connolly SJ, Roberts R, Gent M, for the Canadian Amiodarone Myocardial Infarction Arrhythmia Trial Investigators. Randomized trial of outcome after myocardial infarction in patients with frequent or repetitive ventricular premature depolarisations: CAMIAT. *Lancet* 1997;349: 675–682.

38. Julian DG, Camm AJ, Janse MJ, et al, for the European Myocardial Infarct Amiodarone Trial Investigators. Randomised trial of effect of amiodarone on mortality in patients with left-ventricular dysfunction after recent myocardial infarction: EMIAT. *Lancet* 1997;349:667–674.

39. Gibson RS, Boden WE, Theroux P, et al. Diltiazem and reinfarction in patients with non-Q-wave myocardial infarction. *N Engl J Med* 1986;315: 423–429.

40. The Multicenter Diltiazem Postinfarction Trial Research Group. The effect of diltiazem on

mortality and reinfarction after myocardial infarction. *N Engl J Med* 1988;319:385–392.

41. The Danish Study Group on Verapamil in Myocardial Infarction. Effect of verapamil on mortality and major events after acute myocardial infarction: the Danish verapamil infarction trial II (DAVIT II). *Am J Cardiol* 1990;66:779–785.

42. Hulley S, Grady D, Bush T, et al. Randomized trial of estrogen plus progestin for secondary prevention of coronary heart disease in postmenopausal women. *JAMA* 1998;280: 605–613.

43. Coronary Drug Research Project Research Group. The coronary drug project: initial findings leading to modifications of its research protocol. *JAMA* 1970;214:1303–1313.

44. Daly E, Vessey MP, Hawkins MM, Carson JL, Gough P, Marsh S. Risk of venous thromboembolism in users of hormone replacement therapy. *Lancet* 1996;348:977–980.

45. Newton KM, LaCroix AZ, McKnight B, et al. Estrogen replacement therapy and prognosis after first myocardial infarction. *Am J Epidemiol* 1997; 145:269–277.

46. Sullivan JM, El-Zeky F, Vander Zwaag R, et al. Effect on survival of estrogen replacement therapy after coronary artery bypass grafting. *Am J Cardiol* 1997;79:847–850.

47. The Writing Group for the PEPI Trial. Effects of estrogen or estrogen/progestin regimens on heart disease risk factors in postmenopausal women. *JAMA* 1995;273:199–208.

48. Miettinen TA, Pyorala K, Olsson AG, Musliner TA, Cook TJ, et al. Cholesterol-lowering therapy in women and elderly patients with myocardial infarction or angina pectoris: findings from the Scandinavian Simvastatin Survival Study (4S). *Circulation* 1997;96:4211–4218.

49. LaRosa JC, He J, Vupputuri S. Effect of statins on risk of coronary disease: A meta-analysis of randomized controlled trials. *JAMA* 1999;282: 2340–2346. Search date 1998; primary sources Medline, bibliographies, and authors' reference files.

50. Knatterud GL, Rosenberg Y, Campeau L, et al. Long-term effects on clinical outcomes of aggressive lowering of low-density lipoprotein cholesterol levels and low-dose anticoagulation in the post coronary artery bypass graft trial. Post CABG Investigators. *Circulation* 2000;102: 157–165.

51. Montagne O, Vedel I, Durand-Zaleski I. Assessment of the impact of fibrates and diet on survival and their cost-effectiveness: evidence from randomized, controlled trials in coronary heart disease and health economic evaluations. *Clin Ther* 1999;21:2027–2035. Search date not stated; primary sources Medline, hand search of reference lists, and systematic reviews.

52. Anon. Secondary prevention by raising HDL cholesterol and reducing triglycerides in patients with coronary artery disease: the Bezafibrate Infarction Prevention (BIP) study. *Circulation* 2000;102:21–27.

53. Ericsson CG, Hamsten A, Nilsson J, Grip L, Svane B, de Faire U. Angiographic assessment of effects of bezafibrate on progression of coronary artery disease in young male postinfarction patients. *Lancet* 1996;347:849–853.

54. Bucher HC, Griffith LE, Guyatt G. Systematic review on the risk and benefit of different cholesterol-lowering interventions. *Arterioscler Thromb Vasc Biol* 1999;19:187–195. Search date October 1996; primary sources Medline, Embase, bibliographic searches.

55. Anon. MRC/BHF Heart Protection Study of cholesterol-lowering therapy and of antioxidant vitamin supplementation in a wide range of patients at increased risk of coronary heart disease death: early safety and efficacy experience. *Eur Heart J* 1999;20:725–741.

56. The Women's Health Initiative Study Group. Design of the women's health initiative clinical trial and observational study. *Control Clin Trials* 1998; 19:61–109.

57. Davis BR, Cutler JA Gordon DJ, et al, for the ALLHAT Research Group. Rationale and design for the antihypertensive and lipid lowering treatment to prevent heart attack trial (ALLHAT). *Am J Hypertens* 1996;9:342–360.

58. Flack JM, Neaton J, Grimm R, et al. Blood pressure and mortality among men with prior myocardial infarction. *Circulation* 1995;92; 2437–2445.

59. Dahlof B, Lindholm LH, Hansson L, et al. Morbidity and mortality in the Swedish trial in old patients with hypertension (STOP-hypertension). *Lancet* 1991;338:1281–1285.

60. Medical Research Council Working Party. MRC trial on treatment of hypertension in older adults: principal results. *BMJ* 1992;304:405–412.

61. Systolic Hypertension in Elderly Patients (SHEP) Cooperative Research Group. Prevention of stroke by antihypertensive treatment in older persons with isolated systolic hypertension. *JAMA* 1991; 265:3255–3264.

62. D'Agostini RB, Belanger AJ, Kannel WB, et al. Relationship of low diastolic blood pressure to coronary heart disease death in presence of myocardial infarction: the Framingham study. *BMJ* 1991;303:385–389.

63. Pfeffer MA, Braunwald E, Moye LA, et al, on behalf of the SAVE investigators. Effect of captopril on mortality and morbidity in patients with left ventricular dysfunction after myocardial infarction: results of the survival and ventricular enlargement trial. *N Engl J Med* 1992;327:669–677.

64. NHS Centre for Reviews and Dissemination, University of York. Cholesterol and coronary heart disease: screening and treatment. *Eff Health Care* 1998;4:Number 1. Search date and primary sources not given.

65. Burr ML, Fehily AM, Gilbert JF, et al. Effects of changes in fat, fish, and fibre intakes on death and myocardial reinfarction: diet and reinfarction trial (DART). *Lancet* 1989;2:757–761.

66. Fehily AM, Vaughan-Williams E, Shiels K, et al. The effect of dietary advice on nutrient intakes: evidence from the diet and reinfarction trial (DART). *J Hum Nutr Dietetics* 1989;2:225–235.

67. GISSI-Prevenzione Investigators. Dietary supplementation with n-3 polyunsaturated fatty acids and vitamin E after myocardial infarction: results of the GISSI-Prevenzione. *Lancet* 1999; 354:447–455.

68. De Lorgeril M, Renaud S, Mamelle N, et al. Mediterranean alpha-linolenic acid-rich diet in secondary prevention of coronary heart disease. *Lancet* 1994;343:1454–1459.

69. Clarke R, Frost C, Collins R, et al. Dietary lipids and blood cholesterol: quantitative meta-analysis of metabolic ward studies. *BMJ* 1997;314: 112–117. Search date 1995; primary sources Medline 1960–1995, hand search of reference lists and nutrition journals.

70. Tang JL, Armitage JM, Lancaster T, et al. Systematic review of dietary intervention trials to lower blood total cholesterol in free-living subjects. *BMJ* 1998;316:1213–1220. Search date 1997; primary sources Medline, Human Nutrition, Embase, and Allied and Alternative Medicine 1966–1997, hand searching the *Am J Clin Nutr*, and references of review articles.

Cardiovascular disorders

Secondary prevention of ischaemic cardiac events

71. Brunner E, White I, Thorogood M, et al. Can dietary interventions change diet and cardiovascular risk factors? A meta-analysis of randomized controlled trials. *Am J Public Health* 1997;87:1415–1422. Search date 1993; primary sources Medline 1966 to July 1993, and manual search of selected journals.

72. Ebrahim S, Davey SG. *Health promotion in older people for the prevention of coronary heart disease and stroke.* London: Health Education Authority, 1996.

73. Waters D. Lessons from coronary atherosclerosis "regression" trials. *Cardiol Clin* 1996;14:31–50.

74. Silagy C, Neil A. Garlic as a lipid lowering agent: a meta-analysis. *J R Coll Physicians Lond* 1994;28: 39–45. Search date July 1992; primary sources Medline 1966 to July 1992; Alternative Medicine database; authors of published studies; manufacturers; and hand searched references.

75. Isaacson JL, Moser M, Stein EA, et al. Garlic powder and plasma lipids and lipoproteins. *Arch Intern Med* 1998;158:1189–119.

76. Berthold HK, Sudhop T, von Bergmann K. Effect of a garlic oil preparation on serum lipoproteins and cholesterol metabolism. *JAMA* 1998;279: 1900–1902.

77. Ripsin CM, Keenan JM, Jacobs DR Jr, et al. Oat products and lipid lowering: a meta-analysis. *JAMA* 1992;267:3317–3325. Search date 1991; primary sources Medline 1966–1991; unpublished trials solicited from all known investigators of lipid-oats association.

78. Stephens NG, Parsons A, Schofield PM, et al. Randomised controlled trial of vitamin E in patients with coronary disease: Cambridge heart antioxidant study (CHAOS). *Lancet* 1996;347:781–786.

79. Rapola JM, Virtamo J, Ripatti S, et al. Randomised trial of α-tocopherol and β-carotene supplements on incidence of major coronary events in men with previous myocardial infarction. *Lancet* 1997;349: 1715–1720.

80. The Heart Outcomes Prevention Evaluation Study Investigators. Vitamin E supplementation and cardiovascular events in high-risk patients. The Heart Outcomes Prevention Evaluation Study Investigators. *N Engl J Med* 2000;342:154–160.

81. Boaz M, Smetana S, Weinstein T, et al. Secondary prevention with antioxidants of cardiovascular disease in endstage renal disease (SPACE): randomised placebo-controlled trial. *Lancet* 2000; 356:1213–18.

82. Wilson TS, Datta SB, Murrell JS, Andrews CT. Relation of vitamin C levels to mortality in a geriatric hospital: a study of the effect of vitamin C administration. *Age Aging* 1973;2:163–170.

83. Burr ML, Hurley RJ, Sweetnam PM. Vitamin C supplementation of old people with low blood levels. *Gerontol Clin* 1975;17:236–243.

84. Hunt C, Chakkravorty NK, Annan G. The clinical and biochemical effects of vitamin C supplementation in short-stay hospitalized geriatric patients. *Int J Vitam Nutr Res* 1984;54:65–74.

85. Lonn EM, Yusuf S. Is there a role for antioxidant vitamins in the prevention of cardiovascular diseases? An update on epidemiological and clinical trials data. *Can J Cardiol* 1997;13:957–965. Search date 1996; primary sources Medline 1965–1996; and one reference from 1997.

86. Jha P, Flather M, Lonn E, Farkouh M, Yusuf S. The antioxidant vitamins and cardiovascular disease: a critical review of epidemiologic and clinical trial data. *Ann Intern Med* 1995;123:860–872.

87. Ness AR, Powles JW, Khaw KT. Vitamin C and cardiovascular disease: a systematic review. *J Cardiovasc Risk* 1997;3:513–521. Search date not given; primary sources Medline, experts, and hand searched references.

88. Oldridge NB, Guyatt GH, Fisher MS, Rimm AA. Cardiac rehabilitation after myocardial infarction: combined experience of randomized clinical trials. *JAMA* 1988;260:945–950. Search date not specified; primary sources Medline.

89. O'Connor GT, Buring JE, Yusuf S, et al. An overview of randomized trials of rehabilitation with exercise after myocardial infarction. *Circulation* 1989;80: 234–244. No details of search date or primary sources given.

90. Berlin JA, Colditz GA. A meta-analysis of physical activity in the prevention of coronary heart disease. *Am J Epidemiol* 1990;132:612–628. No details of search date or primary sources given.

91. Wenger NK, Froelicher NS, Smith LK, et al. *Cardiac rehabilitation and secondary prevention.* Rockville, Maryland: Agency for Health Care Policy and Research and National Heart, Lung and Blood Institute, 1995. Search date and primary source not given.

92. US Department of Health and Human Services. *The health benefits of smoking cessation: a report of the surgeon general.* Bethesda, Maryland: US DHSS, 1990.

93. Working Group for the Study of Transdermal Nicotine in Patients with Coronary Artery Disease. Nicotine replacement therapy for patients with coronary artery disease. *Arch Intern Med* 1994; 154:989–995.

94. Joseph AM, Norman SM, Ferry LH, et al. The safety of transdermal nicotine as an aid to smoking cessation in patients with cardiac disease. *N Engl J Med* 1996;335:1792–1798.

95. Burt A, Thornley P, Illingworth D, White P, Shaw TRD, Turner R. Stopping smoking after myocardial infarction. *Lancet* 1974;1:304–306.

96. Linden W, Stossel C, Maurice J. Psychosocial interventions in patients with coronary artery disease: a meta-analysis. *Arch Intern Med* 1996; 156:745–752. No details of search date or primary sources given.

97. US Department of Health and Human Services. Cardiac rehabilitation. AHCPR Publication No 96–0672, 1995;121–128.

98. Hemingway H, Marmot M. Psychosocial factors in the primary and secondary prevention of coronary heart disease: a systematic review. In: Yusuf S, Cairns JA, Camm AJ, Fallen EL, Gersh BJ, eds. *Evidence based cardiology.* London: BMJ Books, 1998. Search date 1996; primary sources Medline 1966–1996; manual searching of bibliographies of retrieved articles and review articles.

99. Yusuf S, Zucker D, Peduzzi P, et al. Effect of coronary artery bypass graft surgery on survival: overview of 10-year results from randomized trials by the coronary artery bypass graft surgery trialists collaboration. *Lancet* 1994;344:563–570. No search date or primary sources given.

100. Davies RF, Goldberg AD, Forman S, et al. Asymptomatic cardiac ischemia pilot (ACIP) study two-year follow-up: outcomes of patients randomized to initial strategies of medical therapy versus revascularization. *Circulation* 1997;95:2037–2043.

101. Bucher HC, Hengstler P, Schindler C, Guyatt GH. Percutaneous transluminal coronary angioplasty versus medical treatment for non-acute coronary heart disease: Meta-analysis of randomised controlled trials. *BMJ* 2000;321:73–77. Search date December 1998; primary sources Medline 1979 to December 1998; Embase 1979 to December 1998; Cochrane Database 1979 to December 1998; Biological Abstracts 1979 to December 1998; Health Periodicals Database 1979 to December 1998; PASCAL 1979 to December 1998; and hand searched references.

102. Pocock SJ, Henderson RA, Clayton T, Lyman GH, Chamberlain DA. Quality of life after coronary angioplasty or continued medical treatment for angina: three-year follow-up in the RITA-2 trial. Randomized Intervention Treatment of Angina. *J Am Coll Cardiol* 2000;35:907–914.

103. RITA-2 Trial Participants. Coronary angioplasty versus medical therapy for angina: the second randomized intervention treatment of angina (RITA-2) trial. *Lancet* 1997;350:461–468.

104. Parisi AF, Folland ED, Hartigan P. A comparison of angioplasty with medical therapy in the treatment of single-vessel coronary artery disease. *N Engl J Med* 1992;326:10–16.

105. Morris KG, Folland ED, Hartigan PM, Parisi AF. Unstable angina in late follow-up of the ACME trial. *Circulation* 1995;92(supplement I):1–725.

106. Pocock SJ, Henderson RA, Rickards AF, et al. Meta-analysis of randomized trials comparing coronary angioplasty with bypass surgery. *Lancet* 1995;346:1184–1189. No details of search date or primary sources given.

107. Rihal CS, Gersh BJ, Yusuf S. Chronic coronary artery disease: coronary artery bypass surgery vs percutaneous transluminal coronary angioplasty vs medical therapy. In: Yusuf S, Cairns JA, Camm JA, Fallen EL, Gersh BJ, eds. *Evidence based cardiology*. London: BMJ Books, 1998.

108. King SB, Kosinski AS, Guyton RA, Lembo NJ, Weintraub WS. Eight-Year Mortality in the Emory Angioplasty Versus Surgery Trial (EAST). *J Am Coll Cardiol* 2000;35:1116–1121.

109. The BARI Investigators. Seven-Year Outcome in the Bypass Angioplasty Revascularization Investigation (BARI) By Treatment and Diabetic Status. *J Am Coll Cardiol* 2000;35:1122–1129.

110. Bypass Angioplasty Revascularization Investigation (BARI) Investigators. Comparison of coronary bypass surgery with angioplasty in patients with multivessel disease. *N Engl J Med* 1996;335:7–225.

111. Hlatky MA, Rogers WJ, Johnstone I, et al. Medical care costs and quality of life after randomization to coronary angioplasty or coronary bypass surgery. *N Engl J Med* 1997; 336:92–99.

112. Währborg P. Quality of life after coronary angioplasty or bypass surgery. *Eur Heart J* 1999; 20:653–658.

113. Serruys PW, de Jaeger P, Kiemeneij F. A comparison of balloon-expandable-stent implantation with balloon angioplasty in patients with coronary artery disease. *N Engl J Med* 1994;33:489–495.

114. Versaci F, Gaspardone A, Tomai F, Crea F, Chiariello L, Gioffre PA. A comparison of coronary-artery stenting with angioplasty for isolated stenosis of the proximal left anterior descending coronary artery. *N Engl J Med* 1997; 336:817–822.

115. Savage MP, Douglas JS, Fischman DL, et al. Stent placement compared with balloon angioplasty for obstructed coronary bypass grafts. *N Engl J Med* 1997;337:740–747.

116. Witkowski A, Ruzyllo W, Gil R, et al. A randomized comparison of elective high-pressure stenting with balloon angioplasty: six-month angiographic and two-year clinical follow-up. On behalf of AS (Angioplasty or Stent) trial investigators. *Am Heart J* 2000;140:264–271.

117. Sirnes P, Golf S, Yngvar M, et al. Stenting in chronic coronary occlusion (SICCO): a randomized controlled trial of adding stent implantation after successful angioplasty. *J Am Coll Cardiol* 1996;28:1444–1451.

118. Rubartelli P, Niccoli L, Verna E, et al. Stent implantation versus balloon angioplasty in chronic coronary occlusions: results from the GISSOC trial. *J Am Coll Cardiol* 1998;32:90–96.

119. Sievert H, Rohde S, Utech A, et al. Stent or angioplasty after recanalization of chronic coronary occlusions? (the SARECCO trial). *Am J Cardiol* 1999;84:386–390.

120. Erbel R, Haude M, Hopp HW, et al. Coronary artery stenting compared with balloon angioplasty for restenosis after initial balloon angioplasty. *N Engl J Med* 1998;23:1682–1688.

121. Schomig A, Neumann EF, Kastrati A, et al. A randomized comparison of antiplatelet and anticoagulation therapy after the placement of intracoronary stents. *N Engl J Med* 1996;334: 1084–1089.

122. Leon MB, Baim DS, Gordon P, et al. Clinical and angiographic results from the stent anticoagulation regimen study (STARS). *Circulation* 1996;94(supplement I):1–685.

Cathie Sudlow

Specialist Registrar in Neurology

Department of Neurology, Derriford Hospital, Plymouth, UK

Eva Lonn

Associate Professor of Medicine

Hamilton General Hospital, Hamilton, Canada

Michael Pignone

Division of General Internal Medicine, University of North Carolina, Chapel Hill, USA

Andrew Ness

Senior Lecturer in Epidemiology

University of Bristol, Bristol, UK

Charanjit Rihal

Consultant Cardiologist

Mayo Clinic and Mayo Foundation, Rochester, USA

Competing interests: None declared.

Secondary prevention of ischaemic cardiac events

TABLE 1	Prognostic groups for people who survive the acute stage of MI (see text, p 162).

Baseline risk	1 year mortality	Clinical markers[2–4]
High	10–50%	Older age; history or previous MI; reduced exercise tolerance (New York Heart Association functional classes II–IV) before admission; clinical signs of heart failure in the first 2 days (Killip classes IIb, III, and IV) or persistent heart failure on days 3–5 after infarction; early increased heart rate; persistent or early appearance of angina at rest or with minimal exertion; and multiple or complex ventricular arrhythmias during monitoring in hospital.
Moderate	10%	–
Low	2–5%	Younger age (< 55 years), no previous MI, an event free course during the first 5 days after MI.[2]

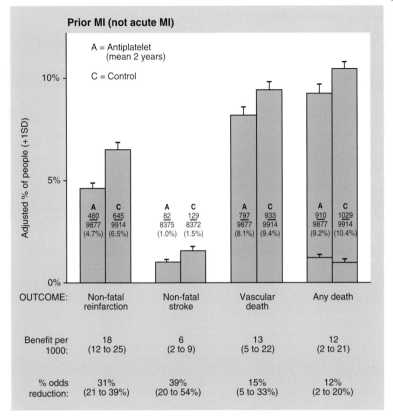

Prior MI (not acute MI)

A = Antiplatelet (mean 2 years)

C = Control

	Non-fatal reinfarction		Non-fatal stroke		Vascular death		Any death	
	A	C	A	C	A	C	A	C
	460	645	82	129	797	933	910	1029
	9877	9914	8375	8372	9877	9914	9877	9914
	(4.7%)	(6.5%)	(1.0%)	(1.5%)	(8.1%)	(9.4%)	(9.2%)	(10.4%)

OUTCOME:

Adjusted % of people (+1SD)

Benefit per 1000:	18 (12 to 25)	6 (2 to 9)	13 (5 to 22)	12 (2 to 21)
% odds reduction:	31% (21 to 39%)	39% (20 to 54%)	15% (5 to 33%)	12% (2 to 20%)

FIGURE 1 The absolute effects of antiplatelet treatment on various outcomes in people with prior MI: results of a systematic review.[10] The columns show the absolute risks over 2 years for each outcome. The error bars represent standard deviations. In the "any death" column, non-vascular deaths are represented by lower horizontal lines (see text, p 163).

Stroke management

Search date May 2001

Gord Gubitz and Peter Sandercock

QUESTIONS

INTERVENTIONS

ACUTE ISCHAEMIC STROKE
Beneficial

Trade off between benefits and harms

Unlikely to be beneficial

Likely to be ineffective or harmful

INTRACEREBRAL HAEMATOMAS
Unknown effectiveness

See glossary, p 202

Key Messages

- Systematic reviews have found that:
  - Stroke rehabilitation units reduce death and severe disability.
  - Thrombolysis reduces the risk of dependency, but increases the risk of death (both from intracranial haemorrhage and from any cause).
  - Early use of aspirin after an ischaemic stroke confirmed by computerised tomography (CT) scan reduces the chance of death and dependency and improves the chance of complete recovery. (We found indirect evidence that aspirin should not be delayed if a CT scan is not readily available within 48 hours. A combined prospective analysis of two large RCTs found that people given aspirin, who were subsequently found to have a haemorrhagic rather than an ischaemic stroke, had similar outcomes to people who were given placebo.)
  - Blood pressure reduction soon after acute ischaemic stroke has not been adequately tested in large scale RCTs and may be harmful.
- One RCT found no evidence that low molecular weight heparin is superior to aspirin alone for the treatment of acute ischemic stroke in people with atrial fibrillation.
- We found no evidence that immediate systemic anticoagulation improved outcome after ischaemic stroke.
- RCTs found no evidence that calcium channel antagonists, lubeluzole, γ-aminobutyric acid (GABA) agonists, glycine antagonists, or N-methyl-D-aspartate (NMDA) antagonists improve clinical outcomes in people with acute ischaemic stroke.

■ We found no evidence of benefit from surgical evacuation of cerebral or cerebellar haematomas.

DEFINITION	Stroke is characterised by rapidly developing clinical symptoms and signs of focal, and at times global, loss of cerebral function lasting more than 24 hours or leading to death, with no apparent cause other than that of vascular origin.[1] Ischaemic stroke is stroke caused by vascular insufficiency (such as cerebrovascular thromboembolism) rather than haemorrhage.
INCIDENCE/ PREVALENCE	Stroke is the third most common cause of death in most developed countries.[2] It is a worldwide problem; about 4.5 million people die from stroke each year. Stroke can occur at any age, but half of all strokes occur in people over 70 years old.[3]
AETIOLOGY/ RISK FACTORS	About 80% of all acute strokes are caused by cerebral infarction, usually resulting from thrombotic or embolic occlusion of a cerebral artery.[4] The remainder are caused either by intracerebral or subarachnoid haemorrhage.
PROGNOSIS	About 10% of all people with acute ischaemic strokes will die within 30 days of stroke onset.[5] Of those who survive the acute event, about 50% will experience some level of disability after 6 months.[6]
AIMS	To minimise impairment, disability, secondary complications, and adverse effects from treatment.
OUTCOMES	Risk of death or dependency (generally assessed as the proportion of people dead or requiring physical assistance for transfers, mobility, dressing, feeding, or toileting 3–6 months after stroke onset);[6] quality of life.
METHODS	*Clinical Evidence* update search and appraisal May 2001.

QUESTION **What are the effects of specialised care in people with stroke?**

One systematic review has found that people with stroke who are managed in specialist stroke rehabilitation units are more likely to be alive and living at home a year after the stroke than those managed in general medical wards, and that stroke unit care reduces time spent in hospital. Observational studies have found that these results are reproducible in routine clinical settings.

Benefits: We found one systematic review (search date 1998, 20 RCTs, 3864 people with stroke) comparing specialised stroke rehabilitation units with conventional care.[7] In most trials, the specialised stroke rehabilitation unit consisted of a designated area or ward, although some trials used a mobile "stroke team". People in these trials were usually transferred to stroke unit care within the first or second week following stroke onset. People cared for in a stroke rehabilitation unit had lower rates of death or dependency after a median follow up of 1 year (RRR 10%, 95% CI 5% to 15%; NNT 16, 95% CI 10 to 43)(see figure 1, p 205).[1] The duration of stay was calculated differently for many of the trials, so the consequent heterogeneity between results limits generalisability. Overall, duration of stay in the stroke unit group was reduced by about 2–11 days. Since the review, two of the included trials have published follow up results. One RCT (220 people) found that care in a combined acute and rehabilitation unit compared with care in general wards increased the proportion of people able to live at home 10 years after their stroke (ARI 11%, 95% CI 1.9% to 20%; NNT 9, 95% CI 5 to 52).[11] The second RCT (220 people) compared treatment in a 15 bed multidisciplinary stroke rehabilitation unit versus treatment in general medical wards.[12] Five years after the stroke, the risk of death or disability for people treated in the stroke unit was reduced (RR 0.91, 95% CI 0.83 to 0.99). We found one additional RCT, which randomised 76 people 2–10 days after their stroke to either an integrated care pathway (see glossary, p 202) or to conventional multidisciplinary care on a stroke rehabilitation unit in the UK.[13] All received similar occupational and physical therapy. Conventional treatment versus the integrated care pathway produced more improvement in the Barthel Index from 4–12 weeks (CI not provided; P < 0.01), and higher scores on the Euroquol (Quality of Life Scale) after 6 months (P < 0.05). It found no significant difference between the two treatments in mortality, duration of hospital stay, or the proportion of people requiring long term institutional care.

Harms: No detrimental effects attributable to stroke units were reported.

Comment: Although the proportional reduction in death or dependency seems larger with thrombolysis (see thrombolysis option below), stroke unit care is applicable to most people with stroke whereas thrombolysis is applicable only to a small proportion. The systematic review did not provide evidence about which aspects of the multidisciplinary approach led to improved outcome, although one limited retrospective analysis of one of the RCTs found that several factors, including early mobilisation, increased use of oxygen, intravenous saline solutions, and antipyretics, might have been responsible.[14] Most of the trials excluded the most mild and severe strokes. Following publication of the systematic review,[7] prospective observational data have been collected in one large series of over 14 000 people in 80 Swedish hospitals.[15] In this series, people admitted to stroke units had reduced dependence at 3 months (RRR 6%, 95% CI 1% to 11%). Although biases are inherent in such observational data, the findings suggest that the results of the meta-analysis may be reproducible in routine clinical settings.

QUESTION What are the effects of medical treatment in acute ischaemic stroke?

OPTION THROMBOLYSIS

We found little evidence on the balance between benefits and harms from thrombolysis in acute ischaemic stroke. One systematic review has found that thrombolysis given soon after acute ischaemic stroke reduces overall risk of death and dependency in the long term, but that this benefit was achieved at the cost of an increased short term risk of fatal intracranial haemorrhage. It remains unclear which people are most likely to benefit or be harmed.

Benefits: We found one systematic review (search date 1999, 17 RCTs, 5216 highly selected people) comparing thrombolysis with placebo given soon after the onset of stroke.[8] All trials used CT or magnetic resonance scanning before randomisation to exclude intracranial haemorrhage or other non-stroke disorders. Results for three different thrombolytic agents (streptokinase, urokinase, and recombinant tissue plasminogen activator) were included, but direct comparison of different thrombolytic drugs was not possible. Two trials used intra-arterial administration and the rest used the intravenous route. Thrombolysis reduced the risk of death or dependency at the end of the studies (ARR 4.2%, 95% CI 1.2% to 7.2%; RRR 7%, 95% CI 3% to 12%; NNT 24, 95% CI 14 to 83) (see figures 1 and 2, p 205).[8] In the subset of trials that assessed intravenous recombinant tissue plasminogen activator, the findings were similar (ARR 5.7%, 95% CI 2.0% to 9.4%; RRR 10%, 95% CI 4% to 16%; NNT 18, 95% CI 11 to 50). One meta-analysis (4 RCTs, individual results of 1292 people with acute ischaemic stroke treated with streptokinase or placebo) found that streptokinase versus placebo had no clear effect on the proportion of people dead or dependent at 3 months, and included the possibility of both substantial benefit or substantial harm (RRR +1%, 95% CI −6% to +8%).[16] People allocated to streptokinase were more likely to be dead after 3 months (RRI 46%, 95% CI 24% to 73%). The combination of aspirin plus streptokinase significantly increased mortality at 3 months ($P = 0.005$), but this did not affect the combined risk of death or severe disability (CI not provided; $P = 0.28$).

Harms: **Fatal intracranial haemorrhage:** In the systematic review, thrombolysis increased fatal intracranial haemorrhage compared with placebo (ARI 4.4%, 95% CI 3.4% to 5.4%; RRI 396%, 95% CI 220% to 668%; NNH 23, 95% CI 19 to 29).[8] In the subset of trials that assessed intravenous recombinant tissue plasminogen activator, the findings were similar (ARI 2.9%, 95% CI 1.7% to 4.1%; RRI 259%, 95% CI 102% to 536%; NNH 34, 95% CI 24 to 59). **Death:** In the systematic review, thrombolysis compared with placebo increased the risk of death by the end of the follow up (ARI 3.3%, 95% CI 1.2% to 5.4%; RRI 23%, 95% CI 10% to 38%; NNH 30, 95% CI 19 to 83).[8] This excess of deaths was offset by fewer people being alive but dependent 6 months after stroke onset. The net effect was a reduction in the number of people who were dead or dependent.

Comment: There was no significant heterogeneity of treatment effect overall, but heterogeneity of results was noted for the outcomes of death, and death or dependency at final follow up among the eight trials of intravenous recombinant tissue plasminogen activator.[8] Explanations may include the combined use of antithrombotic agents (aspirin or heparin within the first 24 h of thrombolysis), stroke severity, the presence of early ischaemic changes on CT scan, and the time from stroke onset to randomisation. A subgroup analysis suggested that thrombolysis may be more beneficial if given within 3 hours of symptom onset, but the duration of the "therapeutic time window" could not be determined reliably. Most of the trial results were of outcome at 3 months; only one trial reported 1 year

Cardiovascular disorders

outcome data.[17] We found little evidence about which people are most and least likely to benefit from thrombolysis. A number of trials of different thrombolytic regimens are underway.[18]

OPTION   ASPIRIN

One systematic review has found that antiplatelet treatment with aspirin started within 48 hours of acute ischaemic stroke reduces the risk of death and dependence, as does the continued long term use of aspirin (see aspirin under stroke prevention, p 215). Most people included in the systematic review had a CT scan to exclude haemorrhage before treatment was started; in such people aspirin was beneficial. Subgroup analysis of two large RCTs found evidence that aspirin should not be delayed if a CT scan is not readily available within 48 hours; people given aspirin who were subsequently found to have a haemorrhagic rather than an ischaemic stroke had similar outcomes to people who were given placebo.

Benefits: **Early use of aspirin:** We found one systematic review (search date 1999, 8 RCTs, 41 325 people with definite or presumed ischaemic stroke), which compared antiplatelet treatment started within 14 days of the stroke versus placebo.[19] Of the data in the systematic review, 98% came from two large RCTs of aspirin 160–300 mg daily started within 48 hours of stroke onset.[9,10] Most people had an ischaemic stroke confirmed by CT scan before randomisation, but people who were conscious could be randomised before CT scan if the stroke was very likely to be ischaemic on clinical grounds. Treatment duration varied from 10–28 days. Aspirin started within the first 48 hours of acute ischaemic stroke reduced death or dependency at 6 months' follow up (RRR 3%, 95% CI 1% to 5%; NNT 77, 95% CI 43 to 333) (see figure 1, p 205) and increased the number of people making a complete recovery (NNT 91, 95% CI 50 to 500). A prospective combined analysis[20] of the two large RCTs[9,10] found a significant reduction in the outcome of further stroke or death with aspirin versus placebo (ARR 0.9%, 95% CI 0.75% to 1.85%; NNT 111, 95% CI 54 to 133). The effect was similar across subgroups (older v younger; male v female; impaired consciousness or not; atrial fibrillation or not; blood pressure; stroke subtype; timing of CT scanning). For the 773 people subsequently found to have had a haemorrhagic stroke rather than an ischaemic stroke, the subgroup analysis found no difference in the outcome of further stroke or death between those who were randomised to aspirin versus placebo (16% v 18%; ARR +2.0%, 95% CI –4.0% to +6.6%).[20] **Long term treatment:** See aspirin under stroke prevention, p 215.

Harms: Aspirin caused an excess of about two intracranial and four extracranial haemorrhages per 1000 people treated, but these small risks were more than offset by the reductions in death and disability from other causes both in the short term[19] and in the long term.[21] Common adverse effects of aspirin (such as dyspepsia and constipation) were dose related.[22]

Comment: We found no clear evidence that any one dose of aspirin is more effective than any other in the treatment of acute ischaemic stroke.

One recent meta-regression analysis of the dose response effect of aspirin on stroke found a uniform effect of aspirin in a range of doses from 50–1500 mg daily.[23] People unable to swallow safely after a stroke may be given aspirin as a suppository.

| OPTION | IMMEDIATE SYSTEMIC ANTICOAGULATION |

One systematic review found no short or long term improvement in acute ischaemic stroke with immediate systemic anticoagulants (unfractionated heparin, low molecular weight heparin, heparinoids, or specific thrombin inhibitors) versus usual care without systemic anticoagulants. Immediate systemic anticoagulants reduce the risk of deep venous thrombosis and pulmonary embolus, but this benefit is offset by a dose dependent risk of intracranial and extracranial haemorrhage. In people with acute ischaemic stroke and atrial fibrillation, one RCT found no evidence that low molecular weight heparin is superior to aspirin alone.

Benefits: **Death or dependency:** We found one systematic review (search date 1999, 21 RCTs, 23 427 people)[24] and two subsequent RCTs.[25,26] The systematic review compared unfractionated heparin, low molecular weight heparin, heparinoids, oral anticoagulants, or specific thrombin inhibitors versus usual care without systemic anticoagulants.[24] Over 80% of the data came from one trial, which randomised people with any severity of stroke to either subcutaneous heparin or placebo, usually after exclusion of haemorrhage by CT scan.[10] The systematic review found no significant difference in the proportion of people dead or dependent in the treatment and control groups at the end of follow up (3–6 months after the stroke: ARR +0.4%, 95% CI −0.9% to +1.7%; RRR 0%, 95% CI −2% to +3%).[24] There was no clear short or long term benefit of anticoagulants in any prespecified subgroups (stroke of presumed cardioembolic origin v others; different anticoagulants). The first subsequent RCT (449 people with acute stroke and atrial fibrillation) found no significant difference between dalteparin (a low molecular weight heparin) versus aspirin for the primary outcome of recurrent ischaemic stroke during the first 14 days (ARI +1.0%, 95% CI −3.6% to +6.2%) or for secondary outcomes, including functional outcome at 3 months.[25] The second RCT randomised 404 people to one of four different doses of the low molecular weight heparin certoparin within 12 hours of stroke onset.[26] There was no difference in neurological outcome between the four groups 3 months after treatment. **Deep venous thrombosis and pulmonary embolism:** We found three systematic reviews.[24,27,28] The first systematic review (search date 1999) included 10 small heterogeneous RCTs (22 000 people), which assessed anticoagulants in 916 people at high risk of deep venous thrombosis after their stroke.[24] Anticoagulation compared with control reduced the risk of deep vein thrombosis (ARR 29%, 95% CI 24% to 35%; RRR 64%, 95% CI 54% to 71%; NNT 3, 95% CI 2 to 4) and reduced symptomatic pulmonary embolism (ARR 0.3%, 95% CI 0.1% to 0.6%; RRR 38%, 95% CI 16% to 54%; NNT 333, 95% CI 167 to 1000). No RCT performed investigations in all people to rule out silent events. The frequency of reported pulmonary emboli was low and varied among RCTs, so there may have been under ascertainment. Two other systematic reviews (search dates 1999, same 5

RCTs in each review, 705 people with acute ischaemic stroke)[27,28] found that low molecular weight heparins or heparinoids versus unfractionated heparin significantly reduced deep venous thrombosis (AR 13% with low molecular weight heparins or heparinoids v 22% with unfractionated heparin; ARR 9%, 95% CI 4.5% to 16%). The number of events was too small to estimate the effects of low molecular weight heparins or heparinoids versus unfractionated heparin on death, intracranial haemorrhage, or functional outcome in survivors.

Harms: One systematic review found that anticoagulation slightly increased symptomatic intracranial haemorrhages within 14 days of starting treatment compared with control (ARI 0.93%, 95% CI 0.68% to 1.18%; RRI 163%, 95% CI 95% to 255%; NNH 108, 95% CI 85 to 147).[24] The large trial of subcutaneous heparin found that this effect was dose dependent (symptomatic intracranial haemorrhage by using medium dose compared with low dose heparin for 14 days; RRI 143%, 95% CI 82% to 204%; NNH 97, 95% CI 68 to 169).[10] The review also found a dose dependent increase in major extracranial haemorrhages after 14 days of treatment with anticoagulants (ARI 0.91%, 95% CI 0.67% to 1.15%; RRI 231%, 95% CI 136% to 365%; NNH 109, 95% CI 87 to 149).[24] The subsequent RCT of dalteparin versus aspirin for people with acute stroke and atrial fibrillation found no difference in adverse events, including symptomatic or asymptomatic intracerebral haemorrhage, progression of symptoms, or early or late death.[25] As in the systematic review,[24] a recent RCT comparing different doses of the low molecular weight heparin certoparin found that intracranial hemorrhage occurred more often in those receiving a higher dose of anticoagulant.[26] However, the overall number of patients experiencing haemorrhagic complications in the RCT may have been artificially lowered, because the study protocol was changed during the trial period so as to exclude patients with early ischaemic changes on CT scan.

Comment: Full publication of the results of a recently completed trial of the low molecular weight heparin tinzaparin is awaited.[29] Alternative treatments to prevent deep venous thrombosis and pulmonary embolism after acute ischaemic stroke include aspirin and compression stockings.

OPTION   BLOOD PRESSURE REDUCTION

One systematic review found no evidence that blood pressure reduction is of benefit in people with acute ischaemic stroke, but suggested that treatment may be harmful.

Benefits: We found one systematic review (search date 1997, 3 RCTs, 113 people with acute stroke) comparing blood pressure lowering treatment with placebo.[30] Several different antihypertensive agents were used. The trials collected insufficient clinical data to allow an analysis of the relation between changes in blood pressure and clinical outcome.

Harms: Two placebo controlled RCTs have suggested that people treated with antihypertensive agents may have a worse clinical outcome and increased mortality.[31,32] The first (295 people with acute ischaemic stroke) compared nimodipine (a calcium channel antagonist) with placebo.[31] The trial was stopped prematurely because of an excess of unfavourable neurological outcomes in the nimodipine treated group. Exploratory analyses confirmed that this negative correlation was related to reductions in mean arterial blood pressure (CI not provided; $P = 0.02$) and diastolic blood pressure ($P = 0.0005$). The second RCT (302 people with acute ischaemic stroke) evaluated β blockers (atenolol or propranolol).[32] There was a non-significant increase in death for people taking β blockers, and no difference in the proportion of people achieving a good outcome. One systematic review (search date 1994, 9 RCTs, 3719 people with acute stroke) compared nimodipine versus placebo; no net benefit was found.[33] A second review (24 RCTs, 6894 people) found a non-significant increase in the risk of death with calcium channel antagonists versus placebo (RRR 8%, 95% CI 1% reduction to 18% increase).[34] Although treatment with calcium channel antagonists in these trials was intended for neuroprotection, blood pressure was lower in the treatment group in several trials.

Comment: Population based studies suggest a direct and continuous association between blood pressure and the risk of recurrent stroke.[35] However, acute blood pressure lowering in acute ischaemic stroke may lead to increased cerebral ischaemia. The systematic review[31] identified several ongoing RCTs and we identified two additional ongoing RCTs not included in the systematic review.[36,37]

OPTION   **NEUROPROTECTIVE AGENTS**

Systematic reviews found no evidence that calcium channel antagonists, GABA agonists, tirilazad, glycine antagonists, or NMDA antagonists improved clinical outcomes in people with acute ischaemic stroke. RCTs found no evidence that lubeluzole improved clinical outcomes in people with acute ischaemic stroke.

Benefits: We found no systematic reviews evaluating the general effectiveness of neuroprotective agents in acute ischaemic stroke. **Calcium channel antagonists:** We found two systematic reviews comparing calcium channel antagonists with placebo.[38,39] The first review (search date 1999, 28 RCTs, 7521 people with acute ischaemic stroke) found that calcium channel antagonists did not significantly reduce the risk of poor outcome (including death) at the end of the follow up period compared with placebo (ARI of poor outcome +4.9%, 95% CI −2.5% to +7.3%; RRI +4%, 95% CI −2% to +9%).[38] The second review (search date 1999)[39] includes one additional RCT (454 people)[40] that was stopped prematurely because of publication of the first review.[38] Inclusion of its data does not change the results of the first review. **GABA agonists:** We found one systematic review (search date 1999, 3 RCTs, 1002 people with acute ischaemic stroke), which found no significant difference between piracetam (a GABA agonist) and control groups for the number of people dead or dependent at the end of follow up (ARI +0.2%, 95% CI −6.0% to +6.4%; RRI 0%, 95% CI −11% to +9%).[41] We found one RCT (1360 people with acute stroke), which identified no significant effect of clomethiazole (a GABA agonist) versus placebo on achievement of functional independence (ARR +1.5%, 95% CI −4.0% to +6.6%; RRR +3.0%, 95% CI −7% to +13%).[42] **Lubeluzole:** We found three RCTs assessing lubeluzole, an inhibitor of presynaptic glutamate release.[43-45] Intention to treat analysis of the first trial (721 people) found that lubeluzole did not significantly reduce mortality at 12 weeks (AR 20.7% with lubeluzole v 25.2% with placebo; ARR 4.5%; P = NS; RRR +18%, 95% CI −7% to +37%).[43] The second RCT (725 people; 365 randomised to lubeluzole, 360 to placebo) also found no significant difference in mortality at 12 weeks with lubeluzole versus placebo (intention to treat analysis: ARR +0.6%, 95% CI −4.8% to +7.4%; RRR +3%, 95% CI −22% to +29%).[44] The third RCT randomised 1786 people (901 treated with lubeluzole, 885 with placebo).[45] Of these, 34% of the lubeluzole group and 33% of the placebo group did not complete the trial. The trial found no overall difference in outcome, defined as a Barthel Index of greater than 70 at 12 weeks' follow up (intention to treat analysis: ARR +3.2%, 95% CI −3.3% to +5.9%). **Glycine antagonists:** We found two RCTs.[46,47] One RCT (1804 conscious people with limb weakness evaluated within 6 h of stroke onset) found no significant difference between gavestinel (GV150526, a glycine antagonist) versus placebo in survival and outcome at 3 months as measured using the Barthel Index (ARR +1.0%, 95% CI −3.5% to +6.0%).[46] The second RCT (1367 people with predefined level of limb weakness and functional independence prior to stroke) also found no significant difference in survival and outcome at 3 months, measured using the Barthel Index (ARI 1.9%, 95% CI −3.8% to +6.4%).[47] **NMDA antagonists:** Two recent RCTs evaluating the NMDA antagonist (see glossary, p 202) CGS19775 found no significant difference in the proportion people with a Barthel Index over 60, but data were limited as the trials were terminated because of adverse outcomes after only 31% of the total planned patient enrolment.[48] **Tirilazad:** We found one systematic review (search date 1998, 6 RCTs, 1757 people) comparing tirilazad, a steroid derivative, with placebo in people with acute ischaemic stroke. Tirilazad was associated with an increase in death and disability at 3 months' follow up when measured using the expanded Barthel Index (ARI 3.9%, 95% CI −0.8% to +8.6%).[49]

Harms: In the systematic review of calcium channel antagonists, indirect and limited comparisons of intravenous versus oral administration found no significant difference in adverse events (ARI of adverse events, iv v oral, +2.3%, 95% CI −0.9% to +3.7%; RRI +17%, 95% CI −3% to +41%).[38] In the systematic review of piracetam, there was a non-significant increase in death with piracetam versus placebo, which was no longer apparent after correction for imbalance in stroke severity.[41] Lubeluzole has also been noted to have adverse outcomes, especially at higher doses. One phase II trial of lubeluzole (232 people) was terminated prematurely because of an excess of deaths in the arm randomised to a higher dosage of drug.[50] This problem has not been noted with the lower drug dosages used in the published phase III studies.[43-45] The trials of CGS19775 were terminated after enrolling 567 people because of greater early mortality in the CGS19775 groups.[48] The systematic review of tirilazad found the drug to be associated with a significant increase in injection site phlebitis (ARI 12.2%, 95% CI 8.7% to 15.7%).[49]

Comment: A systematic review of the effects of lubeluzole is being developed.[51] The effects of the cell membrane precursor citicholine have been evaluated in small trials, and a systematic review is in progress.[52] Systematic reviews are being developed for antioxidants and for excitatory amino acid modulators.[53] Several RCTs are ongoing, including one of intravenous magnesium sulphate[54] and another of diazepam (a GABA agonist).[55]

QUESTION   **What are the effects of surgical treatment for intracerebral haematomas?**

OPTION   **EVACUATION**

We found that the balance between benefits and harms has not been clearly established for the evacuation of supratentorial haematomas. We found no evidence from RCTs on the role of evacuation or ventricular shunting in people with infratentorial haematoma whose consciousness level is declining.

Benefits: **For supratentorial haematomas:** We found three systematic reviews.[56-58] The first review (search date 1998)[56] and second review (search date 1997)[57] both assessed the same four RCTs comparing surgery (craniotomy in three trials and endoscopy in one) versus best medical treatment in 354 people with primary supratentorial intracerebral haemorrhage. The second review also assessed information from case series.[57] Neither review found any significant short or long term differences in death or disability for surgically treated people (ARI +3.3%, 95% CI −5.9% to +12.5%; RRI +5%, 95% CI −7% to +19%). The third review (search date 1999) includes several analyses.[58] The first analysis includes results from seven RCTs (530 people), including two RCTs not included in either of the first two systematic reviews. The overall results are similar to those of the first two systematic reviews, with no significant difference in death or disability for surgically treated people (ARI +3.5%, 95% CI −4.4% to +11.4%). A further analysis of results from only recent, post-CT, well-constructed, balanced trials (5 trials, 224 people in total) did not find a significant difference between the two groups (ARR +9.3%, 95% CI −2.6% to +21.2%). **For infratentorial haematomas:** We found no evidence from systematic reviews or RCTs on the role of surgical evacuation or ventricular shunting.[59]

Harms: The two earlier reviews found that for the 254 people randomised to craniotomy rather than best medical treatment, there was increased death and disability (ARI 12%, 95% CI 1.8% to 22%; RRI 17%, 95% CI 2% to 34%; NNH 8, 95% CI 5 to 56).[56,57] For the 100 people randomised to endoscopy rather than best medical practice, there was no significant effect on death and disability (RRR 24%, 95% CI −2% to +44%). The third systematic review did not evaluate these adverse outcomes.[58]

Comment: Current practice is based on the consensus that people with infratentorial (cerebellar) haematomas whose consciousness level is declining probably benefit from evacuation of the haematoma. The systematic reviews identified several ongoing RCTs assessing the evacuation of supratentorial haematomas.

GLOSSARY

Integrated care pathway A model of care that includes definition of therapeutic goals and specification of a timed plan designed to promote multidisciplinary care, improve discharge planning, and reduce the duration of hospital stay.

NMDA antagonist Glutamate can bind to N-methyl-D-aspartate (NMDA) receptors on cell surfaces. One hypothesis proposed that glutamate released during a stroke can cause further harm to neurones by stimulating the NMDA receptors. NMDA antagonists block these receptors.

REFERENCES

1. Hatano S. Experience from a multicentre stroke register: a preliminary report. *Bull World Health Organ* 1976;54:541–553.

2. Bonita R. Epidemiology of stroke. *Lancet* 1992; 339:342–344.

3. Bamford J, Sandercock P, Dennis M, Warlow C, Jones L, McPherson K. A prospective study of acute cerebrovascular disease in the community: the Oxfordshire community stroke project, 1981–1986. 1. Methodology, demography and incident cases of first ever stroke. *J Neurol Neurosurg Psychiatry* 1988;51:1373–1380.

4. Bamford J, Dennis M, Sandercock P, Burn J, Warlow C. A prospective study of acute cerebrovascular disease in the community: the Oxfordshire community stroke project, 1981–1986. 2. Incidence, case fatality rates and overall outcome at one year of cerebral infarction, primary intracerebral and subarachnoid haemorrhage. *J Neurol Neurosurg Psychiatry* 1990;53:16–22.

5. Bamford J, Dennis M, Sandercock P, Burn J, Warlow C. The frequency, causes and timing of death within 30 days of a first stroke: the Oxfordshire community stroke project. *J Neurol Neurosurg Psychiatry* 1990;53:824–829.

6. Wade DT. Functional abilities after stroke: measurement, natural history and prognosis. *J Neurol Neurosurg Psychiatry* 1987;50:177–182.

7. Stroke Unit Trialists' Collaboration. Organised inpatient (stroke unit) care for stroke. In: The Cochrane Library, Issue 3, 2000. Oxford: Update Software. Search date June 1998; primary sources Cochrane Collaboration Stroke Group, hand searches of reference lists of relevant articles, preliminary findings publicised at stroke conferences, and personal contact with colleagues.

8. Wardlaw JM, del Zoppo G, Yamaguchi T. Thrombolysis for acute ischaemic stroke. In: The Cochrane Library, Issue 3, 2000. Oxford: Update Software. Search date March 1999; primary sources Cochrane Collaboration Stroke Group, Medline, Embase, the Ottawa Stroke Trials Registry, hand searches of references quoted in thrombolysis papers, published abstracts of neurological and cerebrovascular symposia, direct contact with principal investigators of trials, colleagues, and pharmaceutical companies.

9. CAST. Randomised placebo-controlled trial of early aspirin use in 20 000 patients with acute ischaemic stroke. CAST (Chinese Acute Stroke Trial) collaborative group. *Lancet* 1997;349: 1641–1649.

10. International Stroke Trial Collaborative Group. The international stroke trial (IST): a randomised trial of aspirin, heparin, both or neither among 19 435 patients with acute ischaemic stroke. *Lancet* 1997;349:1569–1581.

11. Indredavik B, Bakke RPT, Slordahl SA, Rokseth R, Haheim LL. Stroke unit treatment. 10-year follow-up. *Stroke* 1999;30:1524–1527.

12. Lincoln NB, Husbands S, Trescoli C, Drummond AER, Gladman JRF, Berman P. Five year follow up of a randomised controlled trial of a stroke rehabilitation unit. *BMJ* 2000;320:549.

13. Sulch D, Perez I, Melbourn A, Kalra L. Randomized controlled trial of integrated (managed) care pathway for stroke rehabilitation. *Stroke* 2000;31: 1929–1934.

14. Indredavik B, Bakke RPT, Slordahl SA, Rokseth R, Haheim LL. Treatment in a combined acute and rehabilitation stroke unit. Which aspects are most important. *Stroke* 1999;30:917–923.

15. Stegmayr B, Asplund K, Hulter-Asberg K, et al. Stroke units in their natural habitat: can results of randomized trials be reproduced in routine clinical practice? For the risk-stroke collaboration. *Stroke* 1999;30:709–714.

16. Cornu C, Boutitie F, Candelise L, et al. Streptokinase in acute ischemic stroke: an individual patient data meta-analysis: the thrombolysis in acute stroke pooling project. *Stroke* 2000;31:1555–1560.

17. Kwiatkowski T, Libman R, Frankel M, et al. Effects of tissue plasminogen activator for acute ischemic stroke at one year. National Institute of Neurological Disorders and stroke recombinant tissue plasminogen activator stroke study group. *N Engl J Med* 1999;340:1781–1787.

18. University of Washington Stroke Centre website: http://stroke.wustl.edu/trials.

19. Gubitz G, Sandercock P, Counsell C. Antiplatelet therapy for acute ischaemic stroke. In: The Cochrane Library, Issue 3, 2000. Oxford: Update Software. Search date March 1999; primary sources Cochrane Collaboration Stroke Group, Register of the Antiplatelet Trialists Collaboration, MedStrategy, and contact with pharmaceutical companies marketing antiplatelet agents.

20. Chen Z, Sandercock P, Pan H, et al. Indications for early aspirin use in acute ischemic stroke: a combined analysis of 40 000 randomized patients from the Chinese Acute Stroke Trial and the International Stroke Trial. *Stroke* 2000;31: 1240–1249.

21. Antiplatelet Trialists' Collaboration. Collaborative overview of randomised trials of antiplatelet therapy I: prevention of death, myocardial infarction and stroke by prolonged antiplatelet therapy in various categories of patients. *BMJ* 1994;308:81–106. Search date 1990; primary sources Medline and Current Contents.

22. Slattery J, Warlow CP, Shorrock CJ, Langman MJS. Risks of gastrointestinal bleeding during secondary prevention of vascular events with aspirin – analysis of gastrointestinal bleeding during the UK-TIA trial. *Gut* 1995;37:509–511.

23. Johnson ES, Lanes SF, Wentworth CE, Satterfield MH, Abebe BL, Dicker LW. A metaregression analysis of the dose-response effect of aspirin on stroke. *Arch Intern Med* 1999;159:1248–1253.

24. Gubitz G, Sandercock P, Counsell C, Signorini D. Anticoagulants for acute ischaemic stroke. In: The Cochrane Library, Issue 3, 2000. Oxford: Update Software. Search date March 1999; primary sources Cochrane Collaboration Stroke Group, MedStrategy, Antithrombotic Therapy Trialists' Collaboration Trials Register, and contact with manufacturers of anticoagulants.

25. Berge E, Abdelnoor M, Nakstad P, Sandset P. Low-molecular-weight heparin versus aspirin in people with acute ischaemic stroke and atrial fibrillation: a double-blind randomised study. HAEST Study Group. Heparin in Acute Embolic Stroke Trial. *Lancet* 2000;355:1205–1210.

26. Diener H, Ringelstein E, von Kummer R, et al. Treatment of acute ischemic stroke with the low-molecular-weight heparin certoparin: results of the TOPAS Trial. *Stroke* 2001;32:22–29.

27. Counsell C, Sandercock P. Low-molecular-weight heparins or heparinoids versus standard unfractionated heparin for acute ischaemic stroke. In: The Cochrane Library, Issue 3, 2000. Oxford: Update Software. Search date August 1999; primary sources Cochrane Collaboration Stroke Group, MedStrategy, Antithrombotic Therapy Trialists' Collaboration Trials Register, and contact with manufacturers of anticoagulants.

28. Bath P, Iddenden R, Bath F. Low-molecular-weight heparins and heparinoids in acute ischemic stroke: a meta-analysis of randomized controlled trials. *Stroke* 2000;31:1770–1778. Search date 1999; primary sources Cochrane Stroke Group Database of Trials in Acute Stroke, Cochrane Library, and hand searches of reference lists of identified publications.

29. Bath P for the TAIST Investigators. Tinzaparin in acute ischaemic stroke trial (TAIST). *Cerebrovasc Dis* 2000;10(suppl 2):81.

30. Blood Pressure in Acute Stroke Collaboration (BASC). Interventions for deliberately altering blood pressure in acute stroke. In: The Cochrane Library, Issue 3, 2000. Oxford: Update Software. Search date May 1997; primary sources Cochrane Stroke Group Trials Register, Ottawa Stroke Trials Registry, Medline, Embase, ISI, hand searches of existing review articles, and personal contact with researchers in the field and pharmaceutical companies.

31. Wahlgren NG, MacMahon DG, DeKeyser J, Indredavik B, Ryman T. Intravenous nimodipine west European stroke trial (INWEST) of nimodipine in the treatment of acute ischaemic stroke. *Cerebrovasc Dis* 1994;4:204–210.

32. Barer DH, Cruickshank JM, Ebrahim SB, Mitchell JRA. Low dose beta blockade in acute stroke (BEST trial): an evaluation. *BMJ* 1988;296:737–741.

33. Mohr JP, Orgogozo JM, Harrison MJG, et al. Meta-analysis of oral nimodipine trials in acute ischaemic stroke. *Cerebrovasc Dis* 1994;4:197–203. Search date 1994; primary source Bayer database.

34. Horn J, Orgogozo JM, Limburg M. Review on calcium antagonists in ischaemic stroke; mortality data. *Cerebrovasc Dis* 1998;8(suppl 4):27.

35. Rodgers A, MacMahon S, Gamble G. Blood pressure and risk of stroke patients with cerebrovascular disease. *BMJ* 1996;313:147.

36. Schrader J, Rothemeyer M, Luders S, Kollmann K. Hypertension and stroke – rationale behind the ACCESS trial. *Basic Res Cardiol* 1998;93(suppl 2):69–78.

37. Bath PM, Bath FJ, for the ENOS Investigators. Efficacy of nitric oxide in stroke (ENOS) trial – a prospective large randomised controlled trial in acute stroke. *Cerebrovasc Dis* 2000;10 (Suppl 2):81.

38. Horn J, Limburg M. Calcium antagonists for acute ischemic stroke. In: The Cochrane Library, Issue 3, 2000. Oxford: Update Software. Search date March 1999; primary source Cochrane Stroke Review Group Trials Register.

39. Horn J, Limburg M. Calcium antagonists for ischemic stroke: a systematic review. *Stroke* 2001;32:570–576. Search date May 1999; primary sources Cochrane Collaboration Stroke Group Specialized Register of Controlled Trials, and personal contact with principal investigators and company representatives.

40. Horn J, de Haan R, Vermeulen M, Limburg M. Very Early Nimodipine Use in Stroke (VENUS). A randomized, double-blind, placebo-controlled trail. *Stroke* 2001;32:461–465.

41. Ricci S, Celani MG, Cantisani AT, Righetti E. Piracetam for acute ischaemic stroke. In: The Cochrane Library, Issue 3, 2000. Oxford: Update Software. Search date January 1999; primary sources Cochrane Stroke Review Group Trials Register, Medline, Embase, BIDIS ISI, hand searches of 15 journals, and contact with manufacturers.

42. Wahlgren NG, Ranasinha KW, Rosolacci T, et al. Clomethiazole acute stroke study (CLASS): results of a randomised, controlled trial of clomethiazole versus placebo in 1360 acute stroke patients. *Stroke* 1999;30:21–28.

43. Grotta J, for the US and Canadian Lubeluzole Stroke Study Group. Lubeluzole treatment for acute ischaemic stroke. *Stroke* 1997;28:2338–2346.

44. Diener HC. Multinational randomised controlled trial of lubeluzole in acute ischaemic stroke. *Cerebrovasc Dis* 1998;8:172–181.

45. Diener H, Cortens M, Ford G, et al for the LUB-INT-13 Investigators. Lubeluzole in acute ischemic stroke treatment. A double-blind study with an 8-hour inclusion window comparing a 10-mg daily dose of lubeluzolde with placebo. *Stroke* 2000;31:2543–2551.

46. Lees K, Asplund K, Carolei A, et al. Glycine antagonist (gavestinel) in neuroprotection (GAIN International) in people with acute stroke: a randomised controlled trial. *Lancet* 2000;355:1949–1954.

47. Sacco R, DeRosa J, Haley E Jr, et al. for the GAIN Americas Investigators. Glycine Antagonist in Neuroprotection for Patients with Acute Stroke. GAIN Americas: a randomized controlled trial. *JAMA* 2001;285:1719–1728.

48. Davis S, Lees K, Albers G, et al, for the ASSIST Investigators. Selfotel in acute ischemic stroke. Possible neurotoxic effects of an NMDA antagonist. *Stroke* 2000;31:347–354.

49. Tirilazad International Steering Committee. Tirilazad mesylate inacute ischemic stroke: a systematic review. *Stroke* 2000;31:2257–2265. Search date 1998; primary sources Cochrane Library, hand searches of the reference lists of identified publications, and personal contact with the pharmaceutical company making the drug.

50. Diener H, Hacke W, Hennerici M, Radberg J, Hanston L, De Keyser J, for the Lubeluzole International Study Group. Lubeluzole in acute ischaemic stroke: a double-blind, placebo-controlled phase II trial. *Stroke* 1996;27:76–81.

Cardiovascular disorders

51. Gandolfo C, Conti M. Lubeluzole for acute ischemic stroke [Protocol]. In: The Cochrane Library, Issue 3, 2000. Oxford: Update Software.
52. Saver JL, Wilterdink J. Choline precursors for acute and subacute ischemic and hemorrhagic stroke [Protocol]. In: The Cochrane Library, Issue 3, 2000. Oxford: Update Software.
53. Cochrane Stroke Review Group. Department of Clinical Neurosciences, Western General Hospital, Crewe Road, Edinburgh, UK EH4 2XU. URL: http://www.dcn.ed.ac.uk/csrg.
54. Muir KW, Lees KR. IMAGES. Intravenous magnesium efficacy in stroke trial [abstract]. *Cerebrovasc Dis* 1996;6:75P383.
55. Lodder J, van Raak L, Kessels F, Hilton A. Early GABA-ergic activation study in stroke (EGASIS). *Cerebrovasc Dis* 2000;10(suppl 2):80.
56. Prasad K, Shrivastava A. Surgery for primary supratentorial intracerebral haemorrhage. In: The Cochrane Library, Issue 3, 2000. Oxford: Update Software. Search date August 1998; primary sources Cochrane Collaboration Stroke Group, hand searches of reference lists of all identified trials, specialist journals, and monographs.
57. Hankey G, Hon C. Surgery for primary intracerebral hemorrhage: is it safe and effective? A systematic review of case series and randomised trials. *Stroke* 1997;28:2126–2132. Search date June 1997; primary sources Medline, and hand searches of reference lists of identified articles, published epidemiological studies, and reviews.
58. Fernandes HM, Gregson B, Siddique S, Mendelow AD. Surgery in intracerebral hemorrhage: the uncertainty continues. *Stroke* 2000;31: 2511–2516. Search date October 1999; primary sources Ovid databases (unspecified), Medline, and hand searches of the reference lists of identified articles and relevant cited references.
59. Warlow CP, Dennis MS, van Gijn J, et al, eds. Treatment of primary intracerebral haemorrhage. In: *Stroke: a practical guide to management*. Oxford: Blackwell Science,1996:430–437.

Gord Gubitz
Assistant Professor
Division of Neurology
Dalhousie University
Halifax
Canada

Peter Sandercock
Professor of Neurology
Neurosciences Trials Unit
University of Edinburgh
Edinburgh
UK

Competing interests: GG none declared. PS has given lectures and symposia and received lecture fees and travel expenses from Boehringer Ingelheim, Sanofi, BMJ Publishing Group, and a variety of other companies. PS has also received support from Boehringer Ingelheim and Glaxo Wellcome for trials and research.

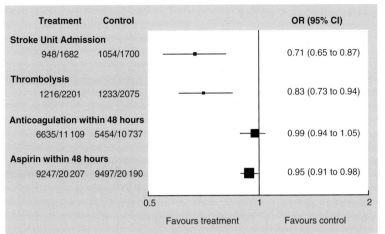

FIGURE 1 Proportional effects on "death or dependency" at the end of scheduled follow up: results of systematic reviews.[7-10] Data refer only to benefits and not to harms (see text, pp 193, 195, 196).

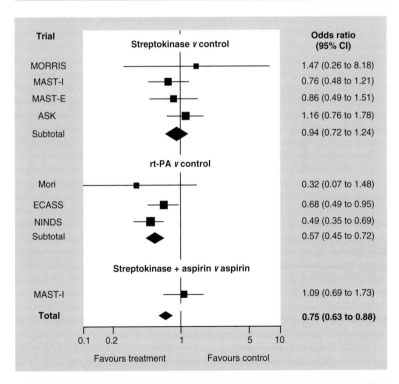

FIGURE 2 Effect of thrombolysis on death and dependency at end of trial: results of review (see text, p 195).[8]

Search date January 2001

Clinical Evidence writers on stroke prevention

Cardiovascular disorders

QUESTIONS

INTERVENTIONS

Key Messages

In people with a prior stroke or TIA

- We found insufficient evidence from RCTs about routine blood pressure reduction.
- RCTs have found that statins may prevent stroke in people with a history of coronary heart disease. We found inconclusive evidence in those with no history of coronary heart disease.
- RCTs have found that routine use of prolonged antiplatelet treatment is beneficial unless there is a clear contraindication, and that aspirin 75 mg daily is as effective as higher doses. We found no good evidence that any other antiplatelet regimen is superior to medium dose aspirin (75–325 mg daily) in the prevention of vascular events.

- RCTs have found that clopidogrel or the combination of aspirin and dipyridamole are safe and effective alternatives to medium dose aspirin.
- One systematic review has found that ticlopidine or clopidogrel reduces the odds of a vascular event compared with aspirin but there was substantial uncertainty about the size of any additional benefit.
- One systematic review found no evidence of benefit from anticoagulation in people in sinus rhythm, but an increased risk of serious bleeding.
- One systematic review has found that carotid endarterectomy reduces the risk of major stroke in people with moderate and severe carotid stenosis provided the risks of imaging and surgery are small.
- We found that the role of percutaneous transluminal angioplasty (PTA) has not been adequately evaluated.

In people with atrial fibrillation and a prior stroke or TIA

- Systematic reviews and RCTs have found that anticoagulants reduce the risk of stroke, provided there is a low risk of bleeding and careful monitoring. Aspirin reduces the risk of stroke, but less effectively than anticoagulants. These findings support the use of aspirin in people with atrial fibrillation and contraindications to anticoagulants.

In people with atrial fibrillation but no other major risk factors for stroke

- Systematic reviews and RCTs have found that anticoagulants are of net benefit, provided there is a low risk of bleeding and careful monitoring. Aspirin is a reasonable alternative in people with contraindications to anticoagulants.

DEFINITION	Prevention in this context is the long term management of people with a prior stroke or transient ischaemic attack (TIA), and of people at high risk of stroke for other reasons such as atrial fibrillation. **Stroke:** See definition under stroke management, p 193. **TIA:** Similar to a mild ischaemic stroke except that symptoms last for less than 24 hours.[1]
INCIDENCE/ PREVALENCE	See incidence/prevalence under stroke management, p 193.
AETIOLOGY/ RISK FACTORS	See aetiology under stroke management, p 193. Risk factors for stroke include prior stroke or TIA, increasing age, hypertension, diabetes, cigarette smoking, and emboli associated with atrial fibrillation, artificial heart valves, or myocardial infarction. The relation with cholesterol is less clear; an overview of prospective studies among healthy middle aged individuals found no association between total cholesterol and overall stroke risk.[2] However, one review of prospective observational studies in eastern Asian people found that cholesterol was positively associated with ischaemic stroke but negatively associated with haemorrhagic stroke.[3]
PROGNOSIS	People with a history of stroke or TIA are at high risk of all vascular events, such as myocardial infarction, but are at particular risk of subsequent stroke (about 10% in the first year and about 5% per year thereafter); see figure 1, p 223, and figure 1 in secondary prevention of ischaemic cardiac events, p 191. People with intermittent atrial fibrillation treated with aspirin should be considered at similar risk of stroke, compared to people with sustained atrial fibrillation treated with aspirin (rate of ischaemic stroke per year, intermittent v sustained, 3.2% v 3.3%).[6]

Stroke prevention

AIMS	To prevent death or disabling stroke, as well as other serious non-fatal outcomes, especially myocardial infarction, with minimal adverse effects from treatment.
OUTCOMES	Rates of death; dependency; myocardial infarction; and stroke.
METHODS	*Clinical Evidence* search and appraisal January 2001.

QUESTION **What are the effects of interventions in people with prior stroke or TIA?**

OPTION **BLOOD PRESSURE REDUCTION**

Cathie Sudlow

We found insufficient evidence for routine blood pressure reduction among people with a prior stroke or TIA, but a large, ongoing RCT will provide further information.

Benefits: We found two overviews[7,8] and three subsequent RCTs.[9-11] One overview of RCTs of antihypertensive treatment (usually comprising a diuretic, a β-blocker, or both), in about 48 000 people with hypertension, most of whom had no history of vascular disease, found that a reduction of about 10–12/5–6 mmHg in systolic/diastolic blood pressure over 2–3 years reduced the risk of stroke (OR 0.62, 95% CI 0.55 to 0.69).[7] A subsequent RCT (4695 elderly people with systolic hypertension) found similar results with a calcium channel antagonist (nitrendipine) versus placebo: a reduction of about 10/5 mmHg over 2 years reduced the risk of stroke (RRR 42%, 95% CI 17% to 60%).[9] In the overview, the proportional effects of treatment on stroke were similar among people with differing degrees of hypertension, among middle aged and elderly people, and among people with or without a prior stroke or TIA.[7] Two of the RCTs (about 500 people) specifically examined blood pressure reduction in people with both hypertension and a prior stroke or TIA. These two RCTs were included in another overview of antihypertensive treatment versus placebo (4 RCTs, about 3000 people with prior stroke or TIA with or without hypertension).[8] Similar, but statistically uncertain, results were obtained: an average diastolic blood pressure reduction of 3 mmHg for about 3 years non-significantly reduced the risk of stroke (OR 0.81, 95% CI 0.61 to 1.01). An unconfirmed preliminary report from a further RCT in China (5665 people with a prior stroke or TIA) comparing a diuretic (indapamide) versus placebo found that reducing diastolic blood pressure by about 2 mm Hg over 2 years significantly reduced stroke incidence (RRR 29%, 95% CI 12% to 42%).[10] We found one large subsequent RCT (9297 people at high risk of vascular disease, including 1000 with prior stroke or TIA, about half had hypertension). It found that about 5 years of ramipril (an angiotensin converting enzyme [ACE] inhibitor) versus placebo reduced the diastolic blood pressure by an average of 2 mm Hg, reduced the risk of stroke (RRR 31%, 95% CI 16% to 44%), and reduced the risk of combined outcome of stroke, myocardial infarction, or cardiovascular death (RRR 22%, 95% CI 14% to 30%). The relative risk reduction was similar among those with or without a prior stroke or TIA, and among those with or without hypertension.[11]

Harms: In people with a history of stroke, reports of an apparently J-shaped relationship between blood pressure and subsequent stroke have led to concerns that blood pressure reduction may actually increase the risk of recurrent stroke, perhaps because of reduced cerebral perfusion.[12] However, preliminary analyses of data from over 15 000 people with a history of cerebrovascular or coronary events included in trials in the overview found a positive relation between diastolic blood pressure and the subsequent risk of stroke; for every 5 mmHg decrease in diastolic blood pressure there was about a 15% proportional reduction in stroke risk. These analyses found no evidence of any threshold below which a lower diastolic blood pressure was not associated with a lower stroke risk.[12,13] The RCTs found no evidence that reducing diastolic blood pressure was hazardous, at least down to about 80 mmHg.[7]

Comment: There is persisting uncertainty about the net effects of blood pressure reduction among people with a previous cerebrovascular event. Further information will be provided by a large RCT that is currently assessing the balance of benefits and risks of treatment with the ACE inhibitor perindopril among 6000 people with a history of stroke or TIA.[8]

OPTION   CHOLESTEROL REDUCTION

We found insufficient evidence about the effects of routinely reducing cholesterol in people with a prior stroke or TIA. Evidence from large RCTs suggests benefit from reducing cholesterol with a statin in people with prior stroke or TIA who also have a definite history of coronary heart disease (see table 1, p 222).

Benefits: **Effects of cholesterol lowering on stroke:** Large RCTs have assessed the effects of reducing cholesterol on coronary heart disease risk, in many thousands of people, both in those with a history of coronary heart disease and in healthy people. These trials did not specifically aim to include people with a prior stroke or TIA, but many reported on stroke as an outcome.[14-16] We found several overviews of these trials, reporting similar findings, and three of these include all of the relevant data.[14,15,17] The overviews found no evidence that reducing mean total cholesterol by about 11% with a fibrate, resin, or dietary regimen significantly altered stroke, but found that reducing mean total cholesterol by about 21% with a statin reduced the relative odds of stroke by 24% (and reduced the relative odds of coronary heart disease by a third) (see table 1, p 222).[14-16] One subsequent, large RCT assessed the effects of treatment designed to raise high density lipoprotein (HDL) cholesterol and lower triglycerides. The RCT (2531 men with coronary heart disease and low HDL cholesterol) compared gemfibrozil versus placebo, given over about 5 years. It found that gemfibrozil increased HDL cholesterol (by about 6%), reduced triglycerides, did not change low density lipoprotein (LDL) cholesterol, and reduced total cholesterol (by about 4%). Compared with placebo, gemfibrozil produced a significant reduction in coronary heart disease (RRR 22%, 95% CI 7% to 35%), but a non-significant reduction in stroke (RRR +25%, 95% CI −6% to +47%).[18] **Effects of cholesterol reduction in people with a prior stroke or TIA:** We found only two small, early RCTs that directly assessed effects of reducing cholesterol in people with a prior stroke or TIA. The drug used (clofibrate in both cases) produced only a small fall in the mean cholesterol, and the results were inconclusive.[19,20]

Harms: The overviews found uncertain effects of statins on fatal stroke (RR 95% CI ranging from an increase of about a half to one third reduction) (see table 1, p 222),[14] possibly because lowering cholesterol may slightly increase the risk of haemorrhagic stroke, which is more likely than ischaemic stroke to be fatal.[3] Only two large scale statin trials reported haemorrhagic stroke separately, and there were too few events (10 events) to draw any conclusions.[21,22]

Comment: A planned prospective overview of individual participant data from all RCTs of cholesterol reduction aims to summarise the effects of reducing cholesterol among different groups of people, including those with a prior stroke or TIA.[23]

| OPTION | ANTIPLATELET TREATMENT |

RCTs have found that prolonged antiplatelet treatment is beneficial for people with a prior (presumed ischaemic) stroke or TIA, unless there is a clear contraindication. We found no clear evidence that any other antiplatelet regimen is superior to medium dose aspirin (75–325 mg daily) in the prevention of vascular events. Aspirin 75 mg daily is as effective as higher doses in the long term prevention of vascular events, but it remains unclear whether doses lower than 75 mg daily are sufficient. RCTs have found that clopidogrel or the combination of aspirin and dipyridamole are safe and effective alternatives to medium dose aspirin.

Benefits: **Antiplatelet treatment versus no antiplatelet treatment:** One systematic review (search date 1990, 70 000 people at high risk of occlusive arterial disease)[5] found that, compared with no antiplatelet treatment, 1 month or more of antiplatelet treatment reduced the risk of a non-fatal myocardial infarction, non-fatal stroke, or vascular death (OR 0.73, 95% CI 0.70 to 0.76). The review included about 10 000 people with a prior (presumed ischaemic) stroke or TIA, among whom about 20 non-fatal strokes, nine non-fatal myocardial infarctions, and 11 vascular deaths were prevented per 1000 people treated with antiplatelet treatment for about 3 years. There was also a clear reduction in all cause mortality (see figure 1, p 223).[5] Subsequent, large RCTs of antiplatelet treatment versus control among several thousand patients with a prior stroke or TIA found similar results.[24-26] **Different daily doses of aspirin:** About two thirds of the RCTs in the systematic review involved an aspirin regimen, and medium dose aspirin (75–325 mg daily) was the most widely tested. Direct comparisons among 2425 high risk people found the effects on vascular events of daily doses of 75–325 mg or 500–1500 mg to be similar.[5] One subsequent RCT (2849 people undergoing carotid endarterectomy) found that lower doses of 81 mg or 325 mg produced a slightly lower rate of stroke, myocardial infarction, or death than higher doses of 650 mg or 1300 mg daily (AR 6.2% with lower doses v AR 8.4 % with higher doses; P = 0.03).[27] Indirect comparisons in the systematic review found that daily doses of less than 160 mg (mostly 75–150 mg), 160–325 mg, and 500–1500 mg had similar effects in preventing vascular events.[5] The inclusion of data from two subsequent large RCTs among high risk people (one of them including almost 1400 people with a prior ischaemic stroke or TIA)[24] assessing a daily dose of exactly 75 mg versus control,[24,28] found that this aspirin dose significantly reduced vascular events (OR 0.71, 95% CI 0.61 to 0.83).[5] We found more limited evidence for effects of doses under 75 mg daily. One RCT (about 6000 people with prior stroke or TIA) found that, compared with placebo, aspirin 50 mg daily reduced the combined outcome of stroke or death (RRR 13%, 95% CI 1% to 25%).[25] A second RCT (about 3000 people with recent TIA or minor ischaemic stroke) directly compared aspirin 30 mg daily versus 283 mg daily, and found no evidence of a difference in effect, although the trial could not rule out a clinically important difference.[29] **Dipyridamole and aspirin:** The systematic review found no clear evidence that any regimen was more effective than medium dose aspirin alone in the prevention of vascular events. It found that adding dipyridamole to aspirin did not seem to produce a reduction in vascular events compared with aspirin alone, but the possibility of a small additional benefit was not excluded.[5] One more recent RCT found that, although adding dipyridamole to aspirin 50 mg daily significantly reduced stroke (RRR about 23%), the combination did not significantly reduce the combined risk of stroke or death (RRR 13%, P = NS).[25] A detailed review of all trials that have assessed the addition of dipyridamole to aspirin is underway.[30] **Thienopyridines (clopidogrel and ticlopidine):** We found one systematic review of RCTs comparing either ticlopidine or clopidogrel with aspirin (search date 1999, 4 RCTs, 22 656 people at high risk of vascular disease, including 9840 with a TIA or ischaemic stroke).[31] Most people were included in a large trial of clopidogrel (75 mg daily) versus aspirin (325 mg daily).[32] Compared with aspirin, the thienopyridines reduced the odds of a vascular event by 9% (OR 0.91, 95% CI 0.84 to 0.98), but there was substantial uncertainty about the size of any additional benefit (11 events prevented per 1000 people treated for about 2 years, 95% CI 2 to 19 events).[31]

Harms: Potentially life threatening bleeding is the most important adverse effect of antiplatelet treatment. **Intracranial haemorrhages:** These are uncommon, but often fatal, and usually cause significant disability in survivors. The systematic review found that any excess risk of intracranial bleeding with antiplatelet treatment was small, at most one or two per 1000 people a year in trials of long term treatment.[5] **Extracranial haemorrhages:** Unlike intracranial events, extracranial bleeds are much less likely to cause permanent disability or death. The 1994 review found that antiplatelet treatment was significantly associated with a small excess of three per 1000 non-fatal major extracranial bleeds, but no clear excess of fatal extracranial bleeds.[5] **Different doses of aspirin:** In a direct randomised comparison, aspirin 1200 mg daily was associated with more gastrointestinal bleeding than 325 mg daily.[33] We found no definite evidence for any clinically relevant variation in gastrointestinal bleeding risk in the range 75–325 mg daily. However, it seems reasonable to choose the lowest conveniently available dose in this range. **Adverse effects of thienopyridines:** The systematic review of thienopyridines versus aspirin found that the thienopyridines caused significantly less gastrointestinal haemorrhage and upper gastrointestinal upset than aspirin. However, they increased the incidence of skin rash and of diarrhoea (ticlopidine by about twofold and clopidogrel by about a third). Ticlopidine (but not clopidogrel) increased the incidence of neutropenia.[31] Observational studies have also found that ticlopidine is associated with thrombocytopenia and thrombotic thrombocytopenic purpura.[34,35] However, we found no definite evidence of an excess of haematological adverse effects with clopidogrel.[36,37] The results of two RCTs of clopidogrel plus aspirin versus ticlopidine plus aspirin in about 1700 people undergoing coronary artery stenting suggested clopidogrel to be superior to ticlopidine in terms of safety and tolerability.[38,39]

Comment: In people with a prior stroke or TIA, the large absolute reductions in serious vascular events produced by antiplatelet treatment far outweighed any absolute hazards.

OPTION	LONG TERM ORAL ANTICOAGULATION FOR PEOPLE IN NORMAL SINUS RHYTHM

Gord Gubitz and Peter Sandercock

One systematic review comparing oral anticoagulants versus placebo found no significant difference in the risk of stroke recurrence after presumed ischaemic stroke in people in normal sinus rhythm. Risk of fatal intracranial and extracranial haemorrhage was increased.

Benefits: We found one systematic review (search date not stated, 9 small RCTs, mean duration 1.8 years) comparing oral anticoagulants (warfarin, dicoumarol, phenindione) versus placebo.[40] The review included 1214 people in normal sinus rhythm with previous non-embolic presumed ischaemic stroke or TIA, and found no clear benefit of anticoagulation on death or dependency (ARR +4%, 95% CI –6% to +14%; RRR +5%, 95% CI –9% to +18%), or on mortality or recurrent stroke.

Harms: By the end of the RCTs, the review found a significantly increased risk of fatal intracranial haemorrhage (ARI 2%, 95% CI 0.4% to 3.6%; RR 2.51, 95% CI 1.12 to 5.60; NNH 49 people treated with anticoagulants over 1.8 years for one additional non-fatal extracranial haemorrhage, 95% CI 27 to 240).[31] The risk of fatal and non-fatal extracranial haemorrhage was also increased by anticoagulants compared with placebo (ARI 5.1%, 95% CI 3.0% to 7.2%; RR 5.86, 95% CI 2.39 to 14.3; NNH 20, 95% CI 14 to 33). **Warfarin versus aspirin:** One RCT (1316 people) compared aspirin versus oral anticoagulant (target international normalised ratio [INR] 3.0 to 4.5 — see glossary, p 218) for about 14 months after TIA or non-disabling stroke.[41] The trial was stopped early because of an excess number of poor outcomes (almost exclusively related to cerebral haemorrhage) in the anticoagulant group compared with control (AR 12.4% anticoagulant v 5.4% control; ARI 7%, 95% CI 4% to 10%; NNH 14, 95% CI 10 to 25).

Comment: The trials in the systematic review all had major problems with their methods, including poor monitoring of anticoagulation.[40] All were completed before introducing routine computerised tomography

(CT) scanning, which means that people with primary haemorrhagic strokes could have been included. The systematic review could not therefore provide a reliable and precise overall estimate of the balance of risk and benefit regarding death or dependency. Most people in the trial comparing warfarin and aspirin did have a CT scan, but an adverse outcome was still seen with anticoagulants. Two further RCTs are in progress: one compares a lower intensity of adjusted dose warfarin (to maintain an INR of 1.4–2.8) with aspirin 325 mg four times daily within 30 days after stroke and treated for at least 2 years,[42] whereas the other assesses warfarin (to maintain an INR of 2.0 to 3.0) versus aspirin (any dose between 30–325 mg) versus aspirin plus dipyridamole (400 mg daily).[43]

OPTION	CAROTID ENDARTERECTOMY FOR PEOPLE WITH RECENT CAROTID TERRITORY ISCHAEMIA

One systematic review has found that carotid endarterectomy reduces the risk of major stroke and death in people with a recent carotid territory TIA or non-disabling ischaemic stroke who have moderate or severe symptomatic stenosis of the ipsilateral carotid artery. People with milder degrees of stenosis do not benefit from endarterectomy. Evidence from two other systematic reviews suggest a possible benefit in people with asymptomatic but severe stenosis, but the results of a new large scale trial are awaited.

Benefits: **People with symptomatic stenosis:** We found one systematic review (search date 1999, 3 RCTs, 6143 people with a recent neurological event in the territory of a stenosed ipsilateral carotid artery) comparing carotid surgery versus control treatment.[44] Ninety six per cent of these data came from two large RCTs.[45,46] Participants were randomised within 4 and 6 months of the onset of vascular symptoms. The trials used different methods to measure degree of stenosis. The trials included 1247 people with severe stenosis (70–99%,[46] 80–99%[45]), 1259 people with moderate stenosis (50–69%,[46] 70–79%[45]), and 3397 people with mild stenosis (< 50%,[46] < 70%[45]). The degree of benefit from surgery was related to the degree of stenosis. For people with severe stenosis, there was a significant decrease in the subsequent risk of major stroke or death (ARR 6.7%, 95% CI 3.2% to 10.0%; RR 0.52, 95% CI 0.37 to 0.73; NNT 15, 95% CI 10 to 31). People with moderate stenosis also benefited (ARR 4.7%, 95% CI 0.8% to 8.7%; RR 0.73, 95% CI 0.56 to 0.95; NNT 21, 95% CI 11 to 125). People with mild stenosis did not benefit from surgery but had an increased risk of stroke (RR 0.80, 95% CI 0.56 to 1.0). In the trial with longer follow up, the annual risk of stroke after 3 years was not significantly different between people who had had surgery and those who had not.[45] In the other trial, people with severe stenosis had a benefit from endarterectomy at 8 years follow up.[47] **People with asymptomatic stenosis:** We found two systematic reviews (search dates both 1998) evaluating carotid endarterectomy for asymptomatic carotid stenosis (no carotid territory TIA or minor stroke within the past few months).[48,49] One review included results from five RCTs (2440 people).[48] The other review included results from 2203 people from four of these five RCTs, after excluding the fifth RCT because of weak methods.[49] Both reviews found similar results. Carotid endarterectomy reduced the risk of perioperative stroke or death or subsequent ipsilateral stroke (for the review of 4 RCTs:[49] AR 4.9% over 3 years in the surgical group v 6.8% in the medical group; ARR 1.9%, 95% CI 0.1% to 3.9%; NNT 52, 95% CI 26 to 1000; for the review of 5 RCTs:[48] 4.7% over 3 years in the surgical group v 7.4% in the medical group; ARR 2.7%, 95% CI 0.8% to 4.6%; NNT 37, 95% CI 22 to 125). Although the risk of perioperative stroke or death from carotid surgery for people with asymptomatic stenosis seems to be lower than in people with symptomatic stenosis, the risk of stroke or death without surgery in asymptomatic people is relatively low and so, for most people, the balance of risk and benefit from surgery remains unclear.[48,49]

Harms: **People with symptomatic stenosis:** The systematic review of endarterectomy for symptomatic stenosis found that carotid surgery was associated with a definite risk of recurrent stroke or death.[44] The relative risk of disabling stroke or death within 30 days of randomisation was 2.5 (95% CI 1.6 to 3.8). A second systematic review (search date 1996, 36 studies) identified several risk factors for operative stroke and death from carotid endarterectomy, including female sex, occlusion of the contralateral internal carotid artery, stenosis of the ipsilateral external carotid artery, and systolic blood pressure greater than 180 mmHg.[50] Endarterectomy is also associated with other postoperative complications, including wound infection (3%), wound haematoma (5%), and lower cranial nerve injury (5–7%). **People with asymptomatic stenosis:** Given the low prevalence of severe carotid stenosis in the general population, there is concern that screening and surgical intervention in asymptomatic people may result in more strokes than it prevents.[51]

Comment: **People with symptomatic stenosis:** The two RCTs contributing most of the data to the systematic review[38,39] used different techniques to measure the degree of carotid stenosis, but conversion charts are available and were used in the systematic review.[44] The trials, as well as observational studies,[4] found that risk of recurrent stroke was highest about the time of the symptomatic event. **People with asymptomatic stenosis:** A large scale trial is ongoing.[52]

OPTION   **CAROTID PERCUTANEOUS TRANSLUMINAL ANGIOPLASTY**

We found that carotid PTA has not been adequately assessed in people with a recent carotid territory TIA or non-disabling ischaemic stroke who have severe stenosis of the ipsilateral carotid artery.

Benefits: We found no systematic review or placebo controlled RCTs. **Carotid PTA:** One RCT (504 people with a recent carotid territory TIA or non-disabling ischaemic stroke with stenosis of the ipsilateral carotid artery) compared "best medical treatment" plus carotid PTA versus "best medical treatment" plus carotid endarterectomy.[53] Too few people were randomised to provide reliable estimates of efficacy. Preliminary results have been published in abstract form, suggesting that rates of stroke or death at 30 days were similar in endarterectomy and PTA groups. Three year outcome results have also been published in abstract form,[54] finding that although there was a significant increase in restenosis in people undergoing PTA (21% v 5% of people undergoing endarterectomy, P < 0.0001), there was no difference between the two groups in rates of disabling stroke or death, or ipsilateral stroke. **Vertebral artery PTA:** The RCT randomised only 16 people between vertebral PTA and best medical treatment. This did not provide enough data for reliable estimates of efficacy.[53]

Harms: We found insufficient randomised data upon which to comment. Analysis of the safety data of the RCT has not yet been published.[53]

Comment: Two ongoing RCTs are comparing carotid endarterectomy versus primary stenting in people with recently symptomatic severe carotid stenosis.[55,56]

QUESTION **What are the effects of anticoagulant and antiplatelet treatment in people with atrial fibrillation?**

Gord Gubitz, Peter Sandercock and Gregory Lip

Systematic reviews have found that people with atrial fibrillation at high risk of stroke (see glossary, p 218) and with no contraindications benefit from anticoagulation. Antiplatelet agents are less effective than warfarin, and are associated with a lower bleeding risk, but are a reasonable alternative if warfarin is contraindicated or if risk of ischaemic stroke is low. The best time to begin anticoagulation after an ischaemic stroke is unclear.

Benefits: Three risk strata have been identified based on evidence derived from one overview of five RCTs,[57] and one subsequent RCT.[58] **People with atrial fibrillation at high risk of stroke, adjusted dose warfarin versus placebo:** We found one overview[50] and two systematic reviews[59,60] examining the effect of warfarin in different groups of people with atrial fibrillation at high risk of stroke. The overview (5 RCTs, 2461 elderly people with atrial fibrillation and a variety of stroke risks) compared warfarin versus placebo.[51] The review found that anticoagulation reduced the risk of stroke over a mean of 5 years (ARR 4.4%, 95% CI 2.8% to 6.0%; RR 0.32, 95% C1 0.21 to 0.5; NNT 23 over 1 year, 95% CI 17 to 36). The first systematic review (search date not stated) identified two RCTs comparing warfarin with placebo in 1053 people with chronic non-rheumatic atrial fibrillation and a history of prior stroke or TIA.[59] Most people (98%) came from one double blind RCT (669 people within 3 months of a minor stroke or TIA),[61] which compared anticoagulant (target INR 2.5 to 4.0) versus aspirin versus placebo. It found that anticoagulants reduced the risk of recurrent stroke over about 2 years (ARR 13.7%, 95% CI 7.3% to 20.1%; RR 0.39, 95% CI 0.25 to 0.63; NNT 7 over 1 year, 95% CI 5 to 14). The second systematic review (search date 1999, 16 RCTs, 9874 people) included six RCTs (2900 people) of adjusted dose warfarin versus placebo (5 RCTs) or versus control (1 RCT) in high risk people (45% had hypertension, 20% had experienced a previous stroke or TIA).[60] These six RCTs included five primary prevention RCTs and one secondary prevention RCT.[62] Target INR varied among RCTs (2.0–2.6 in primary prevention RCTs and 2.9 in the secondary prevention RCT). The results of this systematic review were similar to the others. The meta-analysis found that adjusted dose warfarin reduced the risk of stroke (5 primary prevention RCTs: ARR 4.0%, 95% CI 2.3% to 5.7%; NNT 25, 95% CI 18 to 43. One secondary prevention RCT: ARR 14.5%, 95% CI 7.7% to 21.3%; NNT 7, 95% CI 5 to 13. Combined primary and secondary prevention RCTs: ARR 5.5%, 95% CI 3.7% to 7.3%; NNT 18, 95% CI 14 to 27). **Adjusted dose warfarin versus minidose warfarin:** We found no systematic review or RCTs of low dose warfarin regimens in people with atrial fibrillation and a recent transient ischaemic attack or acute stroke. We found one RCT (1044 people with atrial fibrillation at high risk of stroke), which compared low, fixed dose warfarin (target INR 1.2–1.5) plus aspirin (325 mg per day) with standard adjusted dose warfarin treatment (target INR 2.0–3.0).[58] Adjusted dose warfarin significantly reduced the combined rate of ischaemic stroke or systemic embolism (ARR 6.0%, 95% CI 3.4% to 8.6%; NNT 17, 95% CI 12 to 29) and of disabling or fatal stroke (ARR 3.9%, 95% CI 1.6% to 6.1%; NNT 26, 95% CI 16 to 63). We found three additional RCTs,[63-65] which aimed to evaluate adjusted dose warfarin versus low dose warfarin and aspirin, but were stopped prematurely when the results of the earlier trial[58] were published. Analyses of the optimal anticoagulation intensity for stroke prevention in atrial fibrillation found that stroke risk was substantially increased at INR levels below 2.[62,66] **Adjusted dose warfarin versus aspirin:** We found two systematic reviews of warfarin versus different antiplatelet regimens in people at higher risk of stroke.[60,67] The first systematic review (search date not stated, 1 RCT)[62] found that, in elderly people with atrial fibrillation and a prior history of stroke or TIA, warfarin (target INR 2.5–4.0) versus aspirin (300 mg) reduced the risk of stroke (AR 22.6% for aspirin v 8.9% for warfarin; ARR 14%, 95% CI 7% to 20%; RR 0.39, 95% CI 0.24 to 0.64; NNT 7, 95% CI 5 to 14).[67] The second systematic review (search date 1999, 16 RCTs, 9874 people) included five RCTs (4 primary prevention RCTs and 1 secondary prevention RCT; 2837 people) of adjusted dose warfarin versus aspirin in high risk people (45% had hypertension, 20% had experienced a previous stroke or TIA).[60] Target INR varied among RCTs (2.0–4.5 in primary prevention RCTs, 2.5–4.0 in the secondary prevention RCT). Adjusted dose warfarin versus aspirin reduced the overall risk of stroke (ARR 2.9%, 95% CI 0.9% to 4.8%; NNT 34, 95% CI 21 to 111). The effect varied widely among the five RCTs, none of which were blinded. **Adjusted dose warfarin versus other antiplatelet treatment:** One systematic review (search date 1999) compared adjusted dose warfarin versus other antiplatelet agents such as indobufen.[60] One RCT included in the review (916 people within 15 days of stroke onset) compared warfarin (INR 2.0–3.5) with indobufen.[68] It found no significant difference in the rate of recurrent stroke between the two groups (AR 5% for indobufen v 4% for warfarin; ARR +1.0%, 95% CI −1.7% to +3.7%). **Aspirin versus placebo:** We found one non-systematic review,[69] which included one RCT of people with atrial fibrillation and prior stroke or TIA. Aspirin reduced the risk of stroke, although the confidence interval included the possibility of no benefit (RRR 21%, 95% CI 0% to 38%). **In people with atrial fibrillation at moderate risk of stroke:** See glossary, p 218. We found no RCT that considered this group specifically. **In people with atrial fibrillation at low risk of stroke, anticoagulants:** See glossary, p 218. We found one systematic review and one overview comparing warfarin with placebo in people with atrial fibrillation and a variety of stroke risks.[57,70] Both reviews included the same five RCTs. The overview (2461 people) found that, for people younger than 65 years with atrial fibrillation (but no history of either hypertension, stroke, TIA, or diabetes), the annual stroke rate was the same with warfarin or placebo (1% per year).[57] The systematic review (search date 1999, 2313 people, mean age 69 years, 20% aged over 75 years; 45% had hypertension, 15% diabetes, and 15% a prior history of myocardial infarction) found that warfarin (INR 2.0–2.6) versus placebo reduced fatal and non-fatal ischaemic stroke (ARR 4.0%, 95% CI 2.4% to 5.6%; NNT 25, 95% CI 18 to 42), reduced all ischaemic strokes or intracranial haemorrhage (ARR 4.5%, 95% CI 2.8% to 6.2%; NNT 22, 95% CI 16 to 36), and reduced the combined outcome of disabling or fatal ischaemic stroke or intracranial hemorrhage (ARR 1.8%, 95% CI 0.5% to 3.1%; NNT 56, 95% CI 32 to 200). **Antiplatelet treatment:** We found two systematic reviews.[60,71] The first (search date 1999, 2 RCTs, 1680 people with either paroxysmal or sustained non-valvular atrial fibrillation confirmed by electrocardiogram but without previous stroke or TIA, 30% age > 75 years) compared aspirin with placebo.[71] In primary prevention, aspirin did not significantly reduce ischaemic stroke (OR 0.71, 95% CI 0.46 to 1.10; ARR +1.6%, 95% CI –0.5% to +3.7%), all stroke (OR 0.70, 95% CI 0.45 to 1.08; ARR +1.8%; 95% CI –0.5% to +3.9%), all disabling or fatal stroke (OR 0.88, 95% CI 0.48 to 1.58; ARR +0.4%, 95% CI –1.2% to +2.0%), or the composite end point of stroke, myocardial infarction, or vascular death (OR 0.76, 95% CI 0.54 to 1.05; ARR +2.3%, 95% CI –0.4% to +5.0%). The second systematic review (search date 1999)[60] included three RCTs of primary prevention. The average rate of stroke among people taking placebo was 5.2%. Meta-analysis of the three RCTs found that antiplatelet agents versus placebo reduced the risk of stroke (ARR 2.2%, 95% CI 0.3% to 4.1%; NNT 45, 95% CI 24 to 333).

Harms: The major risk of anticoagulants and antiplatelet agents was haemorrhage. In the overview evaluating elderly people with variable risk factors for stroke, the absolute risk of major bleeding was 1% for placebo, 1% for aspirin, and 1.3% for warfarin.[57] Another systematic review,[60] found the absolute risk of intracranial haemorrhage increased from 0.1% a year with control to 0.3% a year with warfarin, but the difference was not statistically significant. The absolute risks were three times higher in people who had bled previously. Both bleeding and haemorrhagic stroke were more common in people aged over 75 years. The risk of death after a major bleed ranged from 13–33%, and risk of subsequent morbidity in those who survived a major bleed was 15%. The risk of bleeding was associated with an INR greater than 3, fluctuating INRs, and uncontrolled hypertension. In the systematic review evaluating people with prior stroke or TIA, major extracranial bleeding was more frequent with anticoagulation than with placebo (ARI 4.9%, 95% CI 1.6% to 8.2%; RR 6.2, 95% CI 1.4 to 27.1; NNH 20, 95% CI 12 to 63).[59] The studies were too small to define the rate of intracranial haemorrhage (none occurred in the 2 RCTs). In a systematic review comparing anticoagulants and antiplatelet agents, major extracranial bleeding was more frequent with anticoagulation (ARI 4.9%, 95% CI 1.6% to 8.2%; RR 6.4, 95% CI 1.5

to 28.1; NNH 20, 95% CI 12 to 63).[67] The studies were too small to define the rate of intracranial haemorrhage (in one RCT, none of the people on anticoagulant and one person on aspirin had an intracranial bleed). In the systematic review of oral anticoagulants versus placebo in low risk people,[70] the number of intracranial haemorrhages was small (5 in the treatment group and 2 in the control group), with a non-significant increase in the treatment group. Likewise, in the systematic review assessing antiplatelet therapy in low risk people with atrial fibrillation,[71] too few haemorrhages occurred to characterise the effects of aspirin.

Comment: As well as the trade offs between benefits and harms, each person's treatment preferences should be considered when deciding how to treat.[72-77] We found net benefit of anticoagulation for people in atrial fibrillation who have had a TIA or stroke, or who are over 75 years of age and at a high risk of stroke. We found less clear cut evidence for those aged 65–75 years at high risk, and for those with moderate risk (that is, over age 65 not in a high risk group; those under 65 years of age with clinical risk factors), or for those at low risk (under 65 years of age with no other risk factors). The benefits of warfarin in the RCTs may not translate into effectiveness in clinical practice.[78,79] In the RCTs, most strokes in people randomised to warfarin occurred while they were not in fact taking warfarin, or were significantly underanticoagulated at the time of the event. People in the RCTs were highly selected (< 10%, range 3–40% of eligible people were randomised); many were excluded after assessments for the absence of contraindications and physicians' refusal to enter them into the study. Many of the studies were not double blinded and in some there was poor agreement between raters for "soft" neurological end points. The frequent monitoring of warfarin treatment under trial conditions and motivation of people/ investigators was probably more than that seen in usual clinical practice. The best time to start anticoagulation after an ischaemic stroke is unclear. The evidence supports the need to identify the baseline risk of individuals and to use antithrombotic therapy judiciously.

GLOSSARY

International normalised ratio (INR) A value derived from a standardised laboratory test that measures the effect of an anticoagulant like warfarin. The laboratory materials used in the test are calibrated against internationally accepted standard reference preparations, so that variability between laboratories and different reagents is minimised. Normal blood has an INR of 1. Therapeutic anticoagulation often aims to achieve an INR value of 2–3.5.

People at high risk of stroke People of any age with a previous TIA or stroke, or a history of rheumatic vascular disease, coronary artery disease, congestive heart failure, and/or impaired left ventricular function or echocardiography; and people aged 75 years and over with hypertension, diabetes, or both.

People at moderate risk of stroke People over 65 years of age who are not in the high risk group; and people under 65 years of age with clinical risk factors, including diabetes, hypertension, peripheral arterial disease, and ischaemic heart disease.

People at low risk of stroke All other people under 65 years of age with no history of stroke, TIA, emboliam, hypertension, diabetes, or other clinical risk factors.

REFERENCES

1. Hankey GJ, Warlow CP. *Transient ischaemic attacks of the brain and eye.* London: WB Saunders, 1994.

2. Prospective Studies Collaboration. Cholesterol, diastolic blood pressure, and stroke: 13 000 strokes in 450 000 people in 45 prospective cohorts. *Lancet* 1995;346:1647–1653.

3. Eastern Stroke and Coronary Heart Disease Collaborative Research Group. Blood pressure, cholesterol, and stroke in eastern Asia. *Lancet* 1998;352:1801–1807.

4. Warlow CP, Dennis MS, van Gijn J, et al. Predicting recurrent stroke and other serious vascular events. In: *Stroke. A practical guide to management.* Oxford: Blackwell Science, 1996:545–552.

5. Antiplatelet Trialists' Collaboration. Collaborative overview of randomised trials of antiplatelet therapy – I: prevention of death, myocardial infarction, and stroke by prolonged antiplatelet therapy in various categories of patients. *BMJ* 1994;308:81–106. Search date March 1990; primary sources Medline; Current Contents; hand searches of journals, reference lists, and conference proceedings; and contact with authors of trials and manufacturers.

6. Hart RG, Pearce LA, Rothbart RM, McAnulty JH, Asinger RW, Halperin JL. Stroke with intermittent atrial fibrillation: incidence and predictors during aspirin therapy. Stroke Prevention in Atrial fibrillation Investigators. *J Am Coll Cardiol* 2000; 35:183–187.

7. Collins R, MacMahon S. Blood pressure, antihypertensive drug treatment and the risks of stroke and of coronary heart disease. *Br Med Bull* 1994;50:272–298.

8. PROGRESS Management Committee. Blood pressure lowering for the secondary prevention of stroke: rationale and design of PROGRESS. *J Hypertension* 1996;14(suppl 2):41–46.

9. Staessen JA, Fagard R, Thijs L, et al for the Systolic Hypertension in Europe (Syst–Eur) Trial Investigators. Randomised double-blind comparison of placebo and active treatment for older patients with isolated systolic hypertension. *Lancet* 1997;350:757–764.

10. PATS Collaborating Group. Post-stroke antihypertensive treatment study: a preliminary result. *Chinese Med J* 1995;108:710–717.

11. The Heart Outcomes Prevention Evaluation Study Investigators. Effects of an angiotensin-converting-enzyme inhibitor, ramipril, on death from cardiovascular causes, myocardial infarction, and stroke in high-risk patients. *N Engl J Med* 2000; 342:145–152.

12. Rodgers A, MacMahon S, Gamble G, Slattery J, Sandercock P, Warlow C, for the United Kingdom Transient Ischaemic Attack Collaborative Group. Blood pressure and risk of stroke in patients with cerebrovascular disease. *BMJ* 1996;313:147.

13. Neal B, Clark T, MacMahon S, Rodgers A, Baigent C, Collins R, on behalf of the Antithrombotic Trialists' Collaboration. Blood pressure and the risk of recurrent vascular disease. *Am J Hypertension* 1998;11:25A–26A.

14. Hebert PR, Gaziano M, Hennekens CH. An overview of trials of cholesterol lowering and risk of stroke. *Arch Intern Med* 1995;155:50–55.

15. Hebert PR, Gaziano JM, Chan KS, Hennekens CH. Cholesterol lowering with statin drugs, risk of stroke, and total mortality: an overview of randomized trials. *JAMA* 1997;278:313–321. Search date 1995; primary sources not specified, Cholesterol and Current Events (CARE) data added in October 1996.

16. The long-term intervention with pravastatin in ischaemic disease (LIPID) study group. Prevention of cardiovascular events and death with pravastatin in patients with coronary heart disease and a broad range of initial cholesterol levels. *N Engl J Med* 1998;339:1349–1357.

17. Acheson J, Hutchinson EC. Controlled trial of clofibrate in cerebral vascular disease. *Atherosclerosis* 1972;15:177–183.

18. Anonymous. The treatment of cerebrovascular disease with clofibrate. Final report of the Veterans' Administration Cooperative Study of Atherosclerosis, neurology section. *Stroke* 1973; 4:684–693.

19. Di Mascio R, Marchioli R, Tognoni G. Cholesterol reduction and stroke occurrence: an overview of randomized clinical trials. *Cerebrovasc Dis* 2000; 10:85–92.

20. Rubins HB, Robins SJ, Collins D, et al. Gemfibrozil for the secondary prevention of coronary heart disease in men with low levels of high-density lipoprotein cholesterol. *N Engl J Med* 1999;341: 410–418.

21. Plehn JF, Davis BR, Sacks FM, et al for the CARE Investigators. Reduction of stroke incidence after myocardial infarction with pravastatin: the cholesterol and recurrent events (CARE) study. *Circulation* 1999;99:216–223.

22. Scandinavian Simvastatin Survival Study Group. Randomised trial of cholesterol lowering in 4444 patients with coronary heart disease: the Scandinavian simvastatin survival study (4S). *Lancet* 1994;344:1383–1389.

23. Cholesterol Treatment Trialists' Collaboration. Protocol for a prospective collaborative overview of all current and planned randomized trials of cholesterol treatment regimens. *Am J Cardiol* 1995;75:1130–1134.

24. SALT Collaborative Group. Swedish aspirin low-dose trial (SALT) of 75 mg aspirin as secondary prophylaxis after cerebrovascular ischaemic events. *Lancet* 1991;338:1345–1349.

25. Diener HC, Cunha L, Forbes C, Sivenius J, Smets P, Lowenthal A. European secondary prevention study 2: dipyridamole and acetylsalicylic acid in the secondary prevention of stroke. *J Neurol Sci* 1996;143:1–13.

26. Gotoh F, Tohgi H, Hirai S, Terashi A, Fukuuchi Y, Otomo E, et al. Cilostazol Stroke Prevention Study: a placebo-controlled double-blind trial for secondary prevention of cerebral infarction. *J Stroke Cerebrovasc Dis* 2000;9:147:157.

27. Taylor DW, Barnett HJM, Haynes RB, et al, for the ASA and Carotid Endarterectomy (ACE) Trial Collaborators. Low-dose and high-dose acetylsalicylic acid for patients undergoing carotid endarterectomy: a randomised controlled trial. *Lancet* 1999;353:2179–2184.

28. Juul-Möller S, Edvardsson N, Jahnmatz B, Rosen A, Soreneson S, Omblus R, for the Swedish Angina Pectoris Aspirin Trial (SAPAT) Group. Double-blind trial of aspirin in primary prevention of myocardial infarction in patients with stable chronic angina pectoris. *Lancet* 1992;340: 1421–1425.

29. The Dutch TIA Study Group. A comparison of two doses of aspirin (30 mg vs 283 mg a day) in patients after a transient ischaemic attack or minor ischaemic stroke. *N Engl J Med* 1991;325: 1261–1266.

30. Sudlow C, Baigent C, on behalf of the Antithrombotic Trialists' Collaboration. Different antiplatelet regimens in the prevention of vascular events among patients at high risk of stroke: new evidence from the antithrombotic trialists'

Cardiovascular disorders

collaboration. Seventh European Stroke Conference, Edinburgh, May, 1998. *Cerebrovasc Dis* 1998;8(suppl 4):68.

31. Hankey GJ, Sudlow CLM, Dunbabin DW. Thienopyridine derivatives (ticlopidine, clopidogrel) versus aspirin for preventing stroke and other serious vascular events in high vascular risk patients. In: The Cochrane Library, Issue 1, 2001. Oxford: Update Software. Search date March 1999; primary sources Cochrane Stroke Group Trials Register, Antithrombotic Trialists' database, and personal contact with Sanofi pharmacological company.

32. CAPRIE Steering Committee. A randomised, blinded, trial of clopidogrel versus aspirin in patients at risk of ischaemic events. *Lancet* 1996;348:1329–1339.

33. Farrell B, Godwin J, Richards S, Warlow C. The United Kingdom transient ischaemic attack (UK-TIA) aspirin trial: final results. *J Neurol Neurosurg Psychiatry* 1991;54:1044–1054.

34. Moloney BA. An analysis of the side effects of ticlopidine. In: Hass WK, Easton JD, eds. *Ticlopidine, Platelets and Vascular Disease.* New York: Springer, 1993:117–139.

35. Bennett CL, Davidson CJ, Raisch DW, Weinberg PD, Bennett RH, Feldman MD. Thrombotic thrombocytopenic purpura assoicated with ticlopidine in the setting of coronary artery stents and stroke prevention. *Arch Int Med* 1999;159:2524–2528.

36. Bennett CL, Connors JM, Carwile JM, et al. Thrombotic thrombocytopenic purpura associated with clopidogrel. *N Engl J Med* 2000;342:1773–1777.

37. Hankey GJ. Clopidogrel and thrombotic thrombocytopenic purpura. *Lancet* 2000;356:269–270.

38. Müller C, Büttner HJ, Petersen J, Roskamm H. A randomized comparison of clopidogrel and aspirin versus ticlopidine and aspirin after the placement of coronary-artery stents. *Circulation* 2000;101:590–593.

39. Bertrand ME, Rupprecht H-J, Urban P, Gershlick AH, for the CLASSICS Investigators. Double-blind study of the safety of clopidogrel with and without a loading dose in combination with aspirin compared with ticlopidine in combination with aspirin after coronary stenting. The Clopidogrel Aspirin Stent International Cooperative Study (CLASSICS). *Circulation* 2000;102:624–629.

40. Liu M, Counsell C, Sandercock P. Anticoagulants for preventing recurrence following ischaemic stroke or transient ischaemic attack. In: The Cochrane Library, Issue 1, 2001. Oxford: Update Software. Search date not stated; primary sources Cochrane Stroke Group Trials Register, and contact with companies marketing anticoagulant agents.

41. The Stroke Prevention in Reversible Ischaemia Trial (SPIRIT) Study Group. A randomised trial of anticoagulant versus aspirin after cerebral ischemia of presumed arterial origin. *Ann Neurol* 1997;42:857–865.

42. Mohr J for the WARSS Group. Design considerations for the warfarin-antiplatelet recurrent stroke study. *Cerebrovasc Dis* 1995;5:156–157.

43. De Schryvfer E for the ESPRIT Study Group. ESPRIT: mild anticoagulation, acetylsalicylic acid plus dipyridamole or acetylsalicylic acid alone after cerebral ischaemia of arterial origin [abstract]. *Cerebrovasc Dis* 1998;8(suppl 4):83.

44. Cina C, Clase C, Haynes R. Carotid endarterectomy for symptomatic stenosis. In: The Cochrane Library, Issue 1, 2001. Oxford: Update Software. Search date March 1999; primary sources Cochrane Stroke Group Specialised Register of Trials; Medline; Embase; Healthstar; Serline; Cochrane Controlled Trials Register; DARE; Best Evidence.

45. European Carotid Surgery Trialists' Collaborative Group. Randomised trial of endarterectomy for recently symptomatic carotid stenosis: final results of the MRC European carotid surgery trial. *Lancet* 1998;351:1379–1387.

46. North American Symptomatic Carotid Endarterectomy Trial Collaborators. Beneficial effect of carotid endarterectomy in symptomatic patients with high-grade carotid stenosis. *N Engl J Med* 1991;325:445–453.

47. Barnett HJ, Taylor DW, Eliasziw M, et al. Benefit of carotid endarterectomy in patients with symptomatic moderate or severe stenosis. North American symptomatic carotid endarterectomy trial collaborators. *N Engl J Med* 1998;339:1415–1425.

48. Benavente O, Moher D, Pham B. Carotid endarterectomy for asymptomatic carotid stenosis: a meta–analysis. *BMJ* 1998;317:1477–1480. Search date 1998; primary sources Medline; CCTR Ottawa Stroke Trials Register; Current Contents; and hand searching.

49. Chambers BR, You RX, Donnan GA. Carotid endarterectomy for asymptomatic carotid stenosis. In: The Cochrane Library, Issue 1, 2001. Oxford: Update Software. Search date 1998; primary sources Cochrane Stroke Group Trials Register; Medline; Current Contents; hand searches of reference lists; and contact with researchers in the field.

50. Rothwell P, Slattery J, Warlow C. Clinical and angiographic predictors of stroke and death from carotid endarterectomy: systematic review. *BMJ* 1997;315:1571–1577. Search date 1996; primary sources Medline; Cochrane Collaboration Stroke database; and hand searching of reference lists.

51. Whitty C, Sudlow C, Warlow C. Investigating individual subjects and screening populations for asymptomatic carotid stenosis can be harmful. *J Neurol Neurosurg Psychiatry* 1998;64:619–623.

52. Halliday A, Thomas D, Manssfield A. The asymptomatic carotid surgery trial (ACST). Rationale and design. *Eur J Vascular Surg* 1994;8:703–710.

53. Brown MM, for the CAVATAS Investigators. Results of the carotid and vertebral artery transluminal angioplasty study (CAVATAS) [abstract]. *Cerebrovasc Dis* 1998;8(suppl 4):21.

54. Brown M, Pereira A, McCabe D. Carotid and vertebral transluminal angioplasty study (CAVATAS): 3 year outcome data [abstract]. *Cerebrovasc Dis* 1999;9(suppl 1):66.

55. Brown M. The International Carotid Stenting Study [abstract]. *Stroke* 2000;31:2812.

56. Al-Mubarek N, Roubin G, Hobson R, Ferguson R, Brott T, Moore W. Credentialing of Stent Operators for the Carotid Revascularization Endarterectomy vs Stenting Trial (CREST) [abstract]. *Stroke* 2000;31:292.

57. Atrial Fibrillation Investigators. Risk factors for stroke and efficacy of antithrombotic therapy in atrial fibrillation. *Arch Intern Med* 1994;154:1449–1457.

58. Stroke Prevention in Atrial Fibrillation Investigators. Adjusted-dose warfarin versus low-intensity, fixed-dose warfarin plus aspirin for high-risk patients with atrial fibrillation: stroke prevention in atrial fibrillation III randomised clinical trial. *Lancet* 1996;348:633–638.

59. Koudstaal P. Anticoagulants for preventing stroke in patients with non-rheumatic atrial fibrillation and a history of stroke or transient ischemic attacks. In: The Cochrane Library, Issue 1, 2001. Oxford: Update Software. Search date not stated; primary source Cochrane Stroke Group Trials Register, and contact with trialists.

60. Hart R, Benavente O, McBride R, Pearce L. Antithrombotic therapy to prevent stroke in patients with atrial fibrillation: a meta-analysis. Ann Intern Med 1999;131:492–501. Search date 1999; primary sources Medline; Cochrane Database and Antithrombotic Trialists Collaboration.

61. European Atrial Fibrillation Trial Study Group. Secondary prevention in non-rheumatic atrial fibrillation after transient ischaemic attack or minor stroke. Lancet 1993;342:1255.

62. The European Atrial Fibrillation Trial Study Group. Optimal oral anticoagulant therapy in patients with non-rheumatic atrial fibrillation and recent cerebral ischemia. N Engl J Med 1995;333:5–10.

63. Pengo V, Zasso Z, Barbero F, et al. Effectiveness of fixed minidose warfarin in the prevention of thromboembolism and vascular death in nonrheumatic atrial fibrillation. Am J Cardiol 1998; 82:433–437.

64. Gullov A, Koefoed B, Petersen P, et al. Fixed minidose warfarin and aspirin alone and in combination vs adjusted-dose warfarin for stroke prevention in atrial fibrillation. Second Copenhagen Atrial Fibrillation, Aspirin, and Anticoagulation Study. Arch Intern Med 1998; 158:1513–1521.

65. Hellemons B, Langenberg M, Lodder J, et al. Primary prevention of arterial thrombo-embolism in non-rheumatic atrial fibrillation in primary care: randomised controlled trial comparing two intensities of coumarin with aspirin. BMJ 1999; 319:958–964.

66. Hylek EM, Skates SJ, Sheehan MA, Singer DE. An analysis of the lowest effective intensity of prophylactic anticoagulation for patients with non-rheumatic atrial fibrillation. N Engl J Med 1996; 335:540–546.

67. Koudstaal P. Anticoagulants versus antiplatelet therapy for preventing stroke in patients with non-rheumatic atrial fibrillation and a history of stroke or transient ischemic attacks. In: The Cochrane Library, Issue 1, 2001. Oxford: Update Software. Search date not stated; primary source Cochrane Stroke Group Trials Register, and contact with trialists.

68. Morocutti C, Amabile G, Fattapposta F, et al for the SIFA Investigators. Indobufen versus warfarin in the secondary prevention of major vascular events in non-rheumatic atrial fibrillation. Stroke 1997;28:1015–1021.

69. Atrial Fibrillation Investigators. The efficacy of aspirin in patients with atrial fibrillation: analysis of pooled data from 3 randomized trials. Arch Intern Med 1997;157:1237–1240.

70. Benavente O, Hart R, Koudstaal P, Laupacis A, McBride R. Oral anticoagulants for preventing stroke in patients with non-valvular atrial fibrillation and no previous history of stroke or transient ischemic attacks. In: The Cochrane Library, Issue 1, 2001. Oxford: Update Software. Search date 1999; primary sources Cochrane Stroke Group Specialised Register of Trials; Medline; Antithrombotic Trialists Collaboration database; and hand searches of reference lists of relevant articles.

71. Benavente O, Hart R, Koudstaal P, Laupacis A, McBride R. Antiplatelet therapy for preventing stroke in patients with non-valvular atrial fibrillation and no previous history of stroke or transient ischemic attacks. In: The Cochrane Library, Issue 1, 2001. Oxford: Update Software. Search date June 1999; primary sources Medline; Cochrane Register of Trials; and hand searches of reference lists of relevant articles.

72. Lip G. Thromboprophylaxis for atrial fibrillation. Lancet 1999;353:4–6.

73. Ezekowitz M, Levine J. Preventing stroke in patients with atrial fibrillation. JAMA 1999;281: 1830–1835.

74. Hart R, Sherman D, Easton D, Cairns J. Prevention of stroke in patients with non-valvular atrial fibrillation. Neurology 1998;51:674–681.

75. Feinberg W. Anticoagulation for prevention of stroke. Neurology 1998;51(suppl 3):20–22.

76. Albers G. Choice of antithrombotic therapy for stroke prevention in atrial fibrillation. Warfarin, aspirin, or both? Arch Intern Med 1998;158: 1487–1491.

77. Nademanee K, Kosar E. Long-term antithrombotic treatment for atrial fibrillation. Am J Cardiol 1998; 82:37N–42N.

78. Green CJ, Hadorn DC, Bassett K, Kazanjian A. Anticoagulation in chronic non-valvular atrial fibrillation: a critical appraisal and meta-analysis. Can J Cardiol 1997;13:811–815.

79. Blakely J. Anticoagulation in chronic non-valvular atrial fibrillation: appraisal of two meta-analyses. Can J Cardiol 1998;14:945–948.

Cathie Sudlow
Specialist Registrar in Neurology
Department of Neurology
Derriford Hospital
Plymouth
UK

Gord Gubitz
Assistant Professor
Division of Neurology
Dalhousie University
Halifax
Canada

Peter Sandercock
Professor in Neurology
Neurosciences Trials Unit
University of Edinburgh
Edinburgh
UK

Gregory Lip
Consultant Cardiologist and Reader in Medicine
City Hospital
Birmingham
UK

Competing interests: GL is UK principal investigator for the ERAFT Trial (Knoll) and has been reimbursed by various pharmaceutical companies for attending several conferences, running educational programmes and research projects. PS has given lectures and symposia, and received lecture fees and travel expenses from Boehringer Ingelheim, Sanofi, BMJ Publishing Group, and a variety of other companies, and he has received support from Boehringer Ingelheim and GlaxoWellcome for trials and research. GG and CS, none declared.

TABLE 1 Effects of cholesterol lowering on risk of stroke: results of two systematic reviews of RCTs of non-statin and statin interventions in the primary and secondary prevention of coronary heart disease* (see text, pp 209, 210).

Overview	Number of		Mean reduction in cholesterol (%)	Summary OR (95% CI) for active treatment v control	
	Participants	Strokes		Fatal or non-fatal stroke	Fatal stroke
Non-statin interventions					
1995 overview (11 trials)[14]	36 000	435	11%	0.99 (0.82 to 1.21)	1.10 (0.79 to 1.54)
Statin interventions					
1997 overview (14 trials)[15] + LIPID trial[16]	38 000	827	21%	0.76 (0.66 to 0.87)	0.99 (0.67 to 1.45)
Subtotal, primary prevention trials	8 000	108	20%	0.80 (0.54 to 1.16)	–
Subtotal, secondary prevention trials	30 000	719	22%	0.75 (0.65 to 0.87)	–

* The findings of other published overviews are consistent with the results shown here.

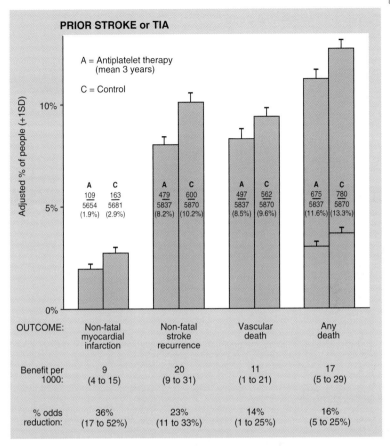

PRIOR STROKE or TIA

A = Antiplatelet therapy
(mean 3 years)

C = Control

	A	C	A	C	A	C	A	C
	109	163	479	600	497	562	675	780
	5654	5681	5837	5870	5837	5870	5837	5870
	(1.9%)	(2.9%)	(8.2%)	(10.2%)	(8.5%)	(9.6%)	(11.6%)	(13.3%)

OUTCOME:	Non-fatal myocardial infarction	Non-fatal stroke recurrence	Vascular death	Any death
Benefit per 1000:	9 (4 to 15)	20 (9 to 31)	11 (1 to 21)	17 (5 to 29)
% odds reduction:	36% (17 to 52%)	23% (11 to 33%)	14% (1 to 25%)	16% (5 to 25%)

FIGURE 1 Absolute effects of antiplatelet treatment on various outcomes in people with a prior stroke or TIA: results of a systematic review.[5] The columns show the absolute risks over 3 years for each outcome; the error bars represent standard deviations. In the "any death" column, non-vascular deaths are represented by lower horizontal lines (see text, pp 207, 210). Adapted with permission.[5]

Thromboembolism

Search date September 2000

David Fitzmaurice, FD Richard Hobbs and Richard McManus

Key Messages

Proximal DVT

- One RCT has found that combined intravenous unfractionated heparin and oral anticoagulant reduce recurrent thromboembolic events in people with proximal deep vein thrombosis (DVT) compared with oral anticoagulants alone.

- Two systematic reviews have found good evidence that longer duration of anticoagulation is associated with significantly fewer recurrent DVTs. One systematic review has found limited evidence that longer duration of anticoagulation is associated with significantly increased risk of major haemorrhage, but the other systematic review has found no significantly increased risk of major haemorrhage.

- Systematic reviews have found that low molecular weight heparin (LMWH) (see glossary, p 233) is at least as effective as unfractionated heparin in reducing the incidence of recurrent thromboembolic disease.

- Systematic reviews have found that LMWH is at least as safe as unfractionated heparin for the treatment of DVT.

Isolated calf vein thrombosis

- One RCT has found that warfarin plus unfractionated heparin reduce the risk of recurrence in isolated calf vein thrombosis compared with unfractionated heparin alone.

- We found insufficient evidence on optimal duration or intensity of anticoagulation.

Pulmonary embolism

- One RCT has found that combined treatment with oral anticoagulant plus intravenous unfractionated heparin reduces mortality compared with unfractionated heparin alone. One RCT found no evidence of a difference in the benefits and harms of LMWH versus unfractionated heparin in people with pulmonary embolism.

Duration of warfarin treatment

- Evidence for intensity and duration of treatment has been extrapolated from studies in people with proximal DVT and any venous thromboembolism.

- Two systematic reviews have found good evidence of a significant reduction in recurrent venous thromboembolism with longer duration of anticoagulation. One systematic review found limited evidence of increased risk of major haemorrhage with longer periods of anticoagulation. The other systematic review found no significantly increased risk of major haemorrhage with longer versus shorter durations of anticoagulation.

- The absolute risk of recurrent venous thromboembolism decreases with time whereas the relative risk reduction with therapy remains constant. Harms of therapy, including major haemorrhage, continue during prolonged treatment. People with thromboembolism have different risk profiles, and it is likely that the optimal duration of anticoagulation will vary between people.

Intensity of warfarin treatment

- One RCT in people with a first episode of idiopathic venous thromboembolism treated for 3 months with warfarin found no significant difference in recurrence between treatment targeted at an international normalised ratio (INR) (see glossary, p 233) of 2.0–3.0 versus an INR of 3.0–4.5. Treatment targeted at the higher INR was associated with a greater risk of bleeding.

Computerised decision support of oral anticoagulation

- We found no RCTs of computerised decision support versus usual management of oral anticoagulation that used clinically important outcomes (major haemorrhage or death). Systematic reviews and RCTs have found limited evidence that computerised decision support of oral anticoagulation improves time spent in the target INR range.

DEFINITION   **Venous thromboembolism** is any thromboembolic event occurring within the venous system, including DVT and pulmonary embolism. **Deep vein thrombosis (DVT)** is a radiologically confirmed partial or total thrombotic occlusion of the deep venous system of the legs sufficient to produce symptoms of pain or swelling. **Proximal DVT** affects the veins above the knee (popliteal, superficial femoral, common femoral, and iliac veins). **Isolated calf vein thrombosis** is confined to the deep veins of the calf and does not affect the veins above the knee. **Pulmonary embolism** is radiologically confirmed partial or total thromboembolic occlusion of pulmonary arteries, sufficient to cause symptoms of breathlessness, chest pain, or both. **Post-thrombotic syndrome** is oedema, ulceration, and impaired viability of the subcutaneous tissues of the leg occurring after DVT. **Recurrence** refers to symptomatic deterioration due to a further (radiologically confirmed) thrombosis, after a previously confirmed thromboembolic event, where there had been an initial partial or total symptomatic improvement. **Extension** refers to a radiologically confirmed new, constant, symptomatic intraluminal filling defect extending from an existing thrombosis.

INCIDENCE/ PREVALENCE
We found no reliable study of the incidence/prevalence of DVT or pulmonary embolism in the UK. A prospective Scandinavian study found an annual incidence of 1.6–1.8 per 1000 people in the general population.[1,2] One post mortem study extrapolated that 600 000 people develop pulmonary embolism each year in the USA, of whom 60 000 die as a result.[3]

AETIOLOGY/ RISK FACTORS
Risk factors for DVT include immobility, surgery (particularly orthopaedic), malignancy, smoking, pregnancy, older age, and inherited or acquired prothrombotic clotting disorders.[4] Evidence for these factors is mainly observational. The oral contraceptive pill is associated with death due to venous thromboembolism (ARI with any combined oral contraception 1 to 3 per million women per year).[5] The principal cause of pulmonary embolism is a DVT.[4]

PROGNOSIS
The annual recurrence rate of symptomatic calf vein thrombosis in people not having surgery is over 25%.[6,7] Between 40–50% of people with symptomatic calf vein thrombosis develop proximal extension.[8] Proximal DVT may cause fatal or non-fatal pulmonary embolism, recurrent venous thrombosis, and the post-thrombotic syndrome. One observational study published in 1946 found a 20% mortality from pulmonary emboli in people in hospital with untreated DVT.[9] One non-systematic review of observational studies found that, in people after surgery who have an asymptomatic calf vein DVT, the rate of fatal pulmonary embolism was 13–15%.[10] The incidence of other complications without treatment is not known. The risk of recurrent venous thrombosis and complications is related to the presence of thrombotic risk factors.[11]

AIMS
To reduce acute symptoms of DVT and to prevent morbidity and mortality associated with thrombus extension, the post-thrombotic syndrome and pulmonary embolisation; to reduce recurrence; and to minimise any adverse effects of treatment.

OUTCOMES
Rates of symptomatic recurrence, post-thrombotic syndrome, symptomatic pulmonary embolism, and death. Proxy outcomes include radiological evidence of clot extension or pulmonary embolism.

METHODS
Clinical Evidence search and appraisal September 2000. Observational studies were used for estimating incidence, prevalence, and adverse event rates. RCTs were included only if cases and outcomes were objectively defined, and if the trial provided dose ranges (with adjusted dosing schedules for oral anticoagulation and unfractionated heparin) and independent, blinded outcome assessment.

OPTION   **ANTICOAGULATION**

We found no RCTs comparing warfarin with placebo. One RCT found that combined warfarin and intravenous unfractionated heparin for initial treatment reduced recurrence of proximal DVT compared with warfarin alone. Two systematic reviews have found that longer duration of anticoagulation is associated with significantly fewer DVT recurrences. Systematic reviews have found that LMWH (see glossary, p 233) is at least as effective as unfractionated heparin in reducing the incidence of recurrent thromboembolic disease. We found evidence from systematic reviews that LMWH is at least as safe as unfractionated heparin for the treatment of DVT.

Benefits: **Warfarin versus placebo:** We found no RCTs. **Warfarin plus heparin versus warfarin alone:** One RCT (120 people with proximal DVT) found that combined intravenous unfractionated heparin plus warfarin reduced recurrence compared with warfarin alone at interim analysis at 6 months, and as a result the trial was stopped (rate of recurrence 12/60 [20%] with warfarin alone v 4/60 [6.7%] with combined treatment, P = 0.058; NNT 8, 95% CI 4 to 71).[12] **Duration of anticoagulation:** We found two systematic reviews. The first systematic review (search date 2000, 4 RCTs, 1500 people)[13] included two RCTs of people with a first episode of venous thromboembolism, one RCT in people with a second episode of venous thromboembolism, and a fourth RCT in people with acute proximal DVT. The periods of treatment compared were different in all four RCTs: 4 weeks versus 3 months, 6 weeks versus 6 months, 3 months versus 27 months, and 6 months versus 4 years. In all RCTs, anticoagulant doses were adjusted to achieve an INR (see glossary, p 233) between 2.0 and 3.0. Individual RCTs found significant protection from thromboembolic complications with prolonged versus shorter treatment (on pooling, 7/758 [0.9%] in the long arm v 91/742 [12%] in the short arm; OR 0.15, 95% CI 0.10 to 0.23). None of the individual RCTs found a significant reduction in mortality. Analysis of pooled results also found no significant reduction in mortality with prolonged versus shorter treatment (OR 0.70, 95% CI 0.45 to 1.09). The second systematic review (search date not stated, 7 RCTs, 2304 people) included three of the same RCTs as the first systematic review plus four RCTs that had been excluded on methodological grounds from the first systematic review (either because of problems with blinding of outcomes or lack of an objective test to confirm thromboembolism).[14] There was wide variation in the duration of short term (3–12 weeks) and longer term (12 weeks–2 years) RCTs. This review also found that longer versus short duration of anticoagulation reduced the risk of recurrent thromboembolism (ARs 74/1156 events per person with longer anticoagulation v 127/1148 with shorter duration; RR 0.60, 95% CI 0.45 to 0.79). **Intensity of anticoagulation:** We found one RCT comparing INR targets of 2.0–3.0 versus 3.0–4.5 for 12 weeks treatment with warfarin following an initial course of intravenous heparin in people with a first episode of idiopathic venous thromboembolism. It found similar recurrence rates at 10 months for both

INR target ranges (recurrence rate 1/47 [2.1%] with lower range v 1/49 [2%] with higher range; P = NS), but found significantly more haemorrhagic events with the higher target range (2/47 [4.3%] v 11/49 [22.4%]; P = 0.015).[15] **Abrupt versus gradual discontinuation of warfarin:** We found one RCT (41 people with DVT), which compared abrupt withdrawal of warfarin versus an additional month of warfarin at a fixed low dose of 1.25 mg/day. It found no significant difference in recurrence rates between the two groups (recurrence in 3 people who stopped warfarin abruptly v 1 person who reduced warfarin gradually).[16] **LMWH versus unfractionated heparin:** We found two systematic reviews confined to symptomatic proximal DVT.[17,18] One (search date 1993, 16 RCTs, 2045 people) found that LMWH reduced thrombus extension compared with unfractionated heparin (ARs not given; OR for thrombus extension 0.45, 95% CI 0.25 to 0.81).[17] The other review (search date 1994, 10 RCTs, 1424 people) found that, compared with unfractionated heparin, low molecular weight heparin reduced symptomatic thromboembolic complications (ARs not given; RR 0.47, 95% CI 0.27 to 0.82) and mortality (RR 0.53, 95% CI 0.31 to 0.90).[18] We also found four systematic reviews comparing LMWH with unfractionated heparin in people with radiologically confirmed symptomatic venous thromboembolism,[19-22] and one subsequent RCT.[23] The first systematic review (search date 1999, 14 RCTs, 4754 people) included five studies (blinded and unblinded, 1636 people) examining proximal thrombosis.[19] Analysis of these trials showed statistically significant reductions in thrombotic complications (LMWH v unfractionated heparin: ARs 39/814 [4.8%] v 64/822 [7.8%]; OR 0.60, 95% CI 0.40 to 0.89). Overall mortality was also reduced (LMWH v unfractionated heparin: ARs 44/814 [5.4%] v 68/822 [8.3%]; OR 0.64, 95% CI 0.43 to 0.93). Eight of the 14 RCTs in the systematic review included people with symptomatic DVT of the leg without symptoms of pulmonary embolism, and these accounted for about 75% of all participants. Analysis of the seven RCTs that concealed treatment allocation found no significant difference between treatments for rates of recurrent venous thromboembolism during treatment (ARs 34/1569 [2.2%] v 43/1595 [2.7%]; OR 0.80, 95% CI 0.51 to 1.26), or at the end of follow up (ARs 75/1671 [4.5%] v 92/1693 [5.4%]; OR 0.82, 95% CI 0.60 to 1.12), or overall mortality (ARs 123/1671 [7.4%] v 150/1694 [8.9%]; OR 0.82, 95% CI 0.64 to 1.05), or major haemorrhage. Wider analysis that included unblinded trials, and so is likely to be more biased, found that LMWH reduced overall mortality and major haemorrhage compared with unfractionated heparin (see harms, p 229). The other three systematic reviews included many of the same trials as the first. Results were similar with no differences between unfractionated heparin and LMWH for recurrent venous thromboembolism or pulmonary embolism, and an unexplained, significant difference in favour of LMWH for total mortality when data were pooled.[20-22] We also found one open RCT not included in the systematic reviews (294 people with acute proximal DVT), which found no significant difference in recurrent DVT rates with intravenous unfractionated heparin in hospital versus LMWH administered subcutaneously twice daily mainly at home (outpatients) or alternatively in hospital versus subcutaneous heparin calcium administered at home (6/98 [6%] with unfractionated heparin v 6/97 [6%] with LMWH v 7/99 [7%] with subcutaneous heparin calcium).[23] See systemic anticoagulation under stroke management, p 197.

Harms: **Warfarin:** Two non-systematic reviews of RCTs and cohort studies found annual bleeding rates of 0–4.8% (fatal bleeding) and 2.4–8.1% (major bleeds).[24,25] Rates depended on how bleeding was defined and the intensity of anticoagulation. No individual study in either review comparing length of anticoagulation found a significant increase in bleeding complications during prolonged versus shorter treatment for venous thromboembolism.[13,14] Both reviews included studies with different periods of treatment and the populations studied had different types of venous thromboembolism (see benefits, p 228). Pooling the results for the first review found that prolonged versus shorter anticoagulation increased the risk of major haemorrhage (19/758 [2.5%] with prolonged anticoagulation v 4/742 [0.5%] with shorter anticoagulation; OR 3.75, 95% CI 1.63 to 8.62). Pooling the results of the second review found a greater risk of major haemorrhage with prolonged versus shorter anticoagulation, but the difference was not significant (10/917 [1.1%] with prolonged treatment v 6/906 [0.7%] with shorter treatment; RR 1.43, 95% CI 0.51 to 4.01). In the RCT of warfarin plus heparin, one person in the combined treatment group committed suicide at 6 months. There were two cancer related deaths, confirmed by post mortem examination, in the group treated with warfarin alone, one in week 11, and the other in week 12.[12]
Heparin: One systematic review (3306 people treated for at least 5 days) found no significant difference in the risk of thrombocytopenia with LMWH versus unfractionated heparin (RR 0.85, 95% CI 0.45 to 1.62).[20] Another systematic review of blinded RCTs found no significant difference in the risk of major haemorrhage with LMWH versus unfractionated heparin in people with venous thromboembolism (ARs 27/1791 [1.5%] v 39/1827 [2.1%]; OR 0.71, 95% CI 0.43 to 1.15).[19] In this systematic review, pooling of blinded and unblinded RCTs found that the risk of major haemorrhage was 1–2% for up to 10 days treatment with either LMWH or unfractionated heparin.[19] Analysis of the five RCTs of people with proximal thrombosis (blinded and unblinded, 1636 people) found a significant reduction in major haemorrhage with LMWH versus unfractionated heparin (ARs 8/814 [1.0%] v 19/822 [2.3%]; OR 0.44, 95% CI 0.21 to 0.95). The other three systematic reviews, covering many of the same trials, found similar significant reductions in major haemorrhage.[20-22] One of the systematic reviews in people with DVT found that, compared with LMWH, unfractionated heparin was associated with higher rates of clinically important bleeding (ARs not given; RR unfractionated v LMWH 2.48, 95% CI 1.27 to 6.67) and death (see benefits, p 228).[11]

Comment: **Studies evaluating harm:** These varied in regard to diagnostic criteria, definitions of adverse events, and intensity of anticoagulation, making interpretation difficult. **Duration of warfarin therapy:** The absolute risk of recurrent venous thromboembolism decreases with time, whereas the relative risk reduction with therapy remains constant. Harms of therapy, including major haemorrhage, continue during prolonged treatment. Individual people have different risk profiles and it is likely that the optimal duration of anticoagulation will vary between people. **Differences between LMWH:** We found no trials comparing different LMWH.

QUESTION	What are the effects of treatment for isolated calf vein thrombosis?

OPTION	ANTICOAGULATION

One RCT found that, in isolated calf vein thrombosis, warfarin plus intravenous unfractionated heparin (INR 2.5–4.2) reduced rates of proximal extension compared with heparin alone. We found insufficient evidence on optimal duration or intensity of anticoagulation.

Benefits: **Anticoagulation:** We found no systematic review and no good placebo controlled RCTs. We found one RCT that compared intravenous unfractionated heparin for at least 5 days with or without 3 months of warfarin. It found that heparin plus warfarin reduced proximal extension of clot at 1 year compared with heparin alone (proximal extension occurred in 1/23 people with heparin plus warfarin v 9/28 people with heparin alone; ARR 28%, 95% CI 8.6% to 47%).[6] **Duration and intensity of anticoagulation:** We found insufficient evidence in people with isolated calf vein thrombosis.

Harms: See harms of anticoagulation, p 229.

Comment: Many reported cases of isolated calf vein thrombosis are asymptomatic but detected radiologically for research purposes. We found very limited evidence on the clinical significance of asymptomatic calf vein thrombosis. Similarly, studies into the incidence of pulmonary embolism associated with isolated calf vein thrombosis detected asymptomatic embolism by ventilation–perfusion scanning, and it is not clear what the clinical significance of these findings are.

QUESTION	What are the effects of treatments for pulmonary embolism?

OPTION	ANTICOAGULATION

One small RCT has found that heparin plus warfarin significantly reduces mortality in people with pulmonary embolism, compared with no anticoagulant treatment. Two RCTs found that LMWH was at least as effective as unfractionated heparin in people with pulmonary embolism.

Benefits: **Anticoagulation:** We found no systematic review. We found one RCT (published 1960; 35 people with pulmonary embolism) comparing heparin plus warfarin with no anticoagulation.[26] It found that anticoagulation reduced mortality (0/16 deaths [0%] with anticoagulation v 5/19 deaths [26%] with no anticoagulation; NNT 4, 95% CI 2 to 16). We found no RCTs of heparin versus placebo, warfarin versus placebo, or heparin plus warfarin versus heparin alone or warfarin alone. **Duration and intensity of anticoagulation:** We found no direct evidence in people with pulmonary embolism alone.

Evidence for intensity and duration of treatment has been extrapolated from studies in people with proximal DVT and any venous thromboembolism. These trials found that bleeding rates were increased by higher INR target ranges (INR 3.0–4.5), but recurrence rates were not significantly different compared with a lower range (INR 2.0–3.0), and that longer courses of anticoagulation reduced recurrence compared with shorter courses (see benefits of anticoagulation under treatments for isolated calf vein thrombosis, p 230). **LMWH versus unfractionated heparin:** We found no systematic review. We found two RCTs. The first (612 people with symptomatic pulmonary embolism who did not receive thrombolysis or embolectomy) found no significant difference in the death rate with subcutaneous LMWH (tinzaparin) versus intravenous heparin (AR 12/304 [3.9%] with tinzaparin v 14/308 [4.5%] with heparin; P = 0.7) or recurrent thromboembolism (5/304 [1.6%] with tinzaparin v 6/308 [1.9%] with heparin; P = 0.8).[27] The second RCT (200 people at study entry with proximal DVT without clinical signs or symptoms of pulmonary embolism but with high probability lung scan findings) found that fixed dose subcutaneous heparin given once daily versus dose adjusted intravenous heparin reduced the number of new episodes of venous thromboembolism (ARs 0/97 [0%] with LMWH v 7/103 [6.8%] with intravenous heparin; P = 0.01).[28]

Harms:
The first RCT comparing LMWH versus unfractionated heparin found no significant difference in the rate of major haemorrhage (3/304 [1.0%] with LMWH v 5/308 [1.6%] with unfractionated heparin; P = 0.5).[27] The second RCT also found no significant difference in the risk of major bleeding with LMWH and intravenous heparin (1/97 [1%] with LMWH v 2/103 [2%] with intravenous heparin; P = 0.6).[28] (See harms of anticoagulants under treatments for proximal DVT, p 229).

Comment:
In the two RCTs,[27,28] the incidence of major haemorrhage was low and the number of people in these RCTs was too small to detect a clinically important difference.

QUESTION **What are the effects of computerised decision support on oral anticoagulation management?**

We found no RCTs of computerised decision support versus usual management of oral anticoagulation that used clinically important outcomes (major haemorrhage or death). Three systematic reviews and three subsequent RCTs have found that computerised decision support in oral anticoagulation improves time spent in the target INR range. Most RCTs were small and brief.

Benefits:
Clinical outcomes: We found no systematic review and no RCTs.
Laboratory outcomes: We found three systematic reviews[29-31] and three subsequent RCTs.[32-34] One systematic review specifically addressed computerised decision support (see glossary, p 233) in oral anticoagulation management and two included oral anticoagulation management in addition to other forms of computerised decision support. The first (search date 1997, 9 RCTs, 1336 people) included eight RCTs using warfarin and one using heparin.[29]

The computer systems advised the doses for initiation of anticoagulation (2 RCTs) and for maintenance of anticoagulation (6 RCTs). Follow up was short (15 days–12 months). Indication for treatment included cardiac diseases and venous thrombosis. The outcome reported by seven of the nine RCTs (1327 people) in the systematic review was the proportion of days within the target range of anticoagulation. The review found that computerised decision support versus usual care increased the time that the INR was in the target range (OR 1.29, 95% CI 1.17 to 1.49). One included trial (small and with the largest effect) introduced significant heterogeneity between the trials and was therefore excluded (OR for remaining RCTs 1.25, 95% CI 1.1 to 1.5). The other two systematic reviews included a wider range of computer support for determining drug dose and included seven[30] and four[31] RCTs of the nine found by the first systematic review.[29] The first subsequent RCT assessed warfarin management after hip replacement (71 people with usual care and 51 people managed with computerised decision support).[32] Only initiation of warfarin was studied. It found no significant difference in the time taken to reach therapeutic levels of anticoagulation (4.7 v 2.8 days). The second RCT compared a specific computerised decision support with physician adjusted dosing in five hospitals.[33] People who were taking warfarin for at least 6 days were selected (285 people) and followed for at least 3 months (results from 254 [89%] were analysed). People managed by computerised decision support spent more time with their INR in the target range than people managed conventionally (63% v 53%; P < 0.05). The third study compared a package of care that included computerised decision support with traditional hospital outpatient management. The intervention was based in primary care: a practice nurse clinic included near patient INR testing and computerised decision support. After 12 months, analysis of 224 people (122 intervention, 102 controls) found more time spent in the target range (69% v 57%; P < 0.001) but no difference in the proportion of tests in range (61% with intervention v 51% with control) or in the point prevalence of tests in range (71% v 62%).[34]

Harms: **Major haemorrhage:** See glossary, p 233. One systematic review RCTs, 1336 people) reported the incidence of major haemorrhage.[29] There were 14 major haemorrhages among 700 (2%) people with computerised decision support and 25 among 636 (3.9%) in the control group. Most of the events occurred in one study making meta-analysis inappropriate. One RCT found no significant difference in overall death rates or serious adverse events with computerised decision support versus usual care.[34]

Comment: We found only limited evidence (from small trials with short follow up of proxy outcomes) on the use of computerised decision support in oral anticoagulation management. Computerised decision support for oral anticoagulation appears at least as effective as human performance in terms of time spent in the target INR range. It is not clear if this will translate to improved clinical outcomes. Larger and longer trials that measure clinical outcomes (particularly harms) are needed.

GLOSSARY

Computerised decision support system A computer program that provides advice on the significance and implications of clinical findings or laboratory results.

International normalised ratio (INR) A value derived from a standardised laboratory test that measures the effect of an anticoagulant. The laboratory materials used in the test are calibrated against internationally accepted standard reference preparations, so that variability between laboratories and different reagents is minimised. Normal blood has an INR of 1. Therapeutic anticoagulation often aims to achieve an INR value of 2–3.5.

Low molecular weight heparins (LMWH) are manufactured from heparin, by using chemical or enzymatic methods. The various formulations of LMWH differ in mean molecular weight, composition, and anticoagulant activity. As a group, LMWHs have distinct properties and it is not yet clear that one LMWH will behave exactly like another. Some subcutaneously administered LMWHs do not require monitoring.

Major haemorrhage Exact definitions vary between studies but usually a major haemorrhage is one involving intracranial, retroperitoneal, joint or muscle bleeding leading directly to death or requiring admission to hospital to stop the bleeding or provide a blood transfusion. All other haemorrhages are classified as minor.

REFERENCES

1. Nordstrom M, Linblad B, Bergqvist D, Kjellstrom. A prospective study of the incidence of deep-vein thrombosis within a defined urban population. *Arch Intern Med* 1992;326:155–160.
2. Hansson PO, Werlin L, Tibblin G, Eriksson H. Deep vein thrombosis and pulmonary embolism in the general population. *Arch Intern Med* 1997;157:1665–1670.
3. Rubinstein I, Murray D, Hoffstein V. Fatal pulmonary emboli in hospitalised patients: an autopsy study. *Arch Intern Med* 1988;148:1425–1426.
4. Hirsh J, Hoak J. Management of deep vein thrombosis and pulmonary embolism. *Circulation* 1996;93:2212–2245.
5. Farley TMM, Meirik O, Chang CL, Marmot MG, Poulter NR. Effects of different progestogens in low oestrogen oral contraceptives on venous thromboembolic disease. *Lancet* 1995;346:1582–1588.
6. Lagerstedt C, Olsson C, Fagher B, Oqvist B, Albrechtsson U. Need for long term anticoagulant treatment in symptomatic calf vein thrombosis. *Lancet* 1985;334:515–518.
7. Lohr J, Kerr T, Lutter K, Cranley R, Spirtoff K, Cranley J. Lower extremity calf thrombosis: to treat or not to treat? *J Vasc Surg* 1991;14:618–623.
8. Kakkar VV, Howe CT, Flanc C, Clarke MB. Natural history of postoperative deep vein thrombosis. *Lancet* 1969;2:230–232.
9. Zilliacus H. On the specific treatment of thrombosis and pulmonary embolism with anticoagulants, with a particular reference to the post thrombotic sequelae. *Acta Med Scand* 1946;170:1–221.
10. Giannoukas AD, Labropoulos N, Burke P, Katsamouris A, Nicolaides AN. Calf deep vein thrombosis: a review of the literature. *Eur J Vasc Endovasc Surg* 1995;10:398–404.
11. Lensing AWA, Prandoni P, Prins MH, Buller HR. Deep-vein thrombosis. *Lancet* 1999;353:479–485.
12. Brandjes DPM, Heijboer H, Buller HR, Rijk M, Jagt H, ten Cate JW. Acenocoumarol and heparin compared with acenocoumarol alone in the initial treatment of proximal-vein thrombosis. *N Engl J Med* 1992;327:1485–1489.
13. Hutten BA, Prins MH. Duration of treatment with vitamin K antagonists in symptomatic venous thromboembolism. In: The Cochrane Library. Issue 4, 2000. Oxford: Update Software. Search date January 2000; primary sources Medline; Embase; hand searching relevant journals, and personal contacts.
14. Pinede L, Duhaut P, Cucherat M, Ninet J, Pasquier J, Boissel JP. Comparison of long versus short duration of anticoagulant therapy after a first episode of venous thromboembolism: a meta-analysis of randomized, controlled trials. *J Intern Med* 2000;247:553–562. Search date not specified; primary sources Medline, Embase, Cochrane Controlled Trials Register, and hand searched reference lists.
15. Hull R, Hirsh J, Jay RM, et al. Different intensities of oral anticoagulant therapy in the treatment of proximal vein thrombosis. *N Engl J Med* 1982;307:1676–1681.
16. Ascani A, Iorio A, Agnelli G. Withdrawal of warfarin after deep vein thrombosis: effects of a low fixed dose on rebound thrombin generation. *Blood Coagul Fibrinolysis* 1999;10:291–295.
17. Leisorovicz A, Simonneau G, Decousous H, Boissel JP. Comparison of efficacy and safety of low molecular weight heparins and unfractionated heparin in initial treatment of deep venous thrombosis: a meta-analysis. *BMJ* 1994;309:299–304. Search date December 1993; primary sources Medline and hand searched references.
18. Lensing AWA, Prins MH, Davidson BL, Hirsh J. Treatment of deep venous thrombosis with low-molecular weight heparins. *Arch Intern Med* 1995;155:601–607. Search date 1994; primary sources Medline 1984 to 1994; manual search and hand searched references.
19. Van den Belt AGM, Prins MH, Lensing AWA, et al. Fixed dose subcutaneous low molecular weight heparins versus adjusted dose unfractionated heparin for venous thromboembolism. In: The Cochrane Library, Issue 4. Oxford: Update Software. Search date July 1999; primary sources Medline, Embase, and LILACS; contact with researchers and pharmaceutical companies; and hand searched references.

20. Dolovich LR, Ginsberg JS, Douketis JD, Holbrook AM, Cheah G. A meta-analysis comparing low-molecular-weight heparins with unfractionated heparin in the treatment of venous thromboembolism. *Arch Intern Med* 2000;160: 181–188. Search date 1996; primary sources Medline; HEALTH; and The Cochrane Library; and hand searched references.

21. Bijsterveld NR, Hettiarachchi R, Peters R, Prins MH, Levi M, Buller HR. Low-molecular weight heparins in venous and arterial thrombotic disease. *Thromb Haemost* 1999;82(suppl 1):139–147. Search date 1999; primary sources Medline 1996 to 1999; Embase 1996 to 1999; principal study investigators; and hand searched references.

22. Rohan JK, Hettiarachchi RJ, Prins MH, Lensing AW, Buller HR. Low molecular weight heparin versus unfractionated heparin in the initial treatment of venous thromboembolism. *Curr Opin Pulmon Med* 1998;4:220–225. Search date not stated; primary sources Medline, Current Contents, Embase.

23. Belcaro G, Nicolaides AN, Cesarone MR, et al. Comparison of low-molecular-weight heparin, administered primarily at home, with unfractionated heparin, administered in hospital, and subcutaneous heparin, administered at home for deep-vein thrombosis. *Angiology* 1999;50: 781–787.

24. Landefeld CS, Beyth RJ. Anticoagulant related bleeding: clinical epidemiology, prediction, and prevention. *Am J Med* 1993;95:315–328.

25. Levine MN, Hirsh J, Landefeld CS, Raskob G. Haemorrhagic complications of anticoagulant treatment. *Chest* 1992;102(suppl):352–363.

26. Barrit DW, Jordan SC. Anticoagulant drugs in the treatment of pulmonary embolism: a controlled trial. *Lancet* 1960;i:1309–1312.

27. Simonneau G, Sors H, Charbonnier B, et al. A comparison of low-molecular weight heparin with unfractionated heparin for acute pulmonary embolism. *N Engl J Med* 1997;337:663–669.

28. Hull RD, Raskob GE, Brant RF, et al. Low-molecular-weight heparin vs heparin in the treatment of patients with pulmonary embolism. American-Canadian Thrombosis Study Group. *Arch Intern Med* 2000;160:229–236.

29. Chatellier G, Colombet I, Degoulet P. An overview of the effect of computer-assisted management of anticoagulant therapy on the quality of anticoagulation. *Int J Med Informatics* 1998;49: 311–320. Search date 1997; primary source Medline.

30. Hunt DL, Haynes RB, Hanna SE, Smith, K. Effects of computer-based clinical decision support systems on physician performance and patient outcomes: a systematic review. *JAMA* 1998;280: 1339–1346. Search date not specified; primary sources Medline, Embase, Inspec, SciSearch, Cochrane Library, and hand searching of reference lists and personal contact with authors.

31. Walton R, Dovey S, Harvey E, Freemantle N. Computer support for determining drug dose: systematic review and meta-analysis. *BMJ* 1999; 318:984–990. Search date 1996, primary sources Specialised Register of Studies from Cochrane Collaboration on Effective Professional Practice, Medline, Embase, hand search of *Therapeutic Drug Monitoring* 1993–1996; contact with experts and pharmaceutical companies.

32. Motykie GD, Mokhtee D, Zebala LP, Caprinin JA, Kudrna JC, Mungall DR. The use of a Bayseian Forecasting Model in the management of warfarin therapy after total hip arthroplasty. *J Arthroplasty* 1999;14:988–993.

33. Poller L, Shiach CR, MacCallum PK, et al. Multicentre randomised study of computerised anticoagulant dosage. European Concerted Action on Anticoagulation *Lancet* 1998;352:1505–1509.

34. Fitzmaurice DA, Hobbs FDR, Murray ET, Holder RL, Allan TF, Rose PE. Oral anticoagulation management in primary care with the use of computerized decision support and near-patient testing. Randomized Controlled Trial. *Arch Intern Med* 2000;160:2343–2348.

David Fitzmaurice
Senior Lecturer

FD Richard Hobbs
Professor

Richard McManus
Clinical Research Fellow

Department of Primary Care and General
Practice
The Medical School
University of Birmingham
Birmingham
UK

Competing interests: RM none declared. FDRH is a member of the European Society of Cardiology (ESC) Working Party on Heart Failure, Treasurer of the British Society for Heart Failure, and Chair of the British Primary Care Cardiovascular Society (PCCS). He has received travel sponsorship and honoraria from a number of multinational biotechnology and pharmaceutical companies with cardiovascular products for plenary talks and attendance at major cardiology scientific congresses and conferences. DF has received reimbursement for attendance at scientific meetings from Leo Laboratories who make tinzaparin, a low molecular weight heparin. The Department of Primary Care and General Practice at the University of Birmingham, where the authors work, has a computerised decision support programme that is commercially available.

Search date November 2000

Madhu Natarajan

Key Messages

- One systematic review of RCTs has found that aspirin reduces the risk of death or myocardial infarction (MI) in people with unstable angina.

- One RCT found that ticlopidine was significantly more effective than conventional treatment (without aspirin) in unstable angina, but was associated with a significant risk of neutropenia.

- RCTs have found that intravenous glycoprotein IIb/IIIa inhibitors may improve outcome in people who undergo early percutaneous interventions when added to aspirin plus heparin, or heparin alone.

- Two RCTs found no significant difference in outcome between oral glycoprotein IIb/IIIa inhibitors versus, or in addition to, aspirin. One RCT has found that orbofiban versus placebo significantly increased mortality at 30 days.

- Two systematic reviews have found that the benefit of adding unfractionated heparin to aspirin is small. One systematic review has found that adding low molecular weight heparins (LMWH) to aspirin significantly reduces the short term rates of death and MI in people with unstable angina. One systematic review found no significant difference in benefits between LMWH and unfractionated heparin. One systematic review comparing short term treatment with LMWH versus unfractionated heparin found no significant difference in the frequency of major bleeding, and found that long term LMWH is associated with a significant increase in the risk of major bleeding compared with placebo.

- RCTs have found that hirudin versus unfractionated heparin in people also taking aspirin reduces short term but not medium term rates of death or MI.
- One systematic review found no evidence that calcium channel blockers prevent death or MI in people with unstable angina.
- We found that the effects of nitrates or β blockers in people with unstable angina have not yet been adequately evaluated.
- Three RCTs found little evidence that routine early invasive treatment reduces mortality compared with initial medical treatment plus, later, more selective intervention.

DEFINITION Unstable angina is distinguished from stable angina, acute MI, and non-cardiac pain, by the pattern (characteristic pain present at rest or on lower levels of activity) or severity (recently increasing intensity, frequency, or duration) of symptoms, and the absence of persistent ST elevation on a resting electrocardiogram (ECG). Unstable angina includes a variety of different clinical patterns: angina at rest of up to 1 week's duration; angina increasing in severity to moderate or severe pain; non-Q wave MI; and post-MI angina continuing for more than 24 hours.

INCIDENCE/ PREVALENCE In industrialised countries the annual incidence of unstable angina is about six of 10 000 people in the general population.

AETIOLOGY/ RISK FACTORS Risk factors are the same as for other manifestations of ischaemic heart disease: older age, previous atheromatous cardiovascular disease, diabetes mellitus, smoking cigarettes, hypertension, hypercholesterolaemia, male sex, and a family history of ischaemic heart disease. Unstable angina can also occur in association with other disorders of the circulation, including heart valve disease, arrhythmia, and cardiomyopathy.

PROGNOSIS In people taking aspirin, the incidence of serious adverse outcomes (such as death, acute MI, or refractory angina requiring emergency revascularisation) is 5–10% within the first 7 days and about 15% at 30 days. Between 5% and 14% of people with unstable angina die in the year after diagnosis, with about half of these deaths occurring within 4 weeks of diagnosis. No single factor identifies people at higher risk of an adverse event. Risk factors include severity of presentation (e.g. duration of pain, rapidity of progression, evidence of heart failure), medical history (e.g. previous unstable angina, acute MI, left ventricular dysfunction), other clinical parameters (e.g. age, diabetes), ECG changes (e.g. severity of ST segment depression, deep T wave inversion, transient ST elevation), biochemical parameters (e.g. troponin concentration), and change in clinical status (e.g. recurrent chest pain, silent ischaemia, haemodynamic instability).

AIMS To relieve pain and ischaemia; to prevent death and MI; to identify people at high risk requiring revascularisation; to facilitate early hospital discharge in people at low and medium risk; to modify risk factors; to prevent death, MI, and recurrent ischaemia after discharge from hospital, with minimum adverse effects.

OUTCOMES Rate of death or MI (often measured at 2, 7, and 30 days, and

6 months after randomisation); adverse effects of treatment. Some RCTs include rates of refractory ischaemia or re-admission for unstable angina.

METHODS   *Clinical Evidence* search and appraisal November 2000.

QUESTION   **What are the effects of antiplatelet treatments?**

OPTION   **ASPIRIN**

One systematic review has found that aspirin alone reduces the risk of death and MI in people with unstable angina. The evidence suggests no added cardiovascular benefit, and possible added harm, from doses of aspirin over 325 mg daily.

Benefits: One systematic review (search date 1990, 145 RCTs, 100 000 people) compared antiplatelet treatment versus placebo.[1] Seven of these trials included a total of 4000 people with unstable angina. The review found that antiplatelet treatment (mostly medium dose aspirin, 75–325 mg daily) reduced the combined outcome of vascular death, MI, or stroke at 6 months (AR 14% on placebo v 9% on antiplatelet treatment; RR 0.65, 95% CI 0.51 to 0.79). This means that 20 people would need to be treated with aspirin rather than placebo to prevent one additional event in 6 months (NNT 20, 95% CI 15 to 34). Individual trials within the systematic review showed consistent benefit from daily aspirin in terms of reduced deaths and MI.

Harms: The review found that people taking doses of aspirin ranging from 75 to 1200 mg daily had no significant adverse events, including gastrointestinal intolerance or bleeding.[1] However, the sum of the evidence suggests no added cardiovascular benefit, and greater incidence of gastrointestinal effects, for aspirin doses greater than 325 mg daily. Some people are allergic to aspirin.

Comment: The systematic review covered a wide range of people with different morbidities and levels of risk. Its results should be generalisable to routine practice.[1] People with unstable angina who are allergic or who do not respond to aspirin will need alternative antiplatelet treatment.

OPTION   **TICLOPIDINE**

One RCT found that ticlopidine was more effective than conventional treatment (without aspirin) in people with unstable angina, but it was associated with a significant risk of reversible neutropenia. Ticlopidine may therefore be an alternative in people who are intolerant of, or allergic to, aspirin.

Benefits: We found no systematic review of ticlopidine in unstable angina. One RCT compared ticlopidine versus conventional treatment without aspirin in 652 people (72% male) with unstable angina treated within 48 hours of admission.[2] At 6 months, there were significantly fewer vascular deaths or non-fatal MI in people taking ticlopidine

(RR compared with control 0.54, 95% CI 0.19 to 0.88; NNT for 6 months 16, 95% CI 9 to 62). We found no trial of ticlopidine versus aspirin in the treatment of unstable angina.

Harms: Reversible neutropenia was reported in 1–2% of people taking ticlopidine. Other adverse effects include diarrhoea and rash.

Comment: Ticlopidine is an alternative for people with unstable angina who are intolerant of, or allergic to, aspirin. A large study is currently comparing clopidogrel plus aspirin versus aspirin alone in this group of people.

OPTION	INTRAVENOUS GLYCOPROTEIN IIB/IIIA PLATELET RECEPTOR INHIBITORS

RCTs have found that adding parenteral glycoprotein IIb/IIIa inhibitors to unfractionated heparin alone or unfractionated heparin plus aspirin reduces deaths and MI. However, this was in the context of high rates of early percutaneous interventions.

Benefits: We found no systematic review, but found three RCTs that assessed adding intravenous glycoprotein IIb/IIIa inhibitors to standard treatment,[3-5] and three RCTs that compared a glycoprotein IIb/IIIa inhibitor versus heparin.[3,5,6] The primary end points varied, but all trials included data on death rates and MI at 30 days (see table 1, p 246). **Added to heparin or aspirin or both:** The first RCT (1915 people with unstable angina or non-Q wave MI) with three treatment arms compared tirofiban, heparin, or both, as an infusion for a mean of 72 hours.[3] The tirofiban alone group was stopped early because of excess mortality at 7 days (AR of death at 7 days, 4.6% with tirofiban alone v 1.1% with heparin alone). The RCT found that compared with heparin alone, tirofiban plus heparin reduced rates of death, MI, or refractory ischaemia (at 7 days, AR 12.9% with tirofiban plus heparin v 17.9% with heparin, RR 0.68, 95% CI 0.53 to 0.88, P = 0.004; at 30 days, AR 18.5% with tirofiban plus heparin v 22.3% with heparin, P = 0.03; at 6 months, AR 27.7% with tirofiban plus heparin v 32.1% with heparin, P = 0.02). Early angiography and intervention were encouraged in this trial. The second RCT (9461 people with unstable angina) compared eptifibatide plus heparin plus aspirin versus heparin plus aspirin. The trial found modest benefit when eptifibatide was added to aspirin and unfractionated heparin (deaths and non-fatal MI at 30 days, eptifibatide 11.6% v placebo 16.7%, P = 0.01). No benefit was seen in people with low rates of intervention with percutaneous transluminal coronary angioplasty (PTCA).[4] The third RCT (2282 people), which included five treatment arms, compared high dose lamifiban with and without heparin versus low dose lamifiban with and without heparin versus heparin plus placebo.[5] The trial found that rates of ischaemic events were similar with high dose lamifiban plus heparin versus heparin plus placebo, but that the combination of low dose lamifiban and heparin reduced ischaemic events (AR of ischaemic event at 6 months, 12.6% with low dose lamifiban plus heparin v 17.9% with heparin plus placebo, P = 0.025). **Versus heparin:** One RCT (3232 people who were already taking aspirin) compared intravenous tirofiban versus heparin for 48 hours.[6] The primary composite end point of death, MI, or refractory ischaemia at

48 hours was significantly lower on tirofiban (AR 3.8% v 5.6%; RR 0.67, 95% CI 0.48 to 0.92), but at 30 days there was no significant difference in the end point of death or MI (see table 1, p 246). The RCT that included five treatment arms (high and low dose lamifiban ± heparin versus heparin plus placebo) was able to compare low and high dose lamifiban alone versus heparin. It found no significant difference in combined outcome of death or non-fatal MI at 30 days between heparin alone, low dose lamifiban alone, or high dose lamifiban alone (AR of death or MI, 11.7% with heparin v 10.6% with low dose lamifiban v 12.0% with high dose lamifiban, P = 0.67).[5] However, at 6 months there were significantly fewer deaths or MI in people on low dose lamifiban alone, compared with high dose lamifiban alone or heparin alone (AR of death or MI, 13.7% with low dose lamifiban v 16.4% with high dose lamifiban v 17.9% with heparin). One further RCT, which included three arms (tirofiban v heparin v both) found that tirofiban alone increased mortality at 7 days compared with other treatments.[3] This arm of the trial was therefore stopped early.[3]

Harms: No significant difference was reported in rates of major bleeding between tirofiban and heparin (AR 0.4% in both groups).[6] When high dose lamifiban was added to heparin, there were significantly more intermediate or major bleeds versus heparin alone (AR 12.1% v 5.5%, P = 0.002), although bleeding rates were similar with low dose lamifiban plus heparin compared with heparin plus placebo.[5] Reversible thrombocytopenia occurred more frequently with tirofiban than with heparin (AR 1.1% v 0.4%, P = 0.04).[6]

Comment: The smaller trial of adding a glycoprotein IIb/IIIa inhibitor to standard treatment[5] suggests that a "dose ceiling" may exist beyond which escalation of dose results in higher bleeding complications with no increase in efficacy.

OPTION	ORAL GLYCOPROTEIN IIB/IIIA PLATELET RECEPTOR INHIBITORS

Two RCTs have found no significant difference in outcome between oral glycoprotein IIb/IIIa inhibitors versus, or in addition to, aspirin. One RCT found that orbofiban versus placebo significantly increased mortality at 30 days.

Benefits: We found no systematic review. **Versus aspirin:** One RCT (9233 people, 75% with non-Q wave MI) compared aspirin versus low dose sibrafiban (designed to achieve ≥ 25% inhibition of platelet aggregation) or high dose sibrafiban (designed to achieve ≥ 50% inhibition of platelet aggregation).[7] The dose of sibrafiban ranged from 3–6 mg. The RCT found no significant difference between aspirin versus sibrafiban in the primary composite end point of death, MI, or severe recurrent ischaemia after 90 days of treatment (aspirin v low dose sibrafiban [9.8%] v [10.1%]; OR 1.03, 95% CI 0.87 to 1.21: aspirin v high dose sibrafiban [9.8%] v [10.1%]; OR 1.03, 95% CI 0.87 to 1.21). **Versus placebo:** One RCT (10 288 people, 60% with non-Q wave MI) compared orbofiban (50 mg twice daily) or orbofiban (50 mg twice daily for 30 days, then 30 mg twice daily thereafter) versus placebo.[8] All people received aspirin prior to randomisation. It found no significant difference between orbofiban versus placebo in the primary composite end point of death, MI, recurrent ischaemia, urgent revascularisation, or stroke after 30 days (orbofiban groups combined v placebo, 9.9% v 10.8%, P = 0.12), or after 10 months (orbofiban fixed dose v placebo, 22.8% v 22.9%, P = 0.59; variable dose v placebo, 23.1% v 22.9%, P = 0.41), but found a significant increase in mortality at 30 days (orbofiban groups combined v placebo, 2.0% v 1.4%, P = 0.02), which did not quite reach significance at 10 months (orbofiban variable dose v placebo, 5.1% v 3.7%, P = 0.09). The unexpected increased mortality resulted in premature termination of the trial.[8]

Harms: The first RCT found that major bleeding was increased in people taking sibrafiban versus placebo, but was only significant for high dose sibrafiban.[7] The second RCT found that major or severe bleeding (excluding intracranial haemorrhage) was significantly increased in both orbofiban groups (fixed dose v placebo, 4.5% v 2.0%, P < 0.0001; variable dose 3.7% v 2.0%, P = 0.0004).[8]

Comment: None.

| QUESTION | What are the effects of antithrombin treatments? |

| OPTION | UNFRACTIONATED HEPARIN |

Two systematic reviews of six small RCTs have found benefit from adding unfractionated heparin to aspirin in people with unstable angina, but this may have occurred by chance.

Benefits: **Added to aspirin:** We found two systematic reviews that met our quality criteria.[9,10] Both included the same six RCTs in 1353 people with unstable angina who were treated with either heparin and aspirin or aspirin alone for 2–7 days. The first review (search date not stated) found that the risk of death or MI during treatment with heparin plus aspirin was less than that for aspirin alone (AR 55/698 [8%] v 68/655 [10%]); but was not significantly different (OR 0.67, 95% CI 0.44 to 1.02).[9] The second review (search date not stated) used a different statistical method for meta-analysis and found a result that just reached statistical significance (OR 0.67, 95% CI 0.45 to 0.99).[10] The first systematic review also found no significant difference between the two groups (from 4 RCTs with data available) in the rate of death or MI at 12 weeks (AR 12% on heparin plus aspirin v 14% on aspirin alone; RR 0.82, 95% CI 0.56 to 1.20).[9] **Versus LMWH:** See benefits of LMWH, p 241.

Harms: Major bleeding occurred in 0.4% of people on aspirin and 1.5% of those on aspirin plus heparin (RR 1.89, 95% CI 0.66 to 5.38).[9]

Comment: In this situation it is not clear which statistical method is preferred.

| OPTION | LOW MOLECULAR WEIGHT HEPARINS |

One systematic review has found that aspirin plus LMWH is more effective than aspirin alone in the first 30 days after an episode of unstable angina. One systematic review found no significant difference in benefits between LMWH and unfractionated heparin. One systematic

review comparing short term treatment with LMWH versus unfractionated heparin found no significant difference in the frequency of major bleeding, and found that long term LMWH is associated with a significant increase in the risk of major bleeding compared with placebo.

Benefits: **Adding LMWH to aspirin:** We found one systematic review (search date not stated, 2 RCTs, 1639 people),[10] which compared LMWH for up to 7 days versus placebo or untreated control. The review found a reduction in death or MI with LMWH (OR 0.34, 95% CI 0.20 to 0.58). The same systematic review found five RCTs (12 099 people) comparing long term LMWH versus placebo. The review found no benefit of long term LMWH given for up to 90 days (OR for death or MI, LMWH v placebo 0.98, 95% CI 0.81 to 1.17). **Versus unfractionated heparin:** We found one systematic review of five RCTs (12 171 people),[10] which compared an equal duration (maximum 8 days) of LMWH versus unfractionated heparin. The review found no significant difference between treatments (OR for death or MI, LMWH v unfractionated heparin 0.88, 95% CI 0.69 to 1.12).

Harms: One systematic review comparing LMWH versus unfractionated heparin found no significant difference in the frequency of major bleeds between treatments (OR 1.00, 95% CI 0.64 to 1.57)[10] (see harms of unfractionated heparin, p 240). Long term LMWH versus placebo significantly increases the risk of major bleeding (OR 2.26, 95% CI 1.63 to 3.14), equivalent to an excess of 12 bleeds for every 1000 people treated.[10]

Comment: LMWH may be more attractive than unfractionated heparin for routine short term use because coagulation monitoring is not required and it can be self administered after discharge.

OPTION   **HIRUDIN**

RCTs have found that in people with unstable angina taking aspirin, rates of death and MI are significantly lower during infusion of hirudin than during infusion of unfractionated heparin. However, no added benefit is found once the infusion stops. Longer durations of hirudin infusion (> 72 hours) are currently being evaluated. Compared with heparin, hirudin causes significantly more major bleeds requiring transfusion but no more life threatening bleeds or haemorrhagic strokes.

Benefits: We found no systematic review. **Versus unfractionated heparin:** Three large RCTs (>19 000 people with unstable angina taking aspirin, compared R-hirudin versus unfractionated heparin given for 2–3 days.[11-13] A pooled analysis of these trials found reduced risk of cardiovascular death or MI at the end of the 72 hour treatment period (AR 233/9615 [2.4%] for hirudin, 315/9446 [3.3%] for heparin; ARR 0.9%, 95% CI 0.5% to 1.3%; RR 0.77, 95% CI 0.61 to 0.86), with some loss of this early benefit at 7 days (RR 0.83, 95% CI 0.73 to 0.94) and 35 days (RR 0.91, 95% CI 0.83 to 1.0).

Harms: In the largest RCT, hirudin versus unfractionated heparin was associated with a significant increase in the need for transfusion (AR 10.2% v 8.4%, P = 0.01), and a trend for increased extracranial haemorrhage (AR 10.2% v 8.6%, P = 0.06) and intracranial haemorrhage (AR 0.2% v 0.02%, P = 0.06).[11] In the second largest RCT, hirudin was associated with an excess of major bleeding (AR 1.2% v 0.7%; RR 1.71, 95% CI 1.13 to 2.58) but no increase in life threatening bleeds or strokes at day 7.[13] The smallest RCT reported no haemorrhagic strokes and no difference in the rate of major bleeds (about 1% in all groups).[12] Hirudin was associated with a higher rate of minor bleeding (AR 16.2% low dose hirudin [LDHir] v 21.3% medium dose hirudin [MDHir] v 10.5% heparin; RR LDHir v heparin 1.54, 95% CI 1.03 to 2.31; RR MDHir v heparin 2.03, 95% CI 1.39 to 2.96).[12]

Comment: Whether longer duration of treatment has greater benefits is the target of future trials (S Yusuf, personal communication). Two of the RCTs gave doses of hirudin in proportion to the body weight, but gave heparin as a fixed dose.[11,12]

QUESTION   **What are the effects of anti-ischaemic treatments?**

OPTION   **NITRATES, β BLOCKERS, AND CALCIUM CHANNEL BLOCKERS**

We found insufficient evidence on the effects of nitrates, β blockers, and calcium channel blockers on rates of death or MI. Short acting dihydropyridine calcium channel blockers may increase mortality.

Benefits: **Nitrates:** We found no systematic reviews or RCTs of nitrates versus placebo in unstable angina. We found one RCT (162 people with unstable angina) of intravenous glyceryl trinitrate versus placebo for 48 hours. Those receiving glyceryl trinitrate had fewer episodes of chest pain, less severe episodes (pain lasting ≥ 20 minutes), and less need for additional sublingual glyceryl trinitrate.[14] We found one RCT (200 people with unstable angina within 6 months of PTCA) comparing intravenous glyceryl trinitrate, heparin, and glyceryl trinitrate plus heparin versus placebo. The trial found that recurrent angina occurred significantly less frequently in people treated with glyceryl trinitrate alone and glyceryl trinitrate plus heparin compared with placebo, but there was no benefit from heparin alone or additional benefit from combination treatment (P < 0.003 for glyceryl trinitrate alone and for glyceryl trinitrate plus heparin v placebo)[15] **β Blockers:** We found no systematic review of β blockers versus placebo in unstable angina. We found two RCTs. The first RCT (338 people with rest angina not receiving β blocker) compared nifedipine, metoprolol, both, or neither versus placebo.[16] The main outcome was recurrent angina or MI within 48 hours. Metoprolol was significantly more effective than nifedipine. The second RCT (81 people with unstable angina on "optimal doses" of nitrates and nifedipine) compared placebo versus at least 160 mg a day of propranolol.[17] The incidence of cardiac death, MI, and requirement for coronary artery bypass grafting or percutaneous coronary interventions at 30 days did not differ significantly between the two groups (propranolol 16/42 v placebo 18/39, P = NS). People taking propranolol had a lower cumulative probability of experiencing recurrent rest angina over the first 4 days of the trial. The mean number of clinical episodes of angina, duration of angina, glyceryl trinitrate requirement, and ischaemic ST changes by continuous ECG monitoring was also lower. **Calcium channel blockers:** We found one systematic review (search date not stated). It found that calcium channel blockers reduced symptoms and ischaemia but had no effect on rates of MI or death.[18]

Harms: Hypotension is a potential adverse effect of nitrates. However, both older and more recent large RCTs in people with other ischaemic conditions showed that nitrates were safe and well tolerated when used judiciously in clinically appropriate doses. Potential adverse effects of β blockers include bradycardia, exacerbation of reactive airways disease, and hypoglycaemia in diabetics. Observational studies have reported increased mortality with short acting dihydro-pyridine calcium channel blockers (such as nifedipine) in people with coronary heart disease.[19,20]

Comment: We found no good evidence that anti-ischaemic drugs (nitrates, β blockers, calcium channel blockers) prevent death or MI. By consensus, until further data are available, intravenous nitrates remain a first line treatment together with heparin and aspirin in unstable angina.

QUESTION What are the effects of invasive treatments?

OPTION EARLY ROUTINE CARDIAC CATHETERISATION AND REVASCULARISATION

RCTs have found that early invasive treatment reduces symptoms and promotes early discharge compared with early conservative treatment in people with unstable angina. However, they found that early invasive treatment did not reduce rates of death and MI. We found insufficient evidence to ascertain whether certain people (e.g. those who are refractory to medical treatment) are more likely than others to benefit from early invasive treatment.

Benefits: We found no systematic review. We found three RCTs comparing early routine angiography/revascularisation versus medical treatment alone.[21-24] The largest, most recent RCT (2457 people with unstable angina) compared early invasive treatment (within the first 7 days) versus non-invasive treatment plus planned coronary angiography, followed by placebo controlled long term dalteparin for 3 months, using a factorial randomisation protocol.[24] All people were initially treated with open label dalteparin or standard heparin for up to 72 hours after admission. In people randomised to invasive treatment, 96% underwent cardiac catheterisation, and 71% underwent revascularisation within the first 10 days. The trial found that compared with early non-invasive treatment, early invasive treatment reduced the risk of the primary end point of combined death and MI at 6 months (113/1207 [9.4%] v 148/1226 [12.1%]; RR 0.78, 95% CI 0.62 to 0.98), but did not significantly reduce mortality at 6 months (23/1207 [1.9%] with early invasive treatment v 36/1226 [2.9%] with non-invasive treatment; RR 0.65, 95% CI 0.39 to 1.09). The trial also found that invasive treatment significantly reduced angina and re-admission rates (presence of angina at 6 months, 256/1174 [22%] with invasive treatment v 455/1177 [39%] with non-invasive treatment; RR 0.56, 95% CI 0.50 to 0.64, P < 0.001; re-admission during 6 month period, 357/1167 [31%] with invasive treatment v 594/1204 [49%] with non-invasive treatment, RR 0.62, 95% CI 0.60 to 0.69, P < 0.001). The second RCT (1473 people with unstable angina presenting within

24 hours of ischaemic chest discomfort) used a factorial design to compare tissue plasminogen activator versus placebo, and early invasive treatment (cardiac catheterisation at 18–48 hours) versus early conservative treatment.[21,22] All people received aspirin and unfractionated heparin. Within 6 weeks, 64% of people randomised to conservative treatment underwent cardiac catheterisation, 26% underwent percutaneous transluminal coronary angioplasty, and 24% underwent coronary artery bypass grafting. At 6 weeks, there was no significant difference in the composite end point of death, MI, or a symptom limited exercise stress test (invasive 18.1% v conservative 16.2%, P = 0.78). However, invasive treatment significantly reduced re-admission (7.8% v 14.1%, P < 0.001), total duration of all re-admissions (total 365 days v 930 days, P < 0.001), and need for antianginal medications (P < 0.02). At 1 year, there was no significant difference in rates of death or MI (invasive 10.8% v conservative 12.2%, P = 0.42), but the lower numbers of repeat hospital admissions and hospital days with invasive treatment persisted. The third and smallest RCT (920 people) compared invasive versus conservative treatment.[23] Over 23 months of follow up (range 12–44 months) there was no significant difference in the combined primary end point of death or MI (RR 0.87, 95% CI 0.68 to 1.10).

Harms: The largest, most recent RCT found that early invasive treatment increased major bleeding compared with early non-invasive treatment, but found no significant difference between treatments for ischaemic or haemorrhagic stroke (major bleeds, AR 1.6% with invasive treatment v 0.7% with non-invasive treatment, P value not given).[24] The second RCT reported no differences in complication rates (death, MI, emergency coronary artery bypass grafting, abrupt vessel closure, haemorrhage, serious hypotension) between invasive and conservative treatment (14% v 13%, P = 0.38).[21,22] In the smallest RCT, people who underwent early invasive treatment were significantly more at risk of death or MI at hospital discharge (36 v 15 people, P = 0.004), 30 days after randomisation (48 v 26 people, P = 0.012), and at 1 year (111 v 85 people, P = 0.05).[23]

Comment: All trials have reported only short term and medium term follow up, so we cannot exclude a long term difference in effect between early invasive and early non-invasive strategies. It is not clear yet whether there are subgroups of people that benefit particularly from either invasive or conservative treatment. Advances in catheterisation and revascularisation technology and periprocedural management may reduce the early risks of invasive treatment in the future.

REFERENCES

1. Antiplatelet Trialists' Collaboration. Collaborative overview of randomised trials of antiplatelet therapy. I: Prevention of death, myocardial infarction, and stroke by prolonged antiplatelet therapy in various categories of patients. *BMJ* 1994;308:81–106. Search date 1990; primary sources Medline, Current Contents.

2. Balsano F, Rizzon P, Violi F, et al, and the Studio della Ticlopidina nell'Angina Instabile Group. Antiplatelet treatment with ticlopidine in unstable angina: a controlled multicentre clinical trial. *Circulation* 1990;82:17–26.

3. PRISM-PLUS Study Investigators. Inhibition of the platelet glycoprotein IIb/IIIa receptor with tirofiban in unstable angina and non-Q-wave myocardial infarction. *N Engl J Med* 1998;338:1488–1497.

4. Pursuit Trial Investigators. Inhibition of platelet glycoprotein IIb/IIIa with eptifibatide in patients with acute coronary syndromes. *N Engl J Med* 1998;339:436–443.

5. PARAGON Investigators. International, randomized, controlled trial of lamifiban (a platelet glycoprotein IIb/IIIa inhibitor), heparin, or both in unstable angina. *Circulation* 1998;97:2386–2395.

6. PRISM Study Investigators. A comparison of aspirin plus tirofiban with aspirin plus heparin for unstable angina. *N Engl J Med* 1998;338:1498–1505.

7. The SYMPHONY Investigators. Sibrafiban versus Aspirin to Yield Maximum Protection from Ischemic Heart Events Post-acute Coronary Syndromes. *Lancet* 2000;355:337–345. Comparison of sibrafiban with aspirin for prevention of cardiovascular events after acute coronary syndromes: a randomised trial.

8. Cannon CP, McCabe CH, Wilcox RG, et al. Oral glycoprotein IIb/IIIa inhibition with orbofiban in patients with unstable coronary syndromes (OPUS-TIMI 16) trial. *Circulation* 2000;102:149–156.

9. Oler A, Whooley MA, Oler J, Grady D. Adding heparin to aspirin reduces the incidence of myocardial infarction and death in patients with unstable angina: a meta-analysis. *JAMA* 1996; 276:811–815. Search date 1995; primary sources Medline 1966 to September 1995, hand search of reference lists, consultation with experts.

10. Eikelboom JW, Anand SS, Malmberg K, et al. Unfractionated heparin and low molecular weight heparin in acute coronary syndrome without ST elevation: a meta-analysis. *Lancet* 2000;355:1936–1942. Search date not stated; primary sources Medline and Embase, reference lists of published papers were scanned, experts canvassed for unpublished trials, personal data.

11. GUSTO IIb Investigators. A comparison of recombinant hirudin with heparin for the treatment of acute coronary syndromes. *N Engl J Med* 1996; 335:775–782.

12. OASIS Investigators. Comparison of the effects of two doses of recombinant hirudin compared with heparin in patients with acute myocardial ischemia without ST elevation: a pilot study. *Circulation* 1997;96:769–777.

13. OASIS-2 Investigators. Effects of recombinant hirudin (lepirudin) compared with heparin on death, myocardial infarction, refractory angina, and revascularisation procedures in patients with acute myocardial ischaemia without ST elevation: a randomised trial. *Lancet* 1999;353:429–38.

14. Karlberg KE, Saldeen T, Wallin R, et al. Intravenous nitroglycerine reduces ischaemia in unstable angina pectoris: a double-blind placebo-controlled study. *J Intern Med* 1998;243:25–31.

15. Douchet S, Malekianpour M, Theroux P, et al. Randomized trial comparing intravenous nitroglycerin and heparin for treatment of unstable angina secondary or restenosis after coronary artery angioplasty. *Circulation* 2000;101: 955–961.

16. HINT Research Group. Early treatment of unstable angina in the coronary care unit: a randomized, double blind, placebo controlled comparison of recurrent ischaemia in patients treated with nifedipine or metoprolol or both. *Br Heart J* 1986; 56:400–413.

17. Gottlieb SO, Weisfeldt ML, Ouyang P, et al. Effect of the addition of propranolol to therapy with nifedipine for unstable angina pectoris: a randomized, double-blind, placebo-controlled trial. *Circulation* 1986;73:331–337.

18. Held PH, Yusuf S, Furberg CD. Calcium channel blockers in acute myocardial infarction and unstable angina: an overview. *BMJ* 1989;299: 1187–1192. Search date not stated; primary sources not specified in detail.

19. Furberg CD, Psaty BM, Meyer JV. Nifedipine: dose-related increase in mortality in patients with coronary heart disease. *Circulation* 1995;92: 1326–1331. Search date and primary sources not specified.

20. WHO-ISH Study. Ad hoc subcommittee of the liaison committee of the World Health Organisation and the International Society of Hypertension: effects of calcium antagonists on the risks of coronary heart disease, cancer and bleeding. *J Hypertens* 1997:15:105–115.

21. The TIMI IIIB Investigators. Effects of tissue plasminogen activator and a comparison of early invasive and conservative strategies in unstable angina and non-Q-wave myocardial infarction. Results of the TIMI IIIB trial. *Circulation* 1994;89: 1545–1556.

22. Anderson V, Cannon CP, Stone PH, et al, for the TIMI IIIB Investigators. One-year results of the thrombolysis in myocardial infarction (TIMI) IIIB clinical trial: a randomized comparison of tissue-type plasminogen activator versus placebo and early invasive versus early conservative strategies in unstable angina and non-Q wave myocardial infarction. *J Am Coll Cardiol* 1995;26: 1643–1650.

23. Boden WE, O'Rourke RA, Crawford MH, et al, for the VANQWISH Trial Investigators. Outcomes in patients with acute non-Q-wave myocardial infarction randomly assigned to an invasive as compared with a conservative management strategy. *N Engl J Med* 1998;338:1785–1792.

24. Yusuf S, Zucker D, Peduzzi P, et al. Effect of coronary artery bypass graft surgery on survival: overview of 10-year results from randomized trials by the coronary artery bypass graft surgery trialists collaboration. *Lancet* 1994;344:563–570.

Madhu Natarajan
Division of Cardiology
McMaster University
Hamilton
Canada

Competing interests: None declared.

Cardiovascular disorders

TABLE 1 Effects of intravenous glycoprotein IIb/IIIa inhibitors in unstable angina and non-Q wave myocardial infarction: results of main RCTs (see text, pp 238, 239).

Trial	Total participants	Comparison	Odds reduction for death or MI at 30 days* (95% CI)	NNT to avoid one additional death or MI at 30 days
PRISM-PLUS[3]	1570	Tirofiban + heparin v heparin alone	30% (4% to 49%)	31
PURSUIT[4]	10 948	Eptifibatide + heparin v heparin alone	11% (1.3% to 20%)	67
PARAGON[5]	2282	Lamifiban + heparin v heparin alone	4% (−32% to +30%)	NA
PRISM[6]	3232	Aspirin + tirofiban v aspirin + heparin	20% (−5% to +39%)	NA

* = 1–OR, equivalent to RRR; NA, not applicable; MI, myocardial infarction.

INTERVENTIONS

Key Messages

- RCTs have found that compression heals venous leg ulcers more effectively than no compression.
- One systematic review has found that oral pentoxifylline (oxpentifylline) versus placebo increases the proportion of ulcers that heal completely.
- One systematic review found that, in the presence of compression, hydrocolloid dressings did not heal venous leg ulcers more effectively than simple, non-adherent dressings.
- We found insufficient evidence to determine whether topical negative pressure, or any particular occlusive or non-occlusive dressing, increased healing or reduced the pain of venous leg ulcers.
- We found limited evidence that human skin equivalent or peri-ulcer injection of granulocyte–macrophage colony stimulating factor may accelerate healing.
- Two RCTs have found that flavonoids increase the rate of healing of venous leg ulcers, but we found no evidence that either stanozolol or rutoside decrease recurrence rates.

Venous leg ulcers

- We found insufficient evidence on the effects of aspirin, intermittent pneumatic compression, oral zinc supplements, ultrasound, low level laser treatment, skin grafting, or vein surgery.
- We found limited evidence that compression prevented recurrence of venous leg ulcers.

DEFINITION	Definitions of leg ulcers vary, but the following is widely used: loss of skin on the leg or foot that takes more than 6 weeks to heal. Some definitions exclude ulcers confined to the foot, whereas others include ulcers on the whole of the lower limb. This review deals with ulcers of venous origin in people without concurrent diabetes mellitus, arterial insufficiency, or rheumatoid arthritis.
INCIDENCE/ PREVALENCE	Between 1.5 and 3/1000 people have active leg ulcers. Prevalence increases with age to about 20/1000 in people aged over 80 years.[1]
AETIOLOGY/ RISK FACTORS	Leg ulceration is strongly associated with venous disease. However, about a fifth of people with leg ulceration have arterial disease, either alone or in combination with venous problems, which may require specialist referral.[1] Venous ulcers (also known as varicose or stasis ulcers) are caused by venous reflux or obstruction, both of which lead to poor venous return and venous hypertension.
PROGNOSIS	People with leg ulcers have a poorer quality of life than age matched controls because of pain, odour, and reduced mobility.[2] In the UK, audits have found wide variation in the types of care (hospital inpatient care, hospital clinics, outpatient clinics, home visits), in the treatments used (topical agents, dressings, bandages, stockings), in healing rates, and in recurrence rates (26–69% in 1 year).[3,4]
AIMS	To promote healing; to reduce recurrence; to improve quality of life, with minimal adverse effects.
OUTCOMES	Ulcer area; number of ulcers healed; number of ulcer free limbs; recurrence rates; number of new ulcer episodes; number of ulcer free weeks or months; number of people who are ulcer free; frequency of dressing/bandage changes; quality of life; adverse effects of treatment.
METHODS	*Clinical Evidence* search and appraisal June 2001. We included RCTs with clinically important and objective outcomes: proportion of wounds healed, healing rates, incidence of new or recurring wounds, infection, and quality of life.

QUESTION   **What are the effects of treatments?**

OPTION   **COMPRESSION**

One systematic review has found that compression heals venous leg ulcers more effectively than no compression. Elastomeric multilayer, high compression bandages, Unna's boot, high compression hosiery, and European short stretch bandages are all effective. We found insufficient evidence to compare different methods of compression.

Benefits: **Compression versus no compression:** We found one recent systematic review (search date 2000, 6 RCTs, 260 people) comparing compression versus no compression.[5] The review found that compression (e.g. short stretch bandages, double layer bandage, and Unna's boot — see glossary, p 256) healed venous leg ulcers more effectively than no compression (e.g. dressing alone). The trials were heterogeneous, using different forms of compression in different settings and populations. The results were not pooled. The results of individual RCTs consistently favoured compression. **Elastomeric versus non-elastomeric multilayer compression:** The systematic review identified three RCTs (273 people) comparing elastomeric multilayer high compression bandages (see glossary, p 255) versus non-elastomeric multilayer compression.[5] Meta-analysis found an increase in the proportion of people whose ulcers healed with 12–15 weeks of high compression treatment versus controls (RRI for healing 54%, 95% CI 19% to 100%; NNT for 12–15 weeks' treatment 5, 95% CI 3 to 12)[5] (see table 1, p 257). **Multilayer high compression versus short stretch regimens:** The systematic review identified four small RCTs (164 people), which found no significant difference between multilayer high compression and short stretch regimens (RRI for healing 10%, 95% CI −22% to +55%).[5] The lack of power in these small studies means that a clinically important difference cannot be excluded. **Multilayer high compression versus single layer bandage:** The systematic review identified four RCTs (280 people) comparing multilayer high compression versus a single layer of bandage.[5] Meta-analysis found an increase in the proportion of ulcers healing with multilayered compression versus controls (RRI 41%, 95% CI 11% to 80%; NNT for variable periods of treatment 6, 95% CI 4 to 18) (see table 1, p 257).

Harms: High levels of compression applied to limbs with insufficient arterial supply, or inexpert application of bandages, can lead to tissue damage and, at worst, amputation.[10] Complication rates were rarely reported in trials.

Comment: People found to be suitable for high compression are those with clinical signs of venous disease (ulcer in the gaiter region, from the upper margin of the malleolus to the bulge of the gastrocnemius; staining of the skin around an ulcer; or eczema), no concurrent diabetes mellitus or rheumatoid arthritis, and adequate arterial supply to the foot as determined by ankle/brachial pressure index. The precise ankle/brachial pressure index below which compression is contraindicated is often quoted as 0.8; however, many trials used the higher cut off of 0.9.[5] Effectiveness is likely to be influenced by the ability of those applying the bandage to generate safe levels of compression. Bandages may be applied by the person with the leg ulcer, their carer, nurse, or doctor. We found no comparisons of healing rates between specialist and non-specialist application of compression. Training improves bandaging technique among nurses.[11] Bandages containing elastomeric fibres can be applied weekly as they maintain their tension over time. Bandages made of wool or cotton, or both, such as short stretch bandages, may need to be reapplied more frequently as they do not maintain their tension.

Cardiovascular disorders

OPTION   INTERMITTENT PNEUMATIC COMPRESSION

Three small RCTs found no evidence of improved healing with intermittent pneumatic compression plus compression bandages versus compression bandages alone.

Benefits: We found one systematic review (search date 1997, 2 RCTs, 67 people) comparing intermittent pneumatic compression (see glossary, p 255) in conjunction with compression (bandages or hosiery) versus compression alone.[12] We found one subsequent RCT (53 people).[13] These trials were all different in design. Pooling of results, using a random effects model, found no difference in healing rates.

Harms: None reported.

Comment: Availability may vary widely between healthcare settings. Treatment can be delivered in the home, in outpatient clinics, or in the hospital ward. Clinical trials have evaluated the use of intermittent pneumatic pressure for 1 hour twice weekly and 3–4 hours daily. Treatment requires resting for 1–4 hours daily, which may reduce quality of life.

OPTION   DRESSINGS AND TOPICAL AGENTS

One RCT has found that bilayer skin replacement versus simple dressings significantly increases complete ulcer healing. Another small RCT has found that infections of granulocyte–macrophage colony stimulating factors versus placebo significantly increase complete healing. We found insufficient evidence on the effects of occlusive or semi-occlusive dressings, simple primary dressings, other topical agents, topical negative pressure, or antimicrobial agents compared with simple primary dressings such as gauze.

Benefits: **Simple low adherent dressings versus occlusive or semi-occlusive dressings:** We found one systematic review (search date 1997, 16 RCTs) comparing occlusive (hydrocolloids) or semi-occlusive dressings (foam, film, alginates) versus simple dressings (such as paraffin-tulle, knitted viscose dressings).[14] Nine of the RCTs compared hydrocolloid dressings versus simple dressings in the presence of compression. A pooled analysis of seven RCTs (714 people) found no evidence of benefit. Two comparisons of foam dressings versus simple dressings; two of film dressings versus simple dressings; and one comparing an alginate versus a simple dressing found no evidence of benefit. However, the RCTs were too small (10–132 people, median 60) to detect anything but a very large difference in effectiveness. **Comparisons between occlusive or semi-occlusive dressings:** The same systematic review identified 12 small RCTs comparing different occlusive or semi-occlusive dressings.[14] There was no significant difference in healing rates between dressings, or insufficient data were provided to calculate their significance. We found one subsequent RCT comparing hydrocolloid and hydrocellular dressings, which found no difference in healing rates.[15] **Topical agents versus inert comparators:** The same systematic review identified 16 RCTs comparing topical agents (such as growth factors, cell suspensions, oxygen free-radical scavengers) versus either placebo preparations or standard care in the treatment of venous leg ulcers.[14] There was insufficient evidence to recommend any topical agent. The studies were small (9–233 people, median 45) and heterogeneous; therefore, results could not be pooled. Five RCTs of topical agents have been published since the systematic review search. One RCT (66 people) of calcitonin (salcatonin) gene related peptide and vasoactive intestinal polypeptide administered by iontophoresis (see glossary, p 255) versus electrical stimulation found no evidence of benefit.[16] One RCT (60 people) compared a 13 week course of injections around the ulcer of granulocyte–macrophage colony stimulating factor 400 μg versus placebo and found an increased proportion of ulcers completely healed (RRI 236%, 95% CI 13% to 1134%; NNT for 6 months' treatment 2, 95% CI 1 to 19) (see table 1, p 257).[7] One RCT (293 people) comparing a cultured allogenic bilayer skin (see glossary, p 255) replacement, which contained both epidermal and dermal components with a non-adherent dressing, found a greater proportion of ulcers healed completely in 6 months with the skin replacement (RRI for the proportion of ulcers healed 29%, 95% CI 4% to 61%; NNT for 6 months' treatment 7, 95% CI 4 to 41) (see table 1, p 257).[8] One RCT (40 people) of topically applied mesoglycan, a profibrinolytic agent, found no evidence of benefit.[17] One RCT (86 people) found no difference after 9 months in time to healing with topical autologous platelet lysate versus placebo.[18] **Topical negative pressure**: We found one systematic review (search date 2000, 2 small RCTs, 34 people).[19] One of the RCTs included some people with venous leg ulcers. It found no clear evidence of benefit of topical negative pressure (see glossary, p 255). **Antimicrobial agents versus placebo or standard care:** We found one systematic review (search date 1997, 14 RCTs) comparing antimicrobial agents versus either placebo agents or standard care.[20] The RCTs were small (25–153 people, median 56), of poor quality, and no firm conclusions could be drawn.

Harms: It is unlikely that low adherent primary wound dressings cause harm, although dressings containing iodine may affect thyroid function if used over large surface areas for extended periods.[21] Many people (50–85%) with venous leg ulcers have contact sensitivity to preservatives, perfumes, or dyes.[22]

Comment: Simple primary dressings maintain a moist environment beneath compression bandages by preventing loss of moisture from the wound.[23]

OPTION	THERAPEUTIC ULTRASOUND

We found insufficient evidence of the effects of therapeutic ultrasound in the treatment of venous leg ulcers.

Benefits: We found one systematic review (search date 1999, 7 RCTs, 470 people) comparing therapeutic ultrasound (see glossary, p 255) versus no ultrasound or sham ultrasound for venous leg ulcers.[24] Ultrasound improved ulcer healing in all studies, but a significant difference was found in only four of the seven RCTs, and heterogeneity precluded pooling the seven RCTs.

Harms: Mild erythema, local pain, and small areas of bleeding have been reported in some trials.

Comment: None.

Cardiovascular disorders

Venous leg ulcers

| OPTION | DRUG TREATMENTS |

One systematic review has found good evidence that oral pentoxifylline (oxpentifylline) versus placebo accelerates the healing of venous leg ulcers. Two RCTs have found that flavonoids increase the rate of healing of venous leg ulcers. We found limited evidence from one RCT that sulodexide accelerated the healing of venous leg ulcers. We found no good evidence on the effects of aspirin or oral zinc supplements.

Benefits: **Pentoxifylline:** We found one systematic review (search date 1999, 9 RCTs).[6] Eight RCTs compared pentoxifylline (1200 mg or 2400 mg daily) versus placebo in venous leg ulcers. The review pooled results from five RCTs, in which compression was standard treatment, and found that more ulcers healed with pentoxifylline than placebo (RRI for healing 30%, 95% CI 10% to 54%; NNT for 6 months' treatment 6, 95% CI 4 to 14). One RCT found no evidence of benefit for pentoxifylline compared with defibrotide (see table 1, p 257). **Flavonoids:** We found two RCTs (245 people) comparing flavonoid 1000 mg daily (900 mg diosmin and 100 mg hesperidin) versus placebo or standard care.[25,26] These RCTs had different lengths of follow up but were similar in other respects. When pooled in a random effects model, flavonoids healed more ulcers than placebo (RRI 80%, 95% CI 20% to 170%). **Thromboxane α_2 antagonists:** We found one RCT (165 people) of an oral thromboxane α_2 antagonist versus placebo for venous leg ulcers. It found no significant difference in the proportion of ulcers healed (54% v 55%).[27] **Oral zinc:** We found one systematic review (search date 1997, 5 RCTs, 151 people) comparing daily doses of 440–660 mg oral zinc sulphate with placebo. The review found no evidence of benefit for oral zinc.[28] **Aspirin:** We found one small RCT of aspirin (300 mg/day, enteric coated) versus placebo. It found that more ulcers healed with aspirin (38% v 0%), but the trial had several weaknesses.[29] **Sulodexide:** We found one RCT (94 people). It found that more ulcers healed after 60 days' treatment with sulodexide (daily im injection for 30 days and then orally for 30 days) in addition to compression therapy than with compression alone (35% v 58%; RRI 61%, 95% CI 3.5% to 163%; NNT 4, 95% CI 2 to 64).[9]

Harms: The systematic review found more adverse effects with pentoxifylline than with placebo, although this was not significant (RR 1.25, 95% CI 0.87 to 1.80). Nearly half of the adverse effects were gastrointestinal (dyspepsia, vomiting, or diarrhoea).[24] Adverse effects of flavonoids, such as gastrointestinal disturbance, were reported in 10% of people.

Comment: Sulodexide is not widely available and daily injections may be unacceptable to some people.

| OPTION | VEIN SURGERY |

We found insufficient evidence of the effects of vein surgery on ulcer healing.

Benefits: We found no systematic review. We found one RCT (47 people) comparing vein surgery (perforator ligation) versus no surgery or surgery plus skin grafting.[30] There was no difference in the proportion of ulcers healed after 1 year or the rate of ulcer healing. The trial was too small to rule out a beneficial effect.

Harms: Vein surgery carries the usual risks of surgery and anaesthesia.

Comment: Several operative approaches are commonly used, including perforator ligation, saphenous vein stripping, and a combination of both procedures.

OPTION SKIN GRAFTING

We found insufficient evidence of the effects of skin grafting on ulcer healing.

Benefits: We found one systematic review (search date 1999, 6 RCTs, 197 people) of skin grafts (autografts or allografts) for venous leg ulcers.[31] In five RCTs people also received compression bandaging; two RCTs (98 people) evaluated split thickness autografts; three RCTs (92 people) evaluated cultured keratinocyte allografts; and one RCT (7 people, 13 ulcers) compared tissue engineered skin (artificial skin) with split thickness skin grafts. We found insufficient evidence to determine whether skin grafting increased the healing of venous ulcers.[31]

Harms: Taking a skin graft leaves a wound that itself requires management and may cause pain. We found no evidence of harm from tissue engineered skin.

Comment: None.

OPTION LOW LEVEL LASER TREATMENT

We found insufficient evidence of the effects of low level laser treatment on ulcer healing.

Benefits: We found two systematic reviews (search dates 1998).[32,33] The larger review (4 RCTs) of laser therapy for venous leg ulcers included the only two RCTs identified by the smaller review.[32] Two RCTs compared low level laser treatment (see glossary, p 255) with sham; one RCT compared laser with ultraviolet therapy; and one RCT compared laser with non-coherent, unpolarised red light. Neither of the two RCTs of laser versus sham found a significant difference in healing rates. There was no significant difference in healing rates with laser when the trials were pooled. A three arm study (30 people) compared laser treatment with laser treatment plus infrared light and with non-coherent, unpolarised red light. Significantly more ulcers healed completely after 9 months' treatment in the group receiving a combination of laser and infrared light compared with non-coherent, unpolarised red light (RRI 140%, 95% CI 22% to 442%; NNT 2, 95% CI 1 to 9). A fourth RCT compared laser and ultraviolet light and found no significant difference.[32]

Harms: Eye protection is required when using some types of laser as the high energy beam may lead to damage of the retina.

Comment: The laser power, wavelength, frequency, duration, and follow up of treatment were different for all the studies.

Venous leg ulcers

QUESTION **What are the effects of interventions to prevent recurrence?**

OPTION **COMPRESSION**

We found limited evidence that compression reduced recurrence but non-compliance with compression is a risk factor for recurrence.

Benefits: **Versus no compression:** We found one systematic review of compression hosiery versus no compression (search date 2000, no identified RCTs),[34] and one subsequent RCT.[35] The RCT (153 people) found that compression stockings worn versus compression stockings not worn reduced recurrence at 6 months (21% v 46%; RRR 54%, 95% CI 24% to 72%; NNT for 6 months' treatment 2, 95% CI 2 to 5).[35] **Versus other forms of compression:** We found one systematic review (search date 2000, 2 RCTs) (see table 1, p 257).[34] One RCT (166 people) compared two brands of UK Class 2 stockings (see comment below) and found no difference in recurrence. The larger RCT (300 people) compared Class 2 and Class 3 stockings (see comment below). With intention to treat analysis, the RCT found no significant reduction in recurrence after 5 years with high compression hosiery (UK Class 3) compared with moderate compression hosiery (UK Class 2). This analysis may underestimate the effectiveness of the Class 3 hosiery because a significant proportion of people changed from Class 3 to Class 2. Both RCTs found that non-compliance with compression hosiery was associated with recurrence.

Harms: The application of high compression to limbs with reduced arterial supply may result in ischaemic tissue damage and, at worst, amputation.[10]

Comment: Compression hosiery is classified according to the magnitude of pressure exerted at the ankle; the UK classification states that Class 2 hosiery is capable of applying 18–24 mm Hg pressure and Class 3 is capable of applying 25–35 mm Hg pressure at the ankle. Other countries use different classification systems. Hosiery reduces venous reflux by locally increasing venous pressure in the legs relative to the rest of the body. This effect only takes place while hosiery is worn. The association between non-compliance with compression and recurrence of venous ulceration provides some indirect evidence of the benefit of compression in prevention. People are advised to wear compression hosiery for life and may be at risk of pressure necrosis from their compression hosiery if they subsequently develop arterial disease. Regular reassessment of the arterial supply is considered good practice, but we found no evidence about the optimal frequency of assessment. Other measures designed to reduce leg oedema, such as resting with the leg elevated, may be useful.

OPTION **SYSTEMIC DRUGS**

We found insufficient evidence on the effects of systemic drugs on ulcer recurrence.

Benefits: We found one systematic review (search date 1997, 2 RCTs, 198 people) of drugs in the prevention of leg ulcer recurrence.[12] The review concluded that there was no evidence that stanozolol or rutoside decreased recurrence rates. One RCT (60 people) of stanozolol versus placebo found no significant difference in recurrence (17% *v* 20%). The other RCT (139 people) of rutoside versus placebo found no significant difference in recurrence (32% *v* 34%).

Harms: Stanozolol is an anabolic steroid; adverse effects included acne, hirsutism, amenorrhoea, oedema, headache, dyspepsia, rash, hair loss, depression, jaundice, and changes in liver enzymes. Tolerance of rutoside was reported to be good; adverse effects included headache, flushing, rashes, and mild gastrointestinal disturbances.[36]

Comment: None.

OPTION **VEIN SURGERY**

We found insufficient evidence on the effects of vein surgery on ulcer recurrence.

Benefits: We found one systematic review (search date 1997, 1 RCT, 30 people).[12] The identified RCT, which was poorly controlled, compared surgery plus compression hosiery versus compression hosiery alone for prevention of recurrence. It found a reduced rate of recurrence when surgery was carried out in addition to the use of compression hosiery (5% *v* 24%; RRR 0.79, 95% CI 0.20 to 0.97).

Harms: Vein surgery has the usual risks of surgery and anaesthesia.

Comment: The results of this trial should be interpreted with caution because it was small and poorly controlled.

GLOSSARY

Cultured allogenic bilayer skin equivalent Also called human skin equivalent. This is made of a lower (dermal) layer of bovine collagen containing living human dermal fibroblasts and an upper (epidermal) layer of living human keratinocytes.

Elastomeric multilayer high compression bandages Usually a layer of padding material followed by one to three additional layers of elastomeric bandages.

Intermittent pneumatic compression External compression applied by inflatable leggings or boots either over, or instead of, compression hosiery or bandages. A pump successively inflates and deflates the boots to promote the return of blood from the tissues. Newer systems have separate compartments in the boots so that the foot is inflated before the ankle, which is inflated before the calf.

Iontophoresis The delivery of an ionic substance by application of an electrical current.

Low level laser treatment Application of treatment energy (< 10 J/cm^2) using lasers of 50 mW or less.

Short stretch bandages Minimally extensible bandages usually made of cotton with few or no elastomeric fibres. They are applied at near full extension to form a semi-rigid bandage.

Therapeutic ultrasound Application of ultrasound to a wound, using a transducer and a water based gel. Prolonged application can lead to heating of the tissues, but when used in wound healing the power used is low and the transducer is constantly moved by the therapist so that the tissue is not significantly heated.

Topical negative pressure Negative pressure (suction) applied to a wound through an open cell dressing (e.g. foam, felt).

Venous leg ulcers

Unna's boot An inner layer of zinc oxide impregnated bandage, which hardens as it dries to form a semi-rigid layer against which the calf muscle can contract. It is usually covered in an elastomeric bandage.

REFERENCES

1. Callam MJ, Ruckley CV, Harper DR, et al. Chronic ulceration of the leg: extent of the problem and provision of care. *BMJ* 1985;290:1855–1856.

2. Roe B, Cullum N, Hamer C. Patients' perceptions of chronic leg ulceration. In: Cullum N, Roe B, eds. *Leg ulcers: nursing management.* Harrow: Scutari,1995:125–134.

3. Roe B, Cullum N. The management of leg ulcers: current nursing practice. In: Cullum N, Roe B, eds. *Leg ulcers: nursing management.* Harrow: Scutari,1995:113–124.

4. Vowden KR, Barker A, Vowden P. Leg ulcer management in a nurse-led, hospital-based clinic. *J Wound Care* 1997;6:233–236.

5. Cullum N, Nelson EA, Fletcher AW, et al. Compression bandages and stockings in the treatment of venous leg ulcers. In: The Cochrane Library, Issue 3, 2000. Oxford: Update Software. Search date May 2000; primary sources 19 electronic databases, hand searches, and personal contacts.

6. Jull AB, Waters J, Arroll B. Oral pentoxifylline for treatment of venous leg ulcers. In: The Cochrane Library, Issue 3, 2000. Oxford: Update Software. Search date 1999; primary sources Cochrane Peripheral Vascular Diseases and Wounds Group, specialised registers, hand searches of reference lists, relevant journals and conference proceedings, personal contact with manufacturer of pentoxifylline, and experts in the field.

7. Da Costa RM, Ribeiro Jesus FM, Aniceto C, et al. Randomized, double-blind, placebo-controlled, dose-ranging study of granulocyte–macrophage colony stimulating factor in patients with chronic venous leg ulcers. *Wound Repair Regen* 1999;7: 17–25.

8. Falanga V, Margolis D, Alvarez O, et al. Rapid healing of venous ulcers and lack of clinical rejection with an allogeneic cultured human skin equivalent. Human Skin Equivalent Investigators Group. *Arch Dermatol* 1998;134:293–300.

9. Scondotto G, Aloisi D, Ferrari P, et al. Treatment of venous leg ulcers with sulodexide. *Angiology* 99;50:883–889.

10. Callam MJ, Ruckley CV, Dale JJ, et al. Hazards of compression treatment of the leg: an estimate from Scottish surgeons. *BMJ* 1987;295:1382.

11. Nelson EA, Ruckley CV, Barbenel J. Improvements in bandaging technique following training. *J Wound Care* 1995;4:181–184.

12. Cullum N, Fletcher A, Semlyen A, et al. Compression therapy for venous leg ulcers. *Qual Health Care* 1997;6:226–231. Search date April 1997; primary sources 18 databases, including Medline, Embase, Cinahl with no restriction on date, hand searches of relevant journals, conference proceedings, and correspondence with experts to obtain unpublished papers.

13. Schuler JJ, Maibenco T, Megerman J, et al. Treatment of chronic venous leg ulcers using sequential gradient intermittent pneumatic compression. *Phlebology* 1996;11:111–116.

14. Bradley M, Cullum N, Nelson EA, et al. Dressings and topical agents for healing of chronic wounds: a systematic review. *Health Technol Assess* 1999;3 No17(Pt2). Search date October 1997; primary sources Cochrane Library, Medline, Embase, and Cinahl.

15. Seeley J, Jensen JL, Hutcherson J. A randomised clinical study comparing a hydrocellular dressing to a hydrocolloid dressing in the management of pressure ulcers. *Ostomy Wound Manage* 1999; 45:39–47.

16. Gherardini G, Gurlek A, Evans GRD, et al. Venous ulcers: improved healing by iontophoretic administration of calcitonin gene-related peptide and vasoactive intestinal polypeptide. *Plast Reconstr Surg* 1998;101:90–93.

17. La Marc G, Pumilia G, Martino A. Effectiveness of mesoglycan topical treatment of leg ulcers in subjects with chronic venous insufficiency. *Minerva Cardioangiol* 1999;47:315–319.

18. Stacey MC, Mata SD, Trengove NJ, Mather CA. Randomised double-blind placebo controlled trial of autologous platelet lysate in venous ulcer healing. *Eur J Endovasc Surg* 2000;20:296–301.

19. Evans D, Land L. Topical negative pressure for treating chronic wounds. In: The Cochrane Library, Issue 2, 2001. Oxford: Update Software. Search date July 2000; primary sources Cochrane Wounds Group Specialised Trials Register, experts, relevant companies, and a hand search.

20. O'Meara S, Cullum N, Majid M, et al. Systematic reviews of wound care management: (3) antimicrobial agents for chronic wounds. *Health Technol Assess* 2000;4(No 21):1–237. Search date October 1997; primary sources Cochrane Library, Medline, Embase, and Cinahl.

21. Thomas S. *Wound management and dressings.* London: Pharmaceutical Press, 1990.

22. Cameron J, Wilson C, Powell S, et al. Contact dermatitis in leg ulcer patients. *Ostomy Wound Manage* 1992;38:10–11.

23. Wu P, Nelson EA, Reid WH, et al. Water vapour transmission rates in burns and chronic leg ulcers: influence of wound dressings and comparison with in vitro evaluation. *Biomaterials* 1996;17: 1373–1377.

24. Flemming K, Cullum N. Therapeutic ultrasound for venous leg ulcers. In: The Cochrane Library, Issue 3, 2000. Oxford: Update Software. Search date 1999; primary sources Cochrane Wounds Group Specialised Trials Register and hand searches of citation lists.

25. Guilhou JJ, Dereure O, Marzin L, et al. Efficacy of Daflon 500 mg in venous leg ulcer healing: a double-blind, randomized, controlled versus placebo trial in 107 patients. *Angiology* 1997;48: 77–85.

26. Glinski W, Chodynicka B, Roszkiewicz J, et al. The beneficial augmentative effect of micronised purified flavonoid fraction (MPFF) on the healing of leg ulcers: an open, multicentre, controlled randomised study. *Phlebology* 1999;14:151–157.

27. Lyon RT, Veith FJ, Bolton L, et al. Clinical benchmark for healing of chronic venous ulcers. Venous Ulcer Study Collaborators. *Am J Surgery* 1998;176:172–175.

28. Wilkinson EAJ, Hawke CI. Does oral zinc aid the healing of chronic leg ulcers? A systematic literature review. *Arch Dermatol* 1998;134: 1556–1560. Search date 1997; primary sources Medline, Embase, Cinahl, Science Citation Index, Biosis, British Diabetic Association Database, Ciscom, Cochrane Controlled Register of Clinical Trials, Dissertation Abstracts, Royal College of Nursing Database, electronic databases of ongoing research, hand searches of wound care journals and conference proceedings, and contact with manufacturer of zinc sulphate tablets.

29. Layton AM, Ibbotson SH, Davies JA, et al. Randomised trial of oral aspirin for chronic venous leg ulcers. *Lancet* 1994;344:164–165.

30. Warburg FE, Danielsen L, Madsen SM, et al. Vein surgery with or without skin grafting versus conservative treatment for leg ulcers. *Acta Dermatol Vereol* 1994;74:307–309.

31. Jones JE, Nelson EA. Skin grafting for venous leg ulcers. In: The Cochrane Library, Issue 3, 2000. Oxford: Update Software. Search date 1999; primary sources Cochrane Wounds Group Specialised Register, hand searches of reference lists, relevant journals, conference proceedings, and personal contact with experts in the field.

32. Flemming K, Cullum N. Laser therapy for venous leg ulcers. In: The Cochrane Library, Issue 3, 2000. Oxford: Update Software. Search date 1998; primary sources 19 electronic databases, hand searches of journals, conference proceedings, and bibliographies.

33. Lucas C, Stanborough RW, Freeman CL, et al. Efficacy of low level laser therapy on wound healing in human subjects: a systematic review. *Lasers Med Sci* 2000;15:84–93. Search date

1998; primary sources Medline, Embase, Cinahl, Cochrane Rehabilitation, and Related Therapies Register of Trials.

34. Cullum N, Nelson EA, Flemming K, Sheldon T. Systematic reviews of wound care management: (5) beds; (6) compression; (7) laser therapy, therapeutic ultrasound, electrotherapy and electromagnetic therapy. *Health Technol Assess* 2001;5(9). Search date April 2000; primary sources Specialised Trials Register of the Cochrane Wounds Group, 19 electronic databases (up to December 1999), and hand searches of relevant journals, conferences and bibliographies of retrieved publications, and personal contact with manufacturers and an advisory panel of experts.

35. Vandongen YK, Stacey MC. Graduated compression elastic stockings reduce lipodermatosclerosis and ulcer recurrence. *Phlebology* 2000;15:33–37.

36. Taylor HM, Rose KE, Twycross RG. A double-blind clinical trial of hydroxyethylrutosides in obstructive arm lymphoedema. *Phlebology* 1993;8(suppl 1):22–28.

E Andrea Nelson
Research Fellow

Nicky Cullum
Reader

Centre for Evidence Based Nursing
University of York, York, UK

June Jones
Clinical Nurse Specialist
North Sefton and West Lancashire
Community Services NHS Trust
Southport
UK

Competing interests: EAN has been reimbursed for attending symposia by Smith and Nephew, Huntleigh Healthcare Ltd, and Convatec. EAN and NC are applicants on a trial of compression bandages for which Beiersdorf UK Ltd is providing trial related education. JJ has been reimbursed for attending symposia by 3M and Convatec.

TABLE 1	NNTs for healing of leg ulcers (see text, pp 249, 251, 252, 254).

Intervention	NNT (95% CI)
Elastomeric multilayer compression v non-elastomeric multilayer compression bandages	5 (3 to 12)[5]
Multilayer high compression v single layer compression bandages	6 (4 to 18)[5]
Pentoxifylline 400 mg three times a day v placebo (concurrent use of compression)	6 (4 to 14)[6]
Peri-ulcer injection of GM–CSF* (400 µg) v placebo	2 (1 to 19)[7]
Cultured allogenic bilayer skin equivalent v non-adherent dressing	7 (4 to 41)[8]
Sulodexide plus compression v compression alone	4 (2 to 64)[29]

*GM–CSF, granulocyte–macrophage colony stimulating factor.

Subject index

Note

When looking up a class of drug, the reader is advised to also look up specific examples of that class of drug where additional entries may be found. The reverse situation also applies. Abbreviations used: CVD – cardiovascular disease; MI – myocardial infarction.

INDEX

Subject index

Subject index

Estimating cardiovascular risk and treatment benefit

Adapted from the New Zealand guidelines on management of dyslipidaemia[1] and raised blood pressure [2] by Rod Jackson

How to use these colour charts

The charts help the estimation of a person's absolute risk of a cardiovascular event and the likely benefit of drug treatment to lower cholesterol or blood pressure. For these charts cardiovascular events include: new angina, myocardial infarction, coronary death, stroke or transient ischaemic attack (TIA), onset of congestive cardiac failure or peripheral vascular syndrome.

There is a group of patients in whom risk can be assumed to be high (>20% in 5 years) without using the charts. They include those with symptomatic cardiovascular disease (angina, myocardial infarction, congestive heart failure, stroke, TIA, and peripheral vascular disease), or left ventricular hypertrophy on ECG.

To estimate a person's absolute five-year risk:
■ Find the table relating to their sex, diabetic status (on insulin, oral hypoglycaemics or fasting blood glucose over 8 mmol/l), smoking status and age. The age shown in the charts is the mean for that category, i.e. age 60 = 55 to 65 years.
■ Within the table find the cell nearest to the person's blood pressure and total cholesterol : HDL ratio. For risk assessment it is enough to use a mean blood pressure based on two readings on each of two occasions, and cholesterol measurements based on one laboratory or two non-fasting Reflotron measurements. More readings are needed to establish the pre-treatment baseline.
■ The colour of the box indicates the person's five-year cardiovascular disease risk (see below).

Notes: (1) People with a strong history of CVD (first degree male relatives with CVD before 55 years, female relatives before 65 years) or obesity (body mass index above 30 kg/m^2) are likely to be at greater risk than the tables indicate. The magnitude of the independent predictive value of these risk factors remains unclear—their presence should influence treatment decisions for patients at borderline treatment levels. (2) If total cholesterol or total cholesterol:HDL ratio is greater than 8 then the risk is at least 15%. (3) Nearly all people aged 75 years or over also have an absolute cardiovascular risk over 15%.

Charts reproduced with permission from The National Heart Foundation of New Zealand. Also available on http://www.nzgg.org.nz/library/gl_complete/bloodpressure/table1.cfm

REFERENCES

1. Dyslipidaemia Advisory Group. 1996 National Heart Foundation clinical guidelines for the assessment and management of dyslipidaemia. *NZ Med J* 1996;109:224–232.
2. National Health Committee. Guidelines for the management of mildly raised blood pressure in New Zealand: Ministry of Health National Health Committee Report, Wellington, 1995.

RISK LEVEL Five-year CVD risk (non-fatal and fatal)		BENEFIT (1) CVD events prevented per 100 treated for five years*	BENEFIT (2) Number needed to treat for five years to prevent one event*
Very High	>30%	>10 per 100	<10
	25–30%	9 per 100	11
	20–25%	7.5 per 100	13
High	15–20%	6 per 100	16
Moderate	10–15%	4 per 100	25
Mild	5–10%	2.5 per 100	40
	2.5–5%	1.25 per 100	80
	<2.5%	<0.8 per 100	>120

*Based on a 20% reduction in total cholesterol or a reduction in blood pressure of 10–15 mmHg systolic or 5–10 mmHg diastolic, which is estimated to reduce CVD risk by about one third over 5 years.

Estimating cardiovascular risk and treatment benefit

RISK LEVEL: MEN

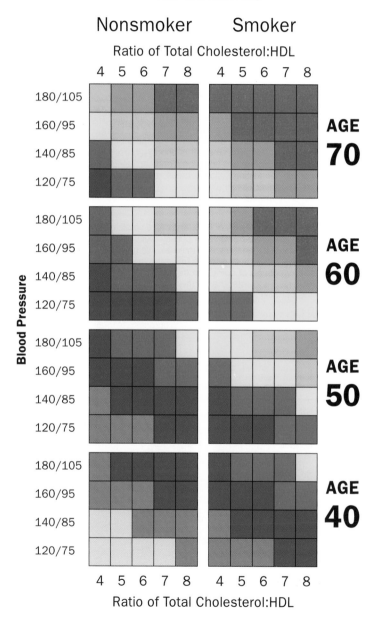

NO DIABETES

Nonsmoker   Smoker

Ratio of Total Cholesterol:HDL

Estimating cardiovascular risk and treatment benefit

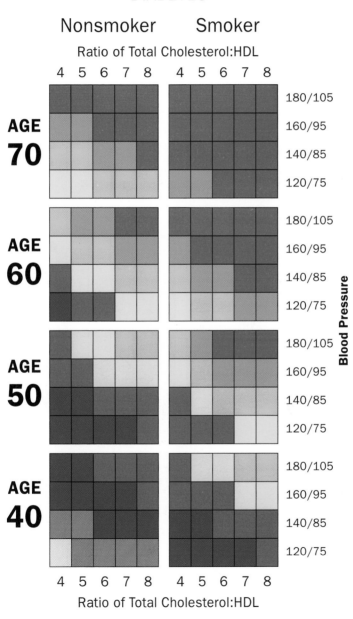

DIABETES

Nonsmoker   Smoker

Ratio of Total Cholesterol:HDL

Blood Pressure

RISK LEVEL: WOMEN

NO DIABETES

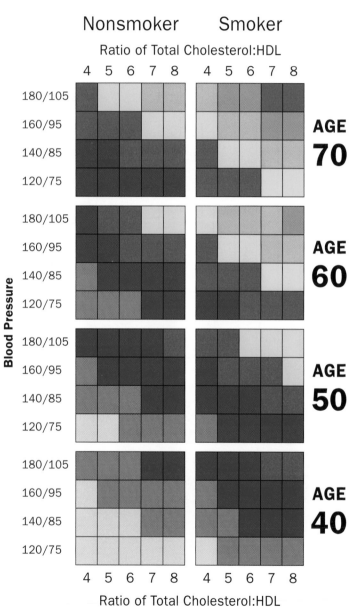

DIABETES

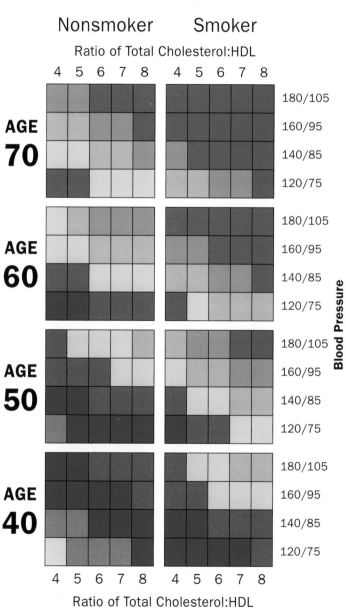

Nonsmoker Smoker

Ratio of Total Cholesterol:HDL

4 5 6 7 8   4 5 6 7 8

AGE 70

180/105
160/95
140/85
120/75

AGE 60

180/105
160/95
140/85
120/75

AGE 50

180/105
160/95
140/85
120/75

AGE 40

180/105
160/95
140/85
120/75

4 5 6 7 8   4 5 6 7 8

Ratio of Total Cholesterol:HDL

Blood Pressure

The number needed to treat: adjusting for baseline risk

Adapted with permission from Chatellier et al, 1996[1]

BACKGROUND

The number needed to treat (NNT) to avoid a single additional adverse outcome is a meaningful way of expressing the benefit of an active treatment over a control. It can be used both to summarise the results of a therapeutic trial or series of trials and to help medical decision making about an individual patient.

If the absolute risk of adverse outcomes in a therapeutic trial is ARC in the control group and ART in the treatment group, then the absolute risk reduction (ARR) is defined as (ARC – ART). The NNT is defined as the inverse of the ARR:

$$NNT = 1/(ARC - ART)$$

Since the Relative Risk Reduction (RRR) is defined as (ARC – ART)/ARC, it follows that NNT, RRR and ARC are related by their definitions in the following way:

$$NNT \times RRR \times ARC = 1$$

This relationship can be used to estimate the likely benefits of a treatment in populations with different levels of baseline risk (that is different levels of ARC). This allows extrapolation of the results of a trial or meta-analysis to people with different baseline risks. Ideally, there should be experimental evidence of the RRR in each population. However in many trials, subgroup analyses show that the RRR is approximately constant in groups of patients with different characteristics. Cook and Sackett therefore proposed that decisions about individual patients could be made by using the NNT calculated from the RRR measured in trials and the baseline risk in the absence of treatment estimated for the individual patient.[2]

The method may not apply to periods of time different to that studied in the original trials.

USING THE NOMOGRAM

The nomogram shown on the next page allows the NNT to be found directly without any calculation: a straight line should be drawn from the point corresponding to the estimated absolute risk for the patient on the left hand scale to the point corresponding to the relative risk reduction stated in a trial or meta-analysis on the central scale. The intercept of this line with the right hand scale gives the NNT. By taking the upper and lower limits of the confidence interval of the RRR, the upper and lower limits of the NNT can be estimated.

REFERENCES

1. Chatellier G, Zapletal E, Lemaitre D, Menard J, Degoulet P. The number needed to treat: a clinically useful nomogram in its proper context. *BMJ* 1996;321:426–429.
2. Cook RJ, Sackett DL. The number needed to treat: a clinically useful measure of treatment effect. *BMJ* 1995;310:452–454.

The number needed to treat

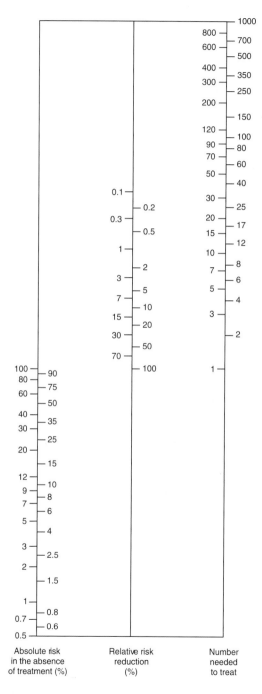

Absolute risk
in the absence
of treatment (%)

Relative risk
reduction
(%)

Number
needed
to treat

FIGURE Nomogram for calculating the number needed to treat.
Published with permission[1]

Also from the BMJ Publishing Group

JOURNALS

Clinical Evidence full edition
The original multidisciplinary version, covering a wide range of specialties.
ISSN: 1462-3846

Subscription price:
Personal - £75/$110;   Student/Nurse - £35/$50;   Institutional - £160/$240

Heart
A leading international clinical journal, which covers all aspects of cardiovascular disease and includes topical, authoritative editorials, comprehensive reviews, and case reports.
ISSN 1355-6037 (print journal)

Subscription price:
Personal print & online - £130/$201;   Personal online only - £80/$125;
Institutional - £309/$476

BOOKS
The full range of cardiology titles published by BMJ Books is available at:
www.cardiology.bmjbooks.com

Evidence-based Cardiology
A ground-breaking text addressing the implementation of evidence-based medicine in the major cardiological subspecialties.
Second Edition
ISBN: 0 7279 1699 8 (due Autumn 2002)
Further details available at: www.evidbasedcardiology.com

Evidence-based Hypertension
Based on central questions the physician needs to ask when managing hypertensive patients.
ISBN: 0 7279 1438 3
£27.50

100 Questions in Cardiology
A compilation of the 100 most frequently asked questions answered by leading cardiologists from the UK and around the world.
ISBN: 0 7279 1489 8
£25.00

For more information on all of these products, and to order online, go to www.bmjpg.com

Clinical evidence
Comment Card

The content of this publication is taken from the full edition of *Clinical Evidence* Issue 6. It is an evolving resource and we welcome any feedback on the current content and suggestions for future editions:

Name: ....

Address: ....

....

....Email: ....

Position

- [ ] Hospital Doctor, Senior
- [ ] Hospital Doctor, Junior
- [ ] GP/Family Physician
- [ ] Pharmacist
- [ ] Nurse
- [ ] PAM
- [ ] Manager
- [ ] Press
- [ ] Researcher
- [ ] Librarian
- [ ] Medical Student
- [ ] Member of Public/ Patient Support Group
- [ ] Other

....

1. Comments concerning the selection of studies

Topic ....

Reference ....

Comment...

....

....

....

2. Suggestions for future editions

....

....

....

....

3. Other comments/questions

....

....

....

....

- [ ] Tick this box if you wish to receive further information on *Clinical Evidence* specialty editions by email

Please return this card free of charge to the address overleaf or email us at: **CEfeedback@bmjgroup.com**

BUSINESS REPLY SERVICE
Licence No LON14537

BMJ Clinical Evidence
BMJ Publishing Group
BMA House
Tavistock Square
LONDON
WC1H 9BR

2